Hospice Inpatient Environments

Hospice
Inpatient
Environments

Compendium and Guidelines

Deborah Allen Carey

VNR VAN NOSTRAND REINHOLD COMPANY
_____________________________________*New York*

Copyright © 1986 by Van Nostrand Reinhold Company Inc.
Library of Congress Catalog Card Number 85-91275
ISBN 0-442-21772-2

Printed in the United States of America

Designed by Karolina Harris

Van Nostrand Reinhold Company Inc.
115 Fifth Avenue
New York, New York 10003

Van Nostrand Reinhold Company Limited
Molly Millars Lane
Wokingham, Berkshire RG11 2PY, England

Van Nostrand Reinhold
480 La Trobe Street
Melbourne, Victoria 3000, Australia

Macmillan of Canada
Division of Canada Publishing Corporation
164 Commander Boulevard
Agincourt, Ontario M1S 3C7, Canada

16 15 14 13 12 11 10 9 8 7 6 5 4 3 2 1

Library of Congress Cataloging in Publication Data

Carey, Deborah Allen.
  Hospice inpatient environments.

  Bibliography: p.
  Includes index.
  1. Hospices (Terminal care)—Planning.
2. Hospice care—Planning. 3. Hospices (Terminal
care)—United States. I. Title.
R726.8.C376 1986   725′.5   85-91275
ISBN 0-442-21772-2

Contents

Preface

The first inkling I had of undertaking work on hospices came, somewhat ironically, from a discussion on birthing centers. A friend was about to embark on her architecture thesis on birthing centers, and we began to trade views on the charged emotional and social significance of birth. Diane commented that birthing centers were a cross between an institution and the home. Moreover, she said, the client needs were unique and the client group large and diverse.

"Aha!" said her professor. "Design for birthing is complex, but consider the design for dying. Now that would be a difficult issue!"

We ended our conversation in agreement that hospice design would be complicated by social factors, the variety of clients, and most especially by the fact that death, unlike birth, is not a joyous occasion.

I quickly became fascinated by the subject. Hospice care, which provides palliative care for the terminally ill and their families, touches on issues of old age, resources, debilitation, social and cultural mores, and material from a wide variety of disciplines. I was free to range over material in anthropology, psychology, sociology, history, medicine, nursing, theology, and philosophy for references to death and dying. The arts, too, promised many hours of investigation. And I knew of at least one architect, Lo-Yi Chan, who had been involved in a hospice facility, in Connecticut.

In what I have since discovered to be a common experience of researchers of this subject, my initial literature search in nonfiction fields turned up little descriptive information on the environments in which people might choose to die. There were numerous articles describing funerals and memorials, but little to explain how the physical enviroment was perceived by the dying, their families, and their caregivers. The inpatient medical environment to which patients come to receive respite, pain management, and symptom control was also inadequately covered. I did find a few passages on St. Christopher's, the well-known British hospice, and on Connecticut, Hillhaven, and other pioneer American freestanding hospice units, but these descriptions had few pictures and almost no drawings.

The novelty of hospice care in the United States, as well as our own emphasis on deinstitutionalization and home care, relegated the topic of inpatient care to a few words in articles that stressed home-care strategies and explained palliative methodology. Not having a local client hospice to question, I had to look further afield.

As a measure of the scarcity of architectural information, there were, in 1981, no comprehensive lists of existing hospices distinguishing inpatient units from *scatterbed*—beds dedicated to hospice care within oncology or other hospital wards—or concentrated settings. I was able, however, to pinpoint probable inpatient hospices from the lists in Kenneth Cohn's *Hospice: Prescription for Terminal Care* (see bibliography) and to correspond with these units by questionnaire and letter.

As responses were returned, the extent of the need for better information became clear. Not only were there more inpatient units than I had expected, but there was also an urgent need on the part of the hospice care providers, architects, and planners to have access to more architectural data. No one had been able to find any more published studies than I had; the research had not been done. Caregivers were especially in need of data because they were in disagreement with their institutional associates about the location for remodels and about other components they had identified as hospice-specific, such as the need for homelike decor, connections to the outdoors, and larger patient rooms with space for family and other visitors.

It became evident that what were considered by medical planners, administrators, and the like to be amenities in hospice design, such as connections to the outdoors and homelike architecture, are, for hospice units, necessities. These homelike and nature concerns, which had been briefly mentioned in the general literature on hospices, were indeed the architectural priorities of the hospice inpatient staff. Moreover, agreement by hospice caregivers and staff on these priorities was found in diverse unit types, from the large freestanding hospices to the smaller remodeled units within hospitals and skilled nursing facilities (SNFs).

The manifestations of these priorities at different hospices and palliative-care units were not, however, uniform. At one unit, homelike concerns were met with donated furniture; at another, the design focused on family rooms and remodeled nursing stations. Few units were able to achieve their ideal designs because of limited budgets and the lack of available information on hospice design. Designers of remodeled units specifically suffered in this respect, for they needed to modify typical hospital space for deinstitutionalized palliative care without architectural data to back up their intentions.

Further conflicts among hospice care providers were also evident in the questionnaires. For example, though multibed rooms are the choice of proponents of the St. Christopher's model of hospice, other hospice caregivers support double or single rooms as superior. Hospices considering inpatient units, lacking data on other U.S. hospices, had no criteria on which to base their decisions. Consequently, many found it necessary to fall back on acute-care or nursing-facility approaches, neither of which is appropriate for the palliative short-term and intermittent inpatient stays of the hospice patient and family.

Questions regarding care also surfaced in the early data. Did the differences between the longer inpatient care of indigents and the short-term respite stays for other hospice patients mean that the architecture itself should be different for each? In some facilities, modified oncology units had hospice beds; did these units provide a better environment for the terminally ill with their segregated hospice areas? Or would a mixture of patients, such as acutely and terminally ill patients, in a completely remodeled oncology unit be a better solution? How much active therapy should be available to the hospice patient? Could an approach be found that would present common design guidelines for these varied palliative-care units without restricting innovation?

To answer these questions, more thorough data and analysis than what I had gathered strictly through the mail would be necessary. Visits to the hospices and the accumulation of on-site photographs and plans were included in my follow-up to the thesis investigation. I developed a model for design guidelines for a spectrum of units and completed the compendium with more detailed data.

This book is designed to bridge the gaps among relevant groups: caregivers, hospice proponents, architects, regulators, families, and patients who might want to know more about inpatient hospices. The core of this effort is Part Two, the Compendium, which provides data on a spectrum of inpatient palliative and hospice-care units. This material is presented so that care providers and others can peruse the solutions and problems of existing units without prejudicial commentary. Architects can glean specific information concerning programmatic design for a range of types of inpatient settings. Photographs and parti drawings are provided to enable readers to get a sense of the environment as a whole, while the environmental and proximity matrices give very specific data on finishes and distances.

Part One was written for caregivers, architects, and planners who want an updated overview of hospice care, the inpatient component, and the role of symbols and rituals in the environment of the dying person. In addition, Part One contains information on the specific users of the inpatient hospice and the dynamics of inpatient care.

Although the material in Part One will undoubtedly be familiar to some hospice caregivers, it condenses information valuable for the design or modification of an inpatient unit. Thus, it is a handy introduction to the hospice for the architect or planner who must know the client before design begins. In addition, since this material places hospice and inpatient care in relation to other kinds of palliative and medical caregiving, it may also be of interest to families, patients, and the medical profession at large.

Caregivers, in turn, might be tempted to leave Part Three, Design Guidelines, to the architects. A quick review, however, should spark the non-designer to consider the implications of a palliative environment, for Part Three was written with both the hospice specialist and architect in mind. The design guidelines are organized in categories that represent the priorities of hospices; the homelike and nature and spiritual concerns so evident in the case studies in Part Two. With guidelines organized to draw examples from the whole range of units, designs for new or remodeled construction stress common intentions, which can be served with a variety of appropriate strategies. Sketches and conceptual diagrams add detailed illustration to the ideas presented in this section.

Part Three also contains a section that focuses specifically on the architectural parameters for the hospice remodeling of a small, parent-based unit. These units have been disregarded in many articles, although they represent the most common architecturally distinct, functionally autonomous inpatient hospices. Finally, the hospice-specific guidelines are supplemented by suggestions for the more typical institutional elements shared with nursing homes and hospitals. In conclusion, the larger issues of hospice design raised in the need to deinstitutionalize caregiving are itemized and discussed.

It is hoped that this material, presented in this three-part scheme, will encourage greater understanding among caregiver, patient and family, and the designer. Hospice is care that serves the "boundless, subtle, fragile, and penetrating needs of its patients and the people they love. . . . Hospice exists to free patients and family from unnecessary restraints, and people involved in it must be ever mindful of that fact" (Bell 1981, 6).

Acknowledgments

I would like to thank the many hospice people who contributed their valuable time and enthusiasm to this work. Special thanks to the staff of the Hospice of the Good Shepherd, Waban, Massachusetts, for their contributions and to the people at Cabrini, Calvary, St. Mary's Hospital for Children in Queens, Dottie Wilson, and to St. Peter's Hospital Hospice in Albany. The architects who were invaluable in compiling information also deserve my deepest thanks.

Without my fellowship from the American Institute of Architects and the American Hospital Association, I would never have completed this work. Thanks to James Jonassen and the staff at the NBBJ Group for their "mentoring."

I would like to acknowledge the contributions of a group of others to this work. They include Dr. Jean Quint Benoliel, Jill Simandl Regan, R.N., Ray Shockey, Stanley Shockey, Dr. Hannelore Wass, and Robert Weisenbach, A.I.A. I would also like to thank my thesis advisors, Elaine LaTourelle and Claus Seligmann, and my parents.

Part One

Hospice Inpatient Care: Setting the Stage

Healing, Papa would tell me,
Is not a science,
But the intuitive art
Of wooing Nature.

        –W. H. Auden

Chapter One

The Hospice Alternative

Since the late 1960s, a profound shift in attitudes toward dying and illness has occurred among consumers and providers of care for the chronically ill (those who have had an illness of long duration, such as heart disease or cancer). Several factors have contributed to this change: the proportional increase in the number of chronically ill patients, as a result of medical advances since 1900; changes in family structure, which often result in the institutionalization of the chronically ill; a new consumerism in the population at large, causing some soul-searching by medical caregivers; and the influence of the British hospice movement, as represented in Britain by Dame Cicely Saunders and made popular in the United States by the work of Dr. Elisabeth Kübler-Ross.

All these factors have focused attention on the issues of death and dying in this culture and produced a concomitant flood of articles, books, and conferences on the subject. Anthropologists, sociologists, medical caregivers, theologians, psychologists, historians, and now architects have added to the burgeoning literature of current thought on death and dying in Western culture. Recently, lawmakers have joined in investigating the health care of the dying in order to establish regulations for safety and payment.

Evaluations of the existing care of the elderly and chronically ill have prompted extensive criticisms of the hospital and the nursing home as places to die. Although most Americans would prefer to die at home, an estimated 80 percent of the American population currently dies in these institutions (Lerner, in Shneidman 1976, 138–62). Hospice care, which is a palliative rather than biomedical treatment, has been employed to help the dying remain at home. Medical and family problems, however, may make home care difficult or impossible. The inpatient hospice unit, as part of a hospital or free-standing facility, seeks to remedy conditions existing within hospitals and nursing homes that are inappropriate for the dying and to facilitate a hospice program of care.

Designers, architects, and hospital planners as well as hospice caregivers and proponents should be reminded of the climate surrounding hospice care and the position of the inpatient unit in order to understand more completely the need for a new program of care and a new building type. As designers, we need to know whom we will serve and how the facility can best help those who will use it. This chapter introduces the demography of patients and discusses social conditions of institutional dying and the hospice movement as a reaction to the existing biomedical model of care and as a part of holistic care and concern. Finally, the role of the inpatient hospice unit is discussed as one part of the hospice movement.

Demographics and Sociology

> There is an old adage that people in general no longer believe but that is well understood by hospital staff, "Never go to the hospital, because hospitals are a place where people die" (Glaser and Strauss 1968, 32).

Not only do people die in hospitals, but today, most people die there instead of in their own homes. The reason for this delegation of care for the dying can be summarized as follows: the increased number of individuals dying from chronic diseases at an advanced age; changes in family structure and corresponding expectations and roles; the organization and operation of contemporary medical care; and decreased dependence upon religious and ethnic ritual.

Since 1900, the primary causes of death have changed from communicable and acute diseases, such as infections, influenza, pneumonia, and tuberculosis, to degenerative diseases "associated with the aging process, heart disease, cancer, and stroke, and by accidental injury" (Lerner, in Shneidman 1976, 130). One of the most dramatic results of this change is the increase in life expectancy. Lerner says that:

> During the first two-thirds of the twentieth century that we have now experienced, life expectancy rose by almost 23 years, an average annual gain of about one third of a year. . . . This is a breathtaking pace compared to any period of human history prior to this century, and it clearly could not be sustained over a long period of time without enormous social disruption (Lerner, in Shneidman 1976, 142).

This gain in life expectancy is not uniform in all subgroups of the population. The poor, for instance, have a much higher comparative mortality at younger ages, with more deaths resulting from childhood diseases, influenza, and pneumonia, as well as more sudden deaths (Lerner, in Shneidman 1976, 152). Therefore, less of this population survives to old age to die of degenerative diseases. In terms of potential hospital users, however, overall statistics show an increase in the number of superannuated patients, as well as an increase in percentage population with long-term chronic illness. Lerner states that the "proportion of all deaths in this country occurring in institutions has been rising steadily, at least for the last two decades and probably for much longer than that. It may now be as high as, or higher than, two thirds of all deaths" (Lerner, in Shneidman 1976, 141). Those institutions have been primarily hospitals and nursing homes. Of those who died at home, almost 50 percent were from heart disease, with cancer, stroke, and accidents composing another 30 percent.

This great proportion of terminally ill people dying in hospitals has profoundly affected the society at large, the family, and the individual. Hospital staff and doctors have become the managers of dying for the whole culture, a role that conflicts with their primary function as life savers and protectors. Hospitals have been organized to deal efficiently with the acutely ill, those patients who need specific medical treatment to cure their disease. Hospitals have made significant inroads in the cure of longer chronic diseases, but the needs of the acknowledged terminally ill person and his family are not best served in institutions whose goal is to cure, not palliate.

Because most doctors are taught to preserve life at all cost, the "care of the terminally ill in the United States has for many years not been differentiated from general acute care, which is the sine qua non of hospital care" (Cohn 1979, 2). Hospitals emphasize curing, not the palliative care necessary for those who are dying. Indeed, the dying are seen in many hospitals as people who cannot be helped. Often, the medical profession may encourage, and even pressure, dying patients to have operations that increase pain and disability on a very slim chance of prolonging existence in a very limited condition (Krant 1973, 24–27). Glaser and Strauss point out that medical caregivers depend on advances in curing, and the profession views death as a failure:

> On the whole, American nurses seem to find it difficult to carry on conversations about death or dying with patients. Only if a patient has already come to terms with death, or if they can honestly assure him he will die "easily," if he is elderly, [do] they find it relatively easy to talk about such topics with him. Unless a patient shows considerable composure about his dying, nurses and physicians lose their composure, except when they are specially trained or specially suited by temperament, or have some unusual empathy with a patient because of a similarity of personal history (Glaser and Strauss 1968, 156).

Philippe Aries, in his commentary "Death Inside Out," discusses another factor in the medical treatment of death.

> Let us note that patients are not blamed (for giving in to dying) in such cases merely because they have demoralized the medical staff, or because of failure to perform their duty, but more seriously because they are considered to have lessened the capacity to resist the sickness itself . . . (Aries 1975, 14).

If dying and death are avoided and stigmatized in the hospital, how are the family and dying affected? "The degree of delegation of responsibility and control over the patient is in the beginning never quite appreciated by the patient or his family, for they are typically rather ignorant of hospital structure, hospital staff, and hospital careers" (Glaser and

Strauss 1968, 33). In *Time for Dying*, Glaser and Strauss discuss the implications of institutional dying in sociological terms:

> The significance of *delegated responsibility* is powerfully suggested by two contrasting situations that we have observed. In the United States, elderly people sometimes refuse to leave home to die in hospitals, and their families often concur in the decision, but when the process of dying involves intricate nursing care or extreme deterioration of bodily functions, the dying person is likely to be sent off to a hospital or nursing home when the family simply can no longer endure the situation. . . . In contrast, families in countries like Greece, Malaya, and Italy frequently still request or insist that their dying relatives be moved from hospital to home when near point of death (Glaser and Strauss 1968, viii).

Glaser and Strauss go on to discuss strategies whereby the behavior of the dying and their families is managed by the order and attitudes of the medical staff; the conflicts become even more severe when the patient and family, of a different ethnic group from the professionals, create a fuss. "Once we observed the nurses intervene in a situation in which a lower-income family noisily carried on right in the room as if the patient were not dying"; the physician was prevailed upon by staff to allow only the mother and father visiting rights to the bedside (Glaser and Strauss 1968, 156). In this situation, the staff imposed their own ethnic values on the patient and family; the family's values were deemed inappropriate and were not allowed. Staff also manages the patient by accepting only behavior it sees as admirable. In their first book on the subject, *Awareness of Dying*, Glaser and Strauss noted that:

> . . . in general, then, the staff appreciates patients who exit with courage and grace not merely because they create fewer scenes and cause less emotional stress, but because they evoke genuine admiration and sympathy, as well as a feeling of professional usefulness (Glaser and Strauss 1965, 89).

The modern American family has been left to deal with the death of its members practically alone. Only the medical profession and some clergy are willing to help. In America, dying is difficult for the individual as well as his family, for many reasons. The dying person and family involved must either accept and manage the hospital environment or choose to go home. Home is not generally perceived as a place in which to recover from a chronic illness, so a decision to bring the terminally ill patient home means that life is essentially over—an extremely difficult decision to make. In addition, the presence of a dying person at home may disturb the daily and life-sustaining activities of the family, a sacrifice not every family is willing to make. Families, too, may perceive that the home does not have enough room for the dying person:

> Although the patient may have shared a room while in good health, usually it is preferable that he be segregated from the family while dying. . . . His presence would be too pervasive, would dominate too much the lives that must go on while he dies (Glaser and Strauss 1968, 190).

There are larger reasons that dying in America is not accepted as a natural part of life. Because most dying takes place in institutions, many Americans never see a person they love die. And, although dying is shown frequently on television news, the image often comes and goes in an instant; the reality of a slow, often debilitating, dying process occurring over many months is not part of television viewing. Unlike most European and Asian countries, too, the continental United States has had no war on home territory in this century, which has drastically reduced the likelihood of civilians witnessing death (Glaser and Strauss 1965, 85).

In *Hospice: Prescription for Terminal Care*, by Kenneth Cohn, the author discusses both the hospital atmosphere and the nursing home as places to die. One of the points he raises is that the dying may have difficulty being surrounded by those who are being cured:

> [dying patients] find it trying to have major surgery and recovery going on all around them, and their presence may be disturbing to other patients as well as to the staff. Patients in separate or single rooms [also] need extra staff if they are not to feel forgotten (Cohn 1979, 81).

Susan Sontag, in her book *Illness as Metaphor*, H. H. Van den Berg, in *The Psychology of the Sickbed*, and Erving Goffman, in his pioneering work *Stigma: Notes on the Management of a Spoiled Identity*, emphasize that hospitals and nursing homes reflect American cultural attitudes toward old age, infirmity, and disease. Americans glorify independence and youth and have a fear of weakness, dependency, infirmity, and disease. We are ashamed of the infirm, or, if we are infirm, we find it difficult to ask for help.

The problems associated with terminal illness are frequently exacerbated, too, if the dying person is placed in a nursing home. There is a slow-moving, timeless quality to the nursing home; it is custodial rather than palliative care. Custodial caregivers are not trained to care for the dying; they have neither the time nor the skills necessary to listen to and help the patient. Nursing-home personnel are most often low paid and physicians' visits are brief and scheduled infrequently. Pain control for the nursing-home patient is not easily managed.

Economic costs for long-term maintenance care are also very high. We find it very expensive to provide nursing-home care at a high standard. This also contributes to the development of an atmosphere not conducive to the care of the terminally ill patient or his family.

The population in American nursing homes is primarily aged, rather than necessarily chronically ill. Some patients may live there for many years, others may die soon after admittance. They may have one or more chronic diseases and limited mobility. Most important, however, patients may have infrequent family visits; some may be virtually abandoned. Glaser and Strauss observe that patients are too often regarded by some staff as "socially, if not biologically dead" (Glaser and Strauss 1968, 59). Because the family may visit but infrequently, the responsibility for care is given over completely to the staff, which may have little room for the views or needs of the patient.

Nonetheless, nursing homes are gradually increasing in importance as places where people die, because more people are living longer and moving into nursing homes as they become elderly.

The Hospice

The hospice movement evolved as an alternative to hospitals and nursing homes as places to die. The movement is gaining momentum in the United States as a reaction to the "cure at any cost" attitude in our acute-care hospitals, to the hospital regulations that have kept the family away from the patient in a crisis situation, and to the attitude of society at large about the place and importance of an individual's death. However, the hospice is not primarily a notion of place; it is a concept of care. Sandol Stoddard calls it a *caring community* (Stoddard 1978, 170).

The United States House of Representatives drafted this definition of the hospice in 1976:

Hospice: a program which provides palliative and supportive care for terminally ill patients and their families, either directly or on a consulting basis with the patient's physician or another community agency such as a Visiting Nurse Association. Originally a medieval name for a way station for pilgrims and travelers where they could be replenished, refreshed, and cared for; used here for an organized program of care for people going through life's last station. The whole family is considered the unit of care, and care extends through the mourning process. Emphasis is placed on symptom control and preparation for and support before and after death, full-scope health services being provided for by an organized interdisciplinary team available on a 24-hour-a-day, seven-day-a-week basis. Hospices originated in England (where there are about 25) and are now appearing in the United States (Rossman 1977, appendix).

As a system for care, the hospice movement addresses the desire of people to die in their own homes, in familiar surroundings with those they love, instead of in the hospital or nursing home. The term hospice is used to differentiate the kind of care provided (palliative) from the care currently given in hospitals (biomedical). This model of compassionate care is not new. In medieval times, the monastery also had a hospice. The gradual divorce of palliative care from medical care is part of the history of scientific medicine and the secularization of society. The monks who provided that first hospice care were barred by the edict of 1163 from performing operations, and the surgery developed later became the profession of barbers and eventually doctors. However, the Catholic orders retained their mission of ministering to the sick and homeless into the twentieth century. It was Sister Mary Aikenhead who founded, in the late nineteenth century in Dublin, a center for the incurably ill and called it a hospice. The old name thereby received its modern specific meaning. Sandol Stoddard explains what occurred next:

Around the turn of the century, a number of other hospices appeared in Great Britain and, in 1892, a "Hostel of God" in London which still exists, but the direct line now leads from Dublin to St. Joseph's Hospice, established by the English Sisters of Charity in London in 1906. After previous training at the Protestant Hospice of St. Luke's (also in London), it was at St. Joseph's during the 1950s and 1960s that Dr. Cicely Saunders further developed her work in pain control, and, together with some of the patients who had inspired and enlightened her during this period, her plans for the founding of St. Christopher's [which then opened in 1967] (Stoddard 1978, 66).

This ministering to the sick and destitute by the Catholic orders had a parallel development in the United States. The Dominican Sisters Congregation of St. Rose of Lima in the U.S. was founded in New York by Rose Hawthorne Lathrop, the daughter of Nathaniel Hawthorne, at the turn of the century. This congregation has seven homes for the incurably ill in the U.S., and considers itself "pre-hospice", meaning that Dr. Saunders's popularizing of the term *hospice* occurred after they had established their homes. The Dominican Sisters say that Dr. Saunders studied their work carefully before establishing St. Christopher's in London.

However, it was Dr. Saunders's work at St. Christopher's, together with the work of Dr. Elisabeth Kübler-Ross, that spurred the development of hospice care in the U.S. The movement here had to grapple with a very different health-care system from that of Great Britain. Whereas community hospitals that function in a neighborhood context are the norm in Great Britain, American hospitals are generally central ones. This, combined with the strikingly different funding and payment situation, the heterogeneous American population, and a notion that "palliative care is against the American way of life" (Lack 1978, 41), encouraged initial hospice programs to emphasize home care. One of the first direct results of Saunders's hospice work was the establishment in 1974 of Hospice, Inc., in New Haven, Connecticut, as a home-care hospice. The rights for hospice designation were eventually transferred to the National Hospice Organization (NHO), a nonprofit group founded in 1977. Hospice, Inc. has since taken the lead in inpatient design by commissioning Lo-Yi Chan to design the Connecticut Hospice, the nation's first architecturally designed freestanding hospice facility, completed in 1980. Their position as a leader in the American hospice field has emphasized the freestanding hospice as a desirable alternative.

Today, however, most American hospices are home-care hospices. Those that elect to receive health-care reimbursement from the federal government have had to make arrangements for inpatient service by contracting with local hospitals or by remodeling their own settings. Medicare will pay for only two or three days of inpatient care during the hospice period (the last six months of life) and so the inpatient aspect of care is severely abbreviated. Currently, Medicare will pay 40 percent of what the government has judged to be the average cost of acute care for the last six months of life.

Eighty percent of this payment goes toward home hospice care.

Many insurance companies are waiting to see what the demand on hospices will be before they provide coverage. Because of these funding problems, some hospices have been billing inpatient coverage under the category of general medical care. However, the advent of diagnostic-related groups for Medicare billing has made this practice very difficult. Diagnostic-related groups (DRGs) no longer allow costs to be hidden within an unitemized category (for example, charging a flat fee of $2,000 for a tonsillectomy without itemizing the separate costs). Any overruns are now paid by the hospital involved and reimbursement funds are not made available until the operation is done.

Thus, hospices are in a difficult position. By law, if they elect to receive Medicare benefits, they are required to have a connection with a hospital or, in some cases, as for respite, to be affiliated with a nursing home for inpatient care, and yet they are offered very little money for both inpatient and home care. Many hospices are waiting to see how Medicare benefits affect other hospices before they elect to receive it.

Medicare standards have done much to improve the record-keeping practices of many hospices, however. Medicare has also attempted to keep in mind the flexible needs of each hospice program, with its differing location and population mix. Common issues, such as the role of the volunteer in hospice care, have also been handled well. Volunteers are essential to low-cost hospice caregiving; restricting their role would not have benefited hospice quality. Volunteers take up the work of many staff members, thereby alleviating some staff burnout. Medicare and government regulations regarding hospices should be adaptable, yet firm enough to ensure quality hospice care. Should the standards become too strict, the hospice will become more and more like the institution it seeks to replace.

The Inpatient Hospice Facility

The need for inpatient care is threefold: to provide a place where medical attention can be concentrated, as, for instance, when adjustments in pain control need to be made; to provide respite care for the family and patient; and to provide compassionate care to indigents and those without family to care for them.

Traditionally, the indigents in this country have been cared for in large wards, frequently nursed by those in the religious orders. At St. Luke's in New York, both indigents and the dying are segregated in large units. Concentrating the dying in certain units has the effect of centralizing palliative care and isolating the terminally ill from those who are recovering, perhaps for the good of both. The advantages of hospital-based hospice care are mainly economic; no new beds need be constructed, multibed rooms are less expensive than private rooms, the doctors and nurses are already there to provide continuity with home care, and insurance can cover the costs. However, there are also disadvantages to hospital-associated hospice care, the primary one being the difficulty of modifying the existing institution. Established patterns of care must be transformed into palliative care. The architecture, too, must be modified if the principles of hospice care are to be met—to provide, for example, a homelike rather than an institutional environment. Despite the difficulties of modifying institutional space, however, it seems that Kenneth Cohn's prediction is correct; that "although British hospices are almost exclusively freestanding, it appears unlikely that United States hospices will emerge as freestanding facilities" (Cohn 1979, 69). As he explains,

> Several additional freestanding facilities will probably be built in the future, but growth of the [hospice] movement will depend on expansion of the home care and the hospital-based models. Home care-based hospices will grow because of the inherent cost-saving features, and hospital-based hospices will proliferate because of the excess of hospital beds available throughout the country (Cohn 1979, 69).

Although one problem with freestanding hospices can be that of continuing care—if the attendant physician makes regular visits to a hospital and must fit the hospice visit into an already busy schedule—the major difficulty with freestanding hospices is the capital costs required to start the program and built the unit. On the other hand, although capital costs are initially high, it is important to realize that the hospice does not have to finance expensive life-saving equipment. Consequently, it does not have to amortize the cost of that technology by a charge against each occupied bed, and hence can charge less per day (Cohn 1979, 86). The main costs of inpatient hospice care are found in the intensive nursing care provided. In Great Britain, for example, "the per-patient cost is about 80 percent of that in a general hospital, with about 85 percent of the budget going to staff salaries" (Cohn 1979, 86).

In addition, the freestanding independent hospice can provide much of what the institution or parent-based hospice cannot. Because it is not associated with a medical facility, it can make the most of the opportunity to develop a homelike environment and play down any acute-care appearance. The independent freestanding facility can contribute to the hospice program of care in many ways, from providing operable windows to designing larger bedrooms. As described by Sandol Stoddard, facility design and hospice principles reinforce each other:

> The hospice inpatient unit must function not as a fortress removed from the rest of society but as a house of life, a place where dying is seen as a natural part of our human pilgrimage, and where death receives consecration and celebration appropriate to this view (Stoddard 1978, 169–70).

The hospice movement has arisen out of a reaction to the existing situation of the dying and their relatives in twentieth-century Britain, Canada, and the United States. It harkens back philosophically to a medieval palliative model and is based upon the premise that the dying need compassionate rather than clinical or biomedical care. The inpatient hospice facility is a small part of the overall movement to care for the dying in their preferred environment, the home. Although the inpatient unit is not the focus of hospice care, it is seen as having the potential to contribute positively to the image and quality of hospice care. Constraints upon the growth and development of the inpatient hospice facility are primarily economic ones; different health-care financing in Britain and the United States seems to point toward a different emphasis on freestanding and remodeled parent-based hospice inpatient units in the two respective countries.

In an address to Yale in 1976, Dr. Cicely Saunders introduced her comments as follows: "I am here from St. Christopher's, which, by the way, is neither a Shangri-La nor a death house" (Saunders, quoted in Stoddard 1978, 95). Summing up the hospice philosophy of palliative care, Saunders continued,

> A patient should no more undergo aggressive treatment, which not only offers no hope of being effective but which may isolate him from all true contact with those around him, than he should merely receive control of symptoms when the underlying cause is still treatable or has once again become so (Saunders, quoted in Stoddard 1978, 95).

Chapter Two

Symbols and Rituals of Death and Dying

Death and dying are part of the philosophical preoccupations of humanity, concerns shared by all cultures throughout time. We struggle to understand why we die, and therefore why we live the way we do, why we live at all, and why the world exists. We try to give meaning to our lives and to our deaths. The hospice, because it deals with dying and death, is part of our culture's answer to these questions.

Every culture has its myths, sustained by traditional rituals and symbols, by which it reaches an understanding of death. Rituals employed at the time of death, dying, or burial reveal a culture's attitude toward the meaning of death and life. Many cultures have a great fear of death, and develop myths and rituals to express or reconcile their fears.

In the Eskimo culture, the fear of death and, seemingly, the idea that death itself is contagious, are manifested by the way in which the dying and dead are handled:

> If a person was expected to die, he was taken into an isolated hut. If he or she died in the dwelling house, everything had to be destroyed. Mourning and taboos, like abstinence from festivals, were connected with death, especially in the case of relatives who had touched the body. The corpse of the deceased was either buried or exposed in the tundra or on the beach. A great part of his personal property was destroyed and placed in the grave (Dupre 1975, 80).

After the death of one of their members, Eskimos will attempt to mollify the spirit world of the dead by naming, during feasts, those who died recently as well as their predecessors. Eskimos generally accord the dead great respect for their perceived power over the living.

As Wilhelm Dupre has noted, in almost all of the Western religions, explanations for the origin of death "culminate in the idea that God withdrew [from mankind] because man did not follow his demands, and that this withdrawal was the beginning of all evil in the present world" (Dupre 1975, 70). This idea is present, for example, in the story of Adam and Eve, who were cast out of the perfect Garden of Eden and caused both evil and death to enter the world because they could not obey God's commands.

The beliefs of a culture that relate to death are part of a larger cosmology in which other events are viewed. In the Hindu religion, death is followed by reincarnation and all events are part of a holy cycle that leads toward the transcendence of all being. Death, therefore, is part of the long journey of existence. The Hindu faithful often pilgrimage to Benares (the city of Shiva, god of transformation and death) and the dead are often cremated there, on the banks of the sacred river Ganges, allowing the spirit to be freed in a holy place. The river symbolizes the journey or passage of the dead.

Journeys are part of other cultural explanations of death as well. In ancient Egyptian belief, the deceased traveled through the otherworld in a solar barge in the company of the sun god, Amen-Ra. In Greek mythology, the souls of the dead were transported across the river Styx in the boat of the ferryman Charon to Hades, the underworld. We speak in this culture of "crossing the bar"; death for us is a journey as well.

Although rituals and myths vary in separate cultures and at different times in the same culture, cultural symbols of death and other transitional events, such as birth, marriage, and puberty, are often very similar. These events, defined as "rites of passage," may have sacred or secular meaning, but there is no culture in which they are ignored (Fried and Fried 1981, 270). The passage from the living state to the world of the dead has symbolic physical correlates: the threshold of a door is one example, and the gate another. As Mircea Eliade writes, ". . . the images of the bridge and the narrow gate . . . suggest the idea of a dangerous passage and, . . . for this reason, frequently occur in initiatory and funerary rituals and mythologies" (Eliade 1959, 181). The symbolism of water, which implies both death and rebirth, is also common. Other symbols that may have universal meaning and are associated with life and death include light, which is seen as favorable, and darkness, viewed as threatening and fearful. Fire is considered both exciting and terrible, and water calming. Seasonal events are also related to stages in life and death. The spring brings renewal and rebirth; fall and winter represent aging and death. These secular symbols are joined with common religious symbols, such as the cross, the passage, paradise, and the circle.

Rituals, symbols, and beliefs associated with death may change over time, or with the influence of more dominant cultures. For example, under the influence of Christianity, the Tlingit Alaskan Indians, who used to cremate their dead, now bury them following a Christian funeral. Instead of burning food and throwing valuables into the fire, as they would have done formerly, they place them in the coffin with the deceased (Fried and Fried 1981, 160). In a related sense, science has affected our sacred and secular understanding of life and death by providing explanations for many phenomena that were previously misunderstood or considered mysterious. However, science is primarily a methodology for establishing fact through replicable experimentation and observation, and cannot give us answers to the meaning of life and death. Yet, as Claude Levi-Strauss has suggested, scientific praxis seems to have "emptied the notions of death and birth of everything not corresponding to mere physiological processes and rendered them [death and birth] unsuitable to convey other meanings" (Levi-Strauss 1966, 264).

Perhaps we humans have given science the burden of making sense of life and death; science has done wonderful things for us. Medical science has delayed death until a very advanced age and saved lives through such inventions as penicillin and through better and faster surgical techniques. To many of us, medicine has taken on magical qualities, for we do not take the time to see how and why it works.

However, science is essentially neutral in man's pursuit of power over nature. And science cannot replace philosophy or religion; we still need to come to terms with the meaning of death and life. Perhaps our infatuation with science as a means to better human life has been tempered by the understanding that science is a tool that can be used to do well or ill, but not the solution to all questions or problems. Similarly, although facts can be established by science, facts are only part of what composes truth. As Gil Elliott has said, "Fact is not superior to myth. Technology is not more efficient than religion. However much factual and technical knowledge we acquire, we shall always have to live with the unpredictable" (Elliott 1976, 132). Death can sometimes be predicted, but its inevitability cannot be countered.

Because hospitals are designed as medical institutions where people are made well, they are not good places to die. Physicians are trained to combat illness with medication, surgery, and testing—scientific procedures designed to arrest and treat disease. However, death itself cannot be treated, nor is it known or understood fully by the living: for the dying, caring is far more important that curing. Likewise, the physical environments of institutional hospitals are not suitable for the dying. One reason is that scientific requirements place strict standards on the physical facility—quantitative criteria take precedence over qualitative considerations. For example, the surfaces within medical institutions must be sanitary; as a result:

> hard shiny materials are chosen instead of materials that mellow with age and generate an atmosphere of warmth . . . [Moreover, hospitals] have grown in scale to such a size that their physical expression is monumental rather than human (Lindheim, Glaser, and Coffin 1977, 13).

Despite their gigantic scale, however, many hospitals still lack adequate space for families and other visitors. This lack of privacy can be a real hardship for the families of terminally ill patients, as well as the families of other patients.

Hospice programs provide an alternative for the dying and their families, and offer an environment in which the dying are neither stigmatized nor feared. Both patient and family are supported through their crisis, which is both personal and cultural. The dying person and his family are encouraged to reach their own conclusions about life and death within an atmosphere that is secure, familiar, and as much like the home as possible.

Homelike hospice architecture is characterized by the addition of elements typical of residential architecture into the institutional context. These elements include symbolic aspects of the home, such as the hearth, as well as functional aspects, such as personalization and duplication of function (that is, rooms that serve several purposes, such as a chapel that doubles as a meditation room or private space). Materials and finishes of the home, such as carpeting, wallpaper, and domestic furnishings, are also part of homelike architecture.

Where else (in addition to symbolic homelike architecture) can hospice caregivers look to find symbols and rituals to help during death and dying? Religious symbols, for one, can be incorporated into the design of the inpatient hospice. Religion traditionally has dealt with the meaning of death, life, and belief, and can be of great help in supporting patients and their loved ones through the processes of dying and grief. However, because people of all faiths will use the inpatient unit, an ecumenical chapel or religious space, with storage for the minister's, rabbi's, or priest's religious articles, is appropriate. Secular symbols of change and transition, such as the narrow gate, the threshold, and the river, may also be appropriate for hospice design. I would recommend that these symbols be used very carefully, however, as we cannot be sure that symbols mean the same things to people from different cultures. Daniel J. Fleming offers the following guidelines for the use of symbols:

We should not allow ourselves to be incapable, still less unwilling, to recognize meaning or beauty in unfamiliar forms. . . .

We must be flexible in attaching different meanings to any given symbol. In the color symbolism of the Renaissance, white stood for purity, joy and life; but in China, white invariably has been the color of mourning. . . .

World symbolism must take account, also, of different psychological climates. That such differences have existed through the centuries is obvious—the mystic emphasis of the medieval mind in contrast to the modern stress on science . . . all the psychological differences of the centuries are present in today's cross section of humanity.

If we are to catch the significance of symbols used in cultures other than our own (and sometimes including our own) we must pass beyond curious observation to intelligent apprehension of inner meaning . . . in terms of environment and tradition.

Last, we must not only realize that our world community is made up of varied tribes, peoples, and tongues, but be aware of certain corrollaries that flow naturally from that fact . . . that each tongue has its favorite metaphors; and that each people has its meaningful representations (Fleming 1955, 103–4).

The hospice is only a partial answer to providing a philosophy for death and life in the modern and scientific age. As Philippe Aries had noted, only with cultural agreement concerning the roles of the individual, nature, evil, and the afterlife will symbols and rituals comfort and explain life and death (Aries 1981, 603). The hospice is a reaction to the anonymity of mass culture; an attempt to establish a caring community of people devoted to a particular concern of human life—human suffering and dying. The hospice movement is concurrent with other movements to promote common interests and community in order to reduce the mass of people to a workable size. Insofar as the hospice is a response to changing cultural values, it may succeed in providing meaningful rituals and symbols for death. Of course, the need for a philosophy that gives meaning to life as well as death is very deep in every culture; the hospice may not provide all the answers. Nonetheless, the hospice's symbolic affect on culture may be considerable. As Carlos Castenada observes, "Every bit of knowledge that becomes power has death as its central force. Death lends the ultimate touch, and whatever is touched by death indeed becomes power" (Castenada, quoted in Kalish and Reynolds 1976, 183). Because it deals with death, the symbols, rituals, and mythmaking potential of the hospice are much greater than most would consciously realize.

Chapter Three

Hospice Users and Programs of Care

This chapter is designed to present to those unfamiliar with inpatient hospice care the basic programs of care, the range of users as well as their problems and needs, and to introduce physical correlates for the functions hospices seek to provide. The material outlined is an overview of the hospice for architects and designers, to display the unique caregiving environment of palliation provided for patients, families, and for the hospice caregivers themselves.

The most current and precise information on the users and actions of the inpatient hospice—that is, the Health Care Financing Administration (HCFA) and the Joint Commission on Accreditation of Hospitals data compiled in the spring and summer of 1983—was not available at the time of this writing. Designers are urged to peruse that data for much more specific details on hospice demographics and caregiving. In addition, the suppositions made in this chapter about hospice users and care programs are intended for general reference only. They present the essential elements of the palliative-care unit. The specific program requirements of any facility or unit design can be found by consulting the caregivers and community.

Identification of Users

Hospice and palliative-care units vary greatly in size and composition. The architecturally distinct and functionally autonomous units that are the focus of this study usually vary from those that serve five or six patients to the large, 200-bed palliative-care hospital. Most of the autonomous units have both home-care and outpatient divisions.

In general, the inpatient unit of a hospice that is architecturally distinct will have a variety of users and support staff: patient and family, administrators and staff, nursing staff, medical director, attending physician, and pharmacist, as well as laundry, food service, and maintenance personnel. In addition, hospice inpatient units often have board members, community resource people, a volunteer coordinator, a social worker, volunteer help, and a chaplain or bereavement counselor. There may be an occupational therapist, physical therapist, or music therapist to assist as well; some units have daycare personnel and even childcare workers. Specialists at some units include ostomy, chemotherapy, and radiation therapists, among others. The home-care component of the hospice may be in-house or contracted to a visiting-nurse service, with same or different staff from that of the hospice inpatient unit. This information can be obtained from each unit, and will vary with the hospice's affiliation and program of care.

Volunteers aiding in hospice care will be drawn from many walks of life, as are the personnel. However, all hospice and palliative caregivers are fully trained and skilled in relieving the suffering and increasing the comfort of the dying. Of course, many of these people will be very sensitive to their profession and generous and patient to others. Hospice volunteers are frequently the survivors of hospice patients, the widowed and the bereaved children. Their experience with personal grief and the program of hospice care makes them uniquely valuable to others facing death.

Hospice patients and their families will enter the inpatient unit for several reasons. Short-term intermittent stays provide time for pain management and symptom control as well as respite from long home care for patient and family. Palliative-care hospitals such as Calvary and Rosary Hill Home tend to have longer inpatient stays for those who are indigent and have no home primary caregiver, or for those whose debilitation is so great there there is no other place for them to stay. Hospices, in contrast, have an average inpatient stay of seventeen days; patients generally die within forty to forty-five days of admission to the program.

To describe the person as a cancer or heart-disease patient would do little to pinpoint all the possible needs of the hospice patient. Hospice patients will be confronting their death, using conscious or unconscious means. Many good references are available that describe the emotional reactions experienced by those diagnosed as terminally ill. Designers should be familiar with the work of Dr. Kübler-Ross (*On Death and Dying*) identifying the possible stages of a person's dealing with dying, including denial and isolation, anger, bargaining, depression, and acceptance (Kübler-Ross 1969).

The greatest fears of the dying include the loss of control, pain, the loss of one's loved ones, and the fear of our reaction to their illness. The dying fear the unknown, financial burdens, and that their lives will have been meaningless. They also fear isolation in their struggle with their illness and death.

The loss and stigma of the dying are legendary. Loss of strength, mobility, weight, and physical change may affect self-image. The dying lose their traditional employment, which affects self-confidence and motivation; they also are about to lose all their loved ones and all they know. Dr. William Gibson, making an address on "The Medical and Psychological Aspects of Terminal Illness," has explained that

> Human value is founded on the principle of self-respect, as well as the freedom to have certain rights that are protected and honored by fellow men. Inclusion in the community requires an individual to be able to communicate, to experience mutuality, and to share the ethical ideas of fidelity, gratitude, reciprocity, justice and love. All of these considerations must be taken seriously, if we are adequately to manage the terminally ill. Total dependency can be viewed as deeply embarrassing and undignified (Gibson 1978, 5).

The confrontation with death is not restricted to the patient only. The patient's family, friends, and staff have a daily struggle to make sense of this extremely difficult and profound issue, in very personal terms. Family may feel guilty, fearful, hurt, or confused about the situation. Staff will inevitably become attached to the patient and also feel grief and loss over their death. These aspects of the hospice confer a solemnity upon the unit, which must be able to absorb the trials of the dying and their loved ones by affirming and accepting the contradictions of human life. This is not to say, however, that hospices require an air of false or undue solemnity; delight and laughter are also a part of life and need a place in the hospice.

Hospice patients usually range in age from sixteen to the elderly. Most hospice units do not take children under sixteen, although St. Peter's Hospice, the St. Rose's Homes, and a few others have accepted child patients. Because children are still growing, their illness may have an unpredictable trajectory; diagnosis may be very difficult. In addition, children are usually in the care of parents who will seldom give up on therapy and who will provide home care. Therefore, although there may be demand for home hospice care, inpatient hospice care is needed less for children. St. Mary's Hospital in Queens is planning a palliative-care unit, which is surveyed in Part Two. In general, the better acute-care hospitals provide places for the family of a dying child (Izumi 1976, 86).

Because men, statistically, do not tend to live as long as women, the oldest patient users of the inpatient unit are likely to be women. The patients will vary in age, marital and family status, and trajectories of illness and debilitation. Many of the dying may have an elderly partner who can provide home care, although quite a few of the oldest may have no surviving family to help them.

Inge Corless, of St. Peter's Hospice, has suggested that location of the facility will determine to some extent the particular demographics of the unit. She has seen that inner city units seem to get "sicker" patients with families in greater distress, a higher percentage of elderly patients with problems such as poverty, a higher percentage of patients without primary caregivers at home, and a higher percentage of well-educated persons. The location will also influence the ethnic and religious base of the patients; however, the affiliation of the hospice does not seem to affect the religious status of the inpatient population.

These factors must be taken into account in the design of the facility. For example, single rooms are appropriate for patients with family and many other visitors; they are inappropriate for severely debilitated patients without family or friends, who cannot easily leave the room to seek company. Ethnic differences in dealing with dying may cause conflict; however, architecture cannot solve a conflict that is best understood and dealt with socially. Projected patient mix and change over time are best left to the individual hospices, which can compare their survey, if necessary, with the comprehensive work of the Hospice of the Good Shepherd (see bibliography).

Debilitation, Care, and Design

The dying are our friends, relatives, and eventually ourselves. The probability of our own death from a chronic illness is very great and behooves us to consider, for a moment, our own perspective on dying from a long-term chronic illness. Identification with the users of the hospice will encourage a fundamental sympathy for design.

The majority of hospice patients die from cancer or heart disease. It has been said, however, that it is important to place physical pain in perspective. It is estimated that 50 percent of cancer patients have little or no physical pain during their illness. Of the remaining 50 percent, 10 percent have mild pain, and half of the remaining 40 percent will need help with intractable pain (Farr 1978, 2). In the hospice, pain control is accomplished through the regular administration of drugs, a description of which is available in virtually every book on hospice care. However, pain control is only part of symptom management. Hospice palliation seeks to mediate the physical discomfort of the patient in many ways. Bathing, changing dressings, and physical closeness (touching and grooming the patient) are part of that symptom management, as are regulating diet, activity, and fluid levels. There are differences in the philosophy of treatment, which may result in some units using suction and oxygen, radiation therapy, and some surgical techniques to alleviate pain and discomfort, as long as they are palliative therapies only.

Debilitation of the individual will vary so much with the trajectory of the illness that each situation deserves a specifically tailored program of care. For example, cancer patients may experience sensory changes, such as nausea under certain lights or sound conditions, and increased or decreased sensitivity to other stimuli. Some hospice patients will be ambulatory, others will be unable to move without assistance; in general, a varied environment that can be modified to suit the needs of the patient will be necessary. Above all, patients need assurance that they will not be abandoned and that staff will try to respond to their complaints with solutions that will work.

The likelihood of progressive disability as well as the awareness of impending death may result in new perceptions on the part of family and patient. Although they may feel, for example, that they will have more control at home, patient or family may not feel safe unless medical and social support are readily available.

The role of the environment in providing comfort in the face of dying and disability is not absolutely clear. On the one hand, hospices have emphasized that caregiving is the most important and significant part of palliation. However, studies at the Royal Victory Hospital Palliative Care Unit suggest that the environment can mitigate or lessen pain in some circumstances, with this effect being "attributable to the difficult to describe environmental influences on the patients' responses to analgesic medication" (Farr 1978, 10). Designers may explore architectural or environmental psychology to obtain parameters for humane design, but should exercise caution before applying the results of psychological experimental data to their designs. As noted by Izumi, although studies of the effects of the environment on the dying patient cover a gamut of experiences and offer important insights on patient reaction, "very few [of these studies] may be considered as information to be used in design" (Izumi 1976, 85). Essentially, many experiments conducted on the effect of the environment on the dying patient cannot be replicated and, thus, cannot be verified. A better approach to design is to consider the existing needs and functional correlates of the hospice. Familiarity with previous design solutions and problems should give the designer a more general basis from which to proceed.

One further note on debilitation. Several units have used debilitation as a basis for their insistence on private or single rooms. Calvary Hospital maintains that their severely debilitated, heterogeneous population must have single bedrooms—all 200 of them. The Certificate of Need at Tacoma General Hospital for remodeled oncology hospice beds also states that single rooms are necessary for all patients, offering the following reasons to support this claim:

- Some patients will have radiation implants, which can affect others nearby;
- Some patients will have infectious diseases;
- There will be immunosuppressed patients, who are at risk of getting infections from others;
- There will be patients who are disruptive, confused, or combative; and
- There will be patients who smoke (Tacoma General Hospital 1981).

It seems that the hospice at Tacoma General treats disease symptoms with active therapies and has a more biomedical program of care than most hospices do.

In the design of a hospice unit, the role of debilitation must be carefully studied and understood. Hospices that seek to minister to the entire person will have different philosophies and designs from those that take a narrower approach, such as treatment of the disease only. The designer must be made aware of the approach of the particular caregivers who will staff the hospice unit.

Program of Care

In general, the activities that occur inside a hospice inpatient unit emanate from the needs of the dying, and include the actions of the primary caregivers, usually nurses, as well as family members, clergy, and friends and visitors. The program characteristics of the Connecticut Hospice are typical of the palliative-care approach adopted by most hospices:

- Coordinated home health care/inpatient care under a central autonomous hospice administration
- Skilled symptom control (physical, sociological, psychological, and spiritual)
- Physician-directed services
- Provision of care by an interdisciplinary team that includes a social worker, nurses, clergy, and several physicians, including the patient's own
- Services available on a 24-hour-a-day, 7-day-a-week, on-call basis, with emphasis on constant availability of medical and nursing skills
- Patient and family regarded as the unit of care
- Bereavement follow-up
- Use of volunteers as an integral part of the interdisciplinary team
- Structured staff support and communication systems
- Patients should be accepted to the program on the basis of health needs, not ability to pay (Lack 1978, 42).

The needs of the dying are primarily the same as for everyone—food, comfort, socializing, privacy, access to diversions (work or play), and choice—but the specifics of their diseases and disabilities and the fact of their dying make these activities more difficult to perform. The trajectory of dying—that is, the speed, disability, and pain involved—varies with each patient. Expectations and fears of the dying and those around them can influence to a large degree the actual behavior of the individuals. Some dying patients are restricted by their diseases, some by their perceptions of their diseases and impending death. The stages of dying, discussed earlier, put special psychological strains on the "normal" activities of the individual. As Glaser and Strauss point out, "with unexpected bodily deterioration, patients panic or begin to lose recognition of themselves as known entities" (Glaser and Strauss 1968, 164). Patients may also go about tying up loose ends, finding faith, or getting family relationships in order. For the dying, the perception of time is often distorted, so that each day takes on a special significance, as noted by Gerda Lerner in *A Death of One's Own:*

> . . . each day seen by itself was an island, existing in its own space and time, longer than any known day because it was irreplaceable . . . . Each day was still, the minutes precious in those golden moments when acceptance brought silence and rest. Yet each day was convulsive, torn with useless thrashing, with resistance and effort . . . . It seemed these months, each longer than the one before it, were a lifetime, an eternity . . . (Lerner 1978, 199).

Much of what occurs in a hospice is the process by which the activities of the dying are expedited by the caregivers, who, because of the disabilties of the patient, must take over the provision of food, comfort, and mobility. The hospice workers, whether nurses, doctors, volunteers, family, or others, are intimately involved in activities and needs that the patient would normally do or satisfy for himself: comfort, privacy, socializing, food, access to diversions, and the right to make choices.

Comfort.

Comfort is a major provision of inpatient hospice care. Many chronic diseases, such as cancer, cause deterioration of strength; treatment may have involved operations that progressively debilitate the body. Colostomies, for example, require the subsequent use of equipment that is awkward, perhaps painful, and sometimes embarrassing for the patient. The disease may cause intense pain as well as a host of distressing symptoms. Pain therapy is a major part of palliative care. To this end, morphine is used in Great Britain and, in the United States, other strong and often addictive drugs are administered regularly to moderate pain. In addition to treating pain, hospice medical staff try to make the patient as comfortable as possible by attending to the patient's physical symptoms. Attending to even seemingly minor problems can make a big difference to the patient, as noted below:

> . . . A hospice nurse can assist in dealing with frequently neglected mouth problems: ill-fitting dentures or cracked mouth, which may accompany medication. Calvary Hospital in the Bronx developed a mouth-care procedure for coating the tongue and dry areas with a bit of mineral oil and milk of magnesia, a procedure which in a very short time can help patients to enjoy eating and drinking again (Rossman 1977, 225).

Providing comfort involves more than attending to the patient's physical condition, however. To comfort the patient emotionally, caregivers listen to the patient and offer counseling and hand-holding. Hospices usually provide several kinds of counseling for family and patient: social counseling, spiritual counseling by clergy, even financial counseling for those with money problems brought on by the expense of long-term illness. In fact, however, physical and emotional caregiving are interrelated. It is difficult to distinguish where physical care and comfort leave off and psychological and emotional care and comfort begin. As Rossman asserts, much nursing care involves brushing hair, stroking and bathing the body, and otherwise providing the comfort that is also physical (Rossman 1977, 225).

As physical comforting involves pillows, diet, movement, and medicines, emotional comforting includes the development of an atmosphere of security and trust, quiet, peacefulness, and warmth. The patient needs to feel that ordinary life complications have fallen away, without judgments or explanations. The patient is not really interested in what the caregivers think, but is very interested in knowing that the caregivers are interested in him and his feelings (Spillane 1978, 9). However, the limits to comforting can be difficult to surmount, as expressed in James Agee's *A Death in the Family:*

> Mary did not speak, and Hannah could not think of a word to say. It was absurd, she realized, but along with everything else, she felt almost a kind of social embarrassment about her speechlessness.
>
> But after all, she thought, what *is* there to say? What earthly help am I, or anyone else? (Agee 1965, 102).

There is comfort in having personal possessions near, in using a convenient telephone to talk, and in having access to the outdoors and religious facilities. Comforting is part of most of the actions of hospice.

Privacy.

Problems of privacy for the terminally ill are severe because of their institutionalization and disease. The dying are, as mentioned before, often debilitated by their illness, yet they have every right to decide their living days. The patient's lack of mobility, the institutional setting, and any embarrassing or difficult problems associated with the patient's illness often make privacy a desirable option. It is expensive to acquire, especially if privacy is equated with the private room. However, the need for privacy is not necessarily solved by private rooms; the relation between the need to socialize and the need to be alone is a complicated one involving family, ethnicity, type of illness, and so on. It is wise to provide a variety of privacy screening devices: varied ward sizes, curtains or handsome screen devices, and the use of separate rooms for special visits.

Other aspects of privacy must also be addressed in the hospice. Access to the bathroom or bathing and elimination facilities should be simple and as much as possible under the patient's control. Of course, the privacy of the patient's thoughts and desires must be respected. This means acoustic privacy is an issue, whether in the case of being overheard or overhearing others.

Socializing.

The socialization of the dying is a matter of both choice and opportunity. Much has already been said about the contemporary dilemma of dying in a hospital, surrounded either by those who are getting better or in an ethos supported by the medical profession; once medical treatment of the illness has been completed, the dying lie like failures to await their fate. Such an environment can do little to comfort the dying. There is often no one to talk to, directly or indirectly, about the facts, the fears, and concerns of the dying individual or their families and friends. The hospice philosophy asserts that this must not be so. The dying have supportive arms, ears, and hearts in the staff of the hospice personnel.

An inpatient unit can provide other avenues for communication as well. Families visiting the hospice may obtain support from others who are experiencing similar feelings. Patients, too, often can help one another and become friends with an honest and satisfying relationship. While socializing often takes an intimate form, birthdays, holidays, and other celebrations also provide deep significance for the dying and their families by enriching life's events. Memorial services and body viewing are another part of the rituals that sustain and comfort.

The physical hospice unit must facilitate this aspect of care; the choice of communication must be maintained. By considering how the bedrooms, common areas, dining and recreation areas, meeting rooms, nurses' stations, and other areas will function, the architect can design space that promotes communication and comfort.

Food.

Food, which would normally be prepared by the patient, is commonly prepared by the hospice staff or by friends or relatives. Hospice palliative care specifies that the patient be involved with and consulted about all aspects of his care. Therefore, meals in the hospice inpatient unit include the serving of favorite foods, in as personal a manner as the patient wishes. Kitchens are to be found in most inpatient units so that the family or friends may prepare or reheat the patient's favorite dishes.

Breakfast is a favorite meal of cancer patients. However, hot breakfast cereal, a soft-boiled egg, or toast with melted butter are difficult to keep hot and fresh if transported long distances or held up along the way. Calvary Hospital solved this problem by installing pantry kitchens on each floor for breakfast food of this nature. Many oncology patients lose their appetite as the day progresses, so that small portions, attractively served, as well as a drink before dinner, can stimulate appetite. Some facilities have courses that are brought around on carts; patients are encouraged to try the soup or a small piece of meat, and the whole routine is given a festive air.

Patients with dry throats need popsicles or juices, which can be kept along with snacks at a nutrition station or a convenient kitchenette. Meals may take place in a dining room or at a central dining table, with linens and other festive details. The ritual of eating and the small pleasures it affords add immeasurably to the quality of hospice life. The sharing of food and breaking of bread together are metaphors for a community of caring. Some patients will be too debilitated to leave their rooms and beds at mealtime, but these occasions can still be made special.

Access to Diversions.

In hospice literature, the importance of providing the patient with access to familiar and pleasant surroundings is stressed. For the sake of convenience, access can be divided into three groups: the provision of suitable space for group and individual activities; appropriate transportation devices, such as movable chairs, beds, or walkers; and access to nature and the outside world.

The availability of suitable space for group and individual activities is very important. Celebrations are a common occurrence, as are memorial services, weekly religious meetings, and daily daycare activities. Privacy necessitates space for quiet reading and contemplation indoors and in gardens. Some patients may wish to work on physical therapy or crafts; however, the short-term respite and symptom control provided by most American inpatient hospices suggests that most activities will be quiet and contemplative. Unlike some hospitals or nursing homes, which may lack appropriate facilities, hospices can provide patients with greater access to their own possessions (such as clothes, pictures, and music), the foods they prefer, as well as people they know and love—or simply people they can trust to care for them.

In addition, the option of access to nature and the daily activities of the community is important. This access could be to a balcony or sunroom, or it may also include gardens or some connection to street life. Operable windows, too, are important, as they connect the hospice patient with the light and the outdoors. On another level, accessibility for the handicapped is of great consequence. At St. Christopher's, the patient's bed is wheeled right to the entrance and to various functions in the hospice, such as chapel and choir. This does not always mean that a short hallway should be designed, but it does mean that an interesting one, offering many views, is desirable. If an individual must be restricted to an environment, it behooves the designer to provide diversion and interest with it.

Kenneth Cohn refers to the quality of life to be maintained for the dying. He includes as aspects of quality,

> Observing the sunrise or sunset from an open window, listening to the birds sing, smelling the flowers, holding a baby, watching the joy of a child opening Christmas gifts, taking a walk in the woods with loved ones (or, if the mood strikes, in solitude), traveling, reading, creating with mind and/or hands, enjoying the infinite activities of an active life (Cohn 1979, 28).

Choice.

Underlying most of the aspects of living mentioned above is the necessity of modifying the institutional environment. The inpatient hospice is a communal living facility. As in communal living situations everywhere, it suffers from the need for schedules and organization of the individuals for the benefit of the whole. However, a major tenet of the hospice movement is the introduction of a large degree of personal choice into an institutional setting. To this end, the architecture should provide an adaptable environment. Temperature and lighting levels will be managed by the patients as much as possible; certainly, windows should be operable and amount of light controllable.

Upon admission to the hospice, patient, family, and staff decide the specific plan for the care of the dying individual and tailor the treatment to suit the patient's needs. Decision making involves selection of food and rooming situation; these choices are enhanced by the variety of accommodations and activities made available. The patient may choose to bring personal items or may opt to smoke. Choice is also encouraged by transition areas that allow for a collecting of thoughts in a space of time, such as alcoves between public and private spaces.

The choice of kind and quality of dying is part of the patient's decision to select hospice care itself. It is emphasized that the program of care in a hospice must be flexible, sensible, and sensitive to the needs of the recipients, so that the hospice will not force its way upon the dying. Twenty-four-hour visiting, pets, the availability of family overnight space, adaptability, personalization, and connection to the outdoors are all part of the ways in which the hospice can provide alternatives.

Needs of Family, Staff, and Visitors.

The needs and behaviors of the dying are mirrored in those of the caregivers and family of the hospice patient. Comfort and privacy, communication, food, diversions, and choice are all needs of the family, friends, volunteers, and staff of the inpatient hospice and patient.

For family members spending time in a hospice, comfort means being alone, if necessary, to grieve, and having staff and others to talk to or sit with. For those who travel to the hospice from a distance, comfort is having a convenient, private telephone for calling home, having daycare facilities for the children, and having a place to lie down. For staff and family, comfort is a bite to eat and a nap, or a conference in a crisis. A good hospice will give the family a sense of security and a sense that all is being done that is necessary and right. Emotional comfort for the staff is another element of good hospice care. Without privacy and retreat areas, staff may become so stressed by the constant death and grieving that they "burn out."

As Mary, a character in Agee's *A Death in the Family*, awaited word of her husband's condition, she lit and relit the kettle for tea; each time, it boiled away. She busied herself making the bed, soothing herself with activity and familiarity (Agee 1965, 91–101). Similarly, family and friends of hospice patients may find it helpful to spend active, productive time with the patient, such as cooking and providing care. The small and repetitive tasks fill up the seemingly endless time.

Socialization and diversions include rituals and celebrations as well as private contemplation or reading. Long waiting hours are broken by music, card playing, and television watching, as well as dining with staff or other visitors. Decoration and outdoor activities are also part of hospice activities. Some family members may wish to help decorate the hospice for holidays or birthdays; all hospice users may choose to stroll or work in the garden. Having convenient access to staff and an environment that is easy and interesting to move about in contributes to the hospice goals of understanding and respect for the dying and their families. Small social activities are of primary importance. Cohn makes the point that "such things as washing the patient's hair, helping the patient to write a letter [and] moving a bed closer to the window to afford a better view of the outdoor activities" are social diversions that provide comfort and contact (Cohn 1979, 73). The architecture should help to facilitate these activities.

The choices made available to the visiting family and friends and staff should be reflected in the architecture of the hospice. With concern for the ambience and image of the hospice, the architect can turn a drab corridor into a warm and pleasant place. The hospice movement encourages involvement with the dying, true concern and care. The choice to visit becomes more tenable in a dignified and pleasant environment.

Additional Hospice Activities

Hospice life also involves the day-to-day running of a unit. The work of the caregivers, staff, and sometimes family involves daily meetings to take samples for medication measurement and change or modify care. In addition, hospice activities include staff correspondence, daily cleaning and maintenance activities, laundry collection, and linen changes. Beds will be lowered and raised, furniture moved, guests and patients greeted, flowers and decorations changed. At some facilities, education of the community involves tours and correspondence, as well as some fund-raising activities.

Charting and billing are also part of daily hospice activity, and those inpatient units that direct home care must schedule visits and volunteer activities. The running of an inpatient facility in these respects is much like any institution, but the flexibility and responsiveness of a hospice regimen make the daily attention to such scheduling very important. The connection of the hospice to the outside world is encouraged and stimulated. Manicurists and hairdressers may visit, and art carts and lending libraries wheeled around to the patients.

Activities Surrounding the Hospice.

The cataloguing of behaviors inside a hospice inpatient facility tells only part of the story of the important design considerations. A hospice is not isolated or excluded from the surrounding community. Good inpatient care extends the realm of care from home to hospital to hospice. Sometimes a patient may return to the hospice several times before dying. The proximity of hospice to home becomes important for visiting and transportation purposes. Likewise, some connection to hospital facilities is essential. Although most hospice patients have finished medical treatment, some may elect to have these services nearby. Perhaps more fundamentally, a good working relationship with a local hospital provides support for the aims of hospice care and continuity of care. The hospice serves as a reminder to the community that death and the dying are among them. If the hospice is situated in a thriving community, the neighborhood itself becomes a reminder to the hospice patients that life goes on about them and that they need not be separated from it until death.

Still in question is the proximity of the hospice to other facilities and services, such as nursing homes. St. Christopher's Hospice has a wing for the indigent or elderly without family, yet there is a reluctance to place these facilities in juxtaposition here in the United States. If the dying are mobile enough to go on day trips from the hospice, what other aspects of community life might they enjoy? Some hospices have incorporated daycare facilities for the children of family and staff. Couldn't proximity to a shopping area, restaurants, or bars be considered? Segregation of the hospice in parklike grounds may provide solitude and opportunities to contemplate nature, but the connection of hospice patients with the daily life of others may be strained.

The rituals of hospice inpatient life are both mundane and sublime, as they represent a slow and natural timelessness. From a perspective that moves from a cup half-empty to one where the fullness of life is revered and cherished, the individual gifts of each member of hospice can be appreciated and accepted. Dying brings fear and sometimes pain, but it also frees. Ritual and celebration make clear that dying is the human condition—no easier now than before, but no stranger to humankind.

Chapter Four

Compendium

The inpatient unit for palliative care has been developed with a special program and philosophy. To understand the special architectural qualities of hospices, we may now turn to the hospices themselves. It is possible to design a hospice inpatient unit without systematic research into fellow units; indeed, until recently, it was necessary to do so, as there were too few examples of comparable facilities. However, the number of American hospice inpatient settings has grown phenomenally in recent years. From the pioneering hospices of Hillhaven, Boonton, and the Connecticut Hospice, the number of freestanding units has now increased to six. The greatest increase in number has been in parent-based hospice facilities, however. These remodeled and converted units form the bulk of this study and support many of the original designs found in the early freestanding units.

The Joint Commission on Accreditation of Hospitals contracted with the federal and state governments to develop standards for hospitals, nursing homes, and now hospices. Hospitals and nursing homes are subject to inspection to determine compliance with Joint Commission standards and eligibility for accreditation and federal reimbursement. Now hospices, too, come under their jurisdiction, although hospices were not subject to inspection for compliance until July 1, 1985, in order to give them time to meet these standards.

As part of their attempt to write standards, the Joint Commission conducted a study to determine, among other things, how many hospices had inpatient units and what those inpatient units consisted of: for example, scattered beds in other units; *architecturally distinct* units within hospitals or skilled nursing facilities (architecturally distinct units de-fined as those with a separate nurses' station); a few designated beds in a hospital ward decorated for hospice use with colored sheets, couches, lounge chairs, tables, artwork of nature scenes, and the like; or freestanding units.

Recent communication from the Joint Commission study suggests that although inpatient accommodation is being supplied through hospices in more and more cases, the architecturally distinct hospice unit is still a minority solution. In Phase II of the study, 720 operational hospice programs were found, but 56 percent of these provided home care only. Thirty-six percent had both home-care and inpatient services; 7 percent provided inpatient care only. A Spring 1983 sample of 375 hospices that offer inpatient care showed that care was provided through scatterbeds a majority of the time. Hospices that used other means had four distinctly different kinds of inpatient settings: mixed oncology and hospice patients in a remodeled combined unit; a separate hospice area within an oncology unit; a hospice area in a medical/surgical unit; and the architecturally distinct and functionally autonomous (or semiautonomous) hospice unit. The Joint Commission has estimated roughly that these architecturally distinct units are a severe minority, representing perhaps 100 hospice programs of a total now well over 1,000.

The architecturally distinct and somewhat autonomous hospice or palliative-care unit is the focus of this study. In this section, these units will be discussed in detail, and generalizations will be made about what has been found in the survey data. In addition, other factors modifying and limiting a palliative-care facility will be laid out, in the hope that designers and caregivers alike will come to know existing units, approaches, and limitations.

Part Two is organized into three chapters. Chapter 4 presents the compendium of existing and planned facilities, with a discussion of methodology, data on specific hospices (in alphabetical order), and several charts that combine the materials.

Chapter 5 compares facilities, with an eye toward rooms and services provided, space planning figures in rough square footages, and detailed information on hospices, organized by type and size. This information will be of interest to the planner and architect, as well as to care providers interested in starting their own inpatient unit. Together, chapters 4 and 5 should provide the reader with a basic understanding of existing hospice unit architecture.

Chapter 6 discusses a variety of specific palliative-care concerns, alternatives in palliative care, and the most basic restraints on current hospice design. This information should help to distinguish the difference between hospice and other forms of health-care architecture, while keeping in mind the practical and economic difficulties of developing a new building type. The newness of hospice care in the United States does not protect it from developing rigidities in approach. The options and constraints mentioned herein are added to address more fully the conditions under which the American hospice is developing its inpatient care and architecture, and to point out the need for designers and architects to remain open to a variety of solutions and approaches.

This section is concluded with a summation of the priorities of hospice architecture found in this survey; these are matched with the intentions of the caregivers as well as the needs of the families and patients. The combination of medical establishment, unconscious patterns in design, and existing resources and limitations makes the development of a completely new kind of institutional facility very difficult, yet the evolution of a hospice building type, at least in terms of intention and services, is both recognizable in this analysis and demonstrably necessary.

No systematic classification of hospice inpatient units has heretofore been available. The architecturally distinct and autonomous facilities are not distinguished in National Hospice Organization literature, nor has the Joint Commission yet separated their functional categories from the architectural classifications necessary to designers and caregivers. As mentioned earlier, the architecturally distinct hospice is a minority in inpatient provision.

Hospice inpatient care, until recently, has been associated with long-term care and is now being found in listings of subacute services. As a location for respite and pain control, the inpatient hospice facility is most often used for short-term and intermittent stays. As such, it represents the middle of a continuum of care bounded by such long-term care facilities as skilled nursing and intermediate care facilities at one end, and the acute-care unit at the other. In the United States, the palliative-care units range from longer-term facilities, where the patient without primary caregiver or funds can find a second home, to the short-term care facilities—designated beds within oncology or medical/surgical units. The short-term, palliative-care units have become the model of American hospice care, with its emphasis on home visiting, primary caregiver, and the United States health-care financing system.

In this sample of hospices and palliative units, no such distinction has been brought to bear. The palliative care of the terminally ill requires flexibility and variety in approach and design. The continuum of care represented by hospice-combined home and inpatient service, with patient and family considered the unit of care, is also represented in the variety of inpatient settings. The values and philosophies of palliative care for the dying underlie the design of every type of unit in the continuum. This survey was undertaken in order to find the common architectural parameters of these shared values, as well as the differences evident in scale and economics. Further investigation into the intentions and existing conditions was pursued in order to sort out the more successful examples of particularly "hospice-like" settings from those units less able to realize their values and priorities.

This compendium should give the planner, designer, or hospice proponent an overview of existing and planned inpatient hospice and palliative-care facilities in the United States, providing data about many hospices that have had little or no publicity up to this time. I have tried to describe the buildings and units so that the stated intentions of the designer do not mask the actual physical environment. Of course, there is no substitute for first-hand observation, especially for obtaining a feeling of the place and the people who enliven and enrich the environment. Nevertheless, it is hoped that this systematic and uniform treatment of a new kind of health-care facility will serve to identify the hospice genre and contribute to more options and better design in the future.

Method

The hospices discussed in this chapter are examples of planned and existing architecturally separate units of the freestanding as well as parent-based types. The greatest coverage is devoted to facilities visited by the author in the fall of 1982; all examples, however, have contributing value as intentionally designed hospice space. It is very difficult to locate existing inpatient hospices that are architecturally distinct, that are more than a few patient rooms at the end of a corridor, decorated with colored sheets and carpeting. I wrote to facilities listed in Kenneth Cohn's *Hospice: Prescription for Terminal Care;* the Health Care Financing Administration and New York State demonstration project listings were also helpful. In addition, I consulted the National Hospice Organization's *Hospices Coast to Coast,* although hospices in this directory are not classified by unit type, but by whether they have contracted for inpatient care.

Initially, I sent the hospices one of two brief questionnaires; one if I was sure that they had a distinct inpatient unit, another if I was not sure. I then sent contacts and facilities a longer follow-up questionnaire. I developed other forms for those units that I visited. From these written documents and contributed plan drawings, I established the details of the unit and found two levels of completeness. The facilities that provided the most data form the first group of twenty-one hospices and palliative-care units.

The second group of twenty-seven hospices and palliative-care facilities includes those for whom information was less complete, in which questionnaires were partially filled out or plans were not submitted. This group also includes some units for which information was gathered through detailed articles or data gathered from others' visits. This group also includes several British facilities and a Canadian hospice unit. These hospices are mentioned or discussed in the chapters that follow the compendium but are not the primary focus of the book, as their survey data were incomplete.

To present the specific data of the first group, the development of special forms was necessary. Information was divided into three categories: general data and a list of architectural or program components, with approximate room sizes and number; a proximity matrix of the general areas of the unit; and a descriptive or environmental matrix for selected areas of the unit. In addition, most facilities have general notes about the unique contributions of the unit. Hospices have been illustrated with photographic documentation whenever possible, and plans and parts have been reproduced for a graphic portrayal of the organization.

In this survey, examples are included of virtually every type of hospice inpatient unit with an architecturally distinct form. The geographic range and environment have been represented, as have sponsorship types. The research represents two years of correspondence and contacts, ending in spring 1983.

The families and hospice patients were not, unfortunately, involved to any extent in the data collection. There were several reasons for excluding them from the survey, the most important one being that patient and family privacy during hospice care should not be compromised or disturbed by questions about the hospice environment. In addition, patients and family are frequently not aware of the qualities of the environment that contribute to their well-being during times of stress. Also, patients may be so grateful to have quality care that they offer no criticism of their environment. Other patients may be too debilitated during their stay at the hospice to answer such post-occupancy questions. Thus, it is difficult to get a representative sample of patient opinion concerning their environment during inpatient stays.

It is important to recognize the phenomenal contributions of the hospice caregivers, who took time and effort from other important duties to contribute to this documentation. It should be stressed that the survey could not have been done without their voluntary help and advice. The intentions of the caregivers and their opinions on hospice care form the bulk of the information in this study.

• BELLIN HOSPICE PROGRAM

744 South Webster Street
P.O. Box 1700
Green Bay, Wisconsin 54305

Classification: Hospice in acute-care hospital
Sponsoring agencies: Bellin Hospital/Home Health Care Agency
Type: Separate inhouse unit
Area served: Green Bay and environs
Inpatient population: 10 maximum; mostly Catholic
Established: N/A
Scope of work involved: formerly acute-care wing
    Architect: Somerville Associates, Inc.
           2020 Riverside Drive
           Green Bay, Wisconsin 54301
Cost of work: N/A
  Build: N/A
  Furnishings: N/A
Comprehensive intention of building selection and/or design: N/A
General intention: Private, homelike family space with residential decor
Location: Upper-floor hospital wing (second floor)
Description:
  Community image: part of community hospital
  Interior image: warm, comfortable, homelike wing
Other:
  Changes (quoted from Bellin staff response to questionnaire): "Bigger patient rooms, no wards, private rest space for staff, chapel on the unit. A design with a lounge in the center and private rooms around the outside is ideal because it offers companionship and ability to withdraw when necessary."
Users:
  Outpatient staff: N/A
  Volunteers: N/A
  Inpatient staff: N/A
  Outpatients served: N/A
  Inpatient average population: N/A
  Inpatient average length of stay: N/A
  Family visitors per week: N/A
Services rendered: Home and inpatient care

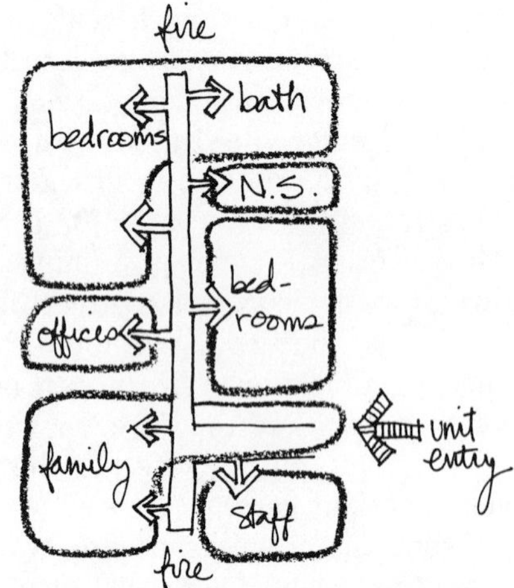

Parti drawing of Bellin Hospice

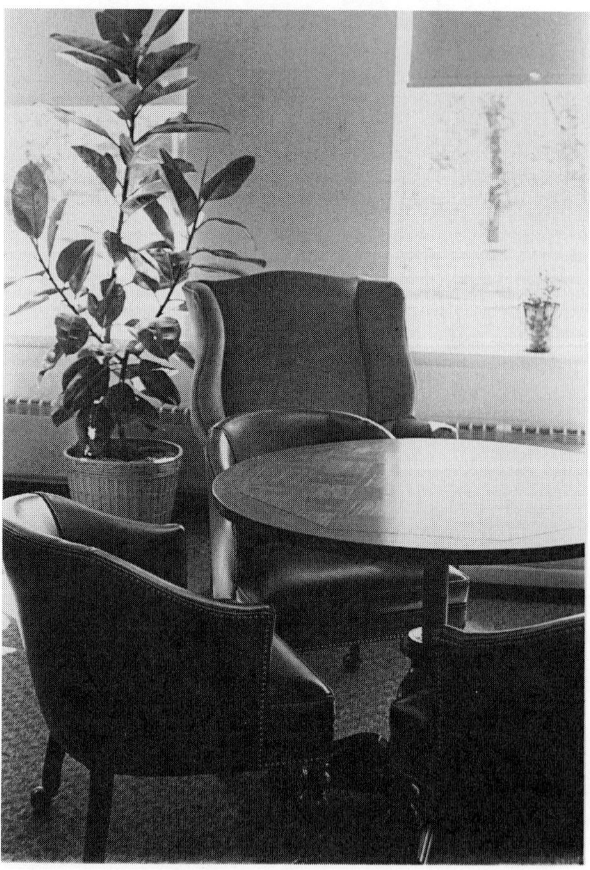

Patient room, Bellin Hospice

BELLIN HOSPICE: ARCHITECTURAL COMPONENTS

Architectural Components	Notes	Wing/Total Number	Rough Dimensions or Size, Square Feet
1. Patient room	Single at each end	2	11′ × 17′
	Other (Four)	2	17′ × 30′
Bathrooms	Handicap (with tub)	1	180
2. Family lounge		1	448
Child area	None		
Eating area	In lounge		
Other	Kitchenette	1	70
Family private room	None		
Family other	None		
Bathrooms	Unit W.C. (m/f)	2	25 (ea.)
Conference	Lounge area in patient room (4)	2	
3. Garden	None		
Gardening area	None		
Chapel	Off unit		
Transition room	Multipurpose	1	11′ × 17′
Meditation room	None		
Chaplain office	None		
4. Nurses' station		1	162
Medication room		1	52
Nurses' retreat	None		
Staff rooms	Locker and storage	1	162
Bathrooms	None		
5. Daycare	None		
Childcare	None		
Massage	None		
Physical therapy	Off unit		
Occupational therapy	None		
Library	None		
Music/reading	See lounge		
Barbershop	None		
Tavern	None		
Store	None		
Game room	See lounge		
6. Kitchen facilities	None		
Unit dining	None		
Other dining	See lounge		
Nutrition station	None		
Kitchenette	See lounge		
7. Offices			
Director/manager		1	218
Nurse coordinator	None		
Social work coordinator	None		
Boardroom	None		
Conference room	None		

BELLIN HOSPICE: ARCHITECTURAL COMPONENTS (*cont'd.*)

Architectural Components	Notes	Wing/Total Number	Rough Dimensions or Size, Square Feet
Volunteer coordinator	None		
Business office	None		
Files	None		
Other	Home-care coordinator	1	218
8. Entry, front door	N/A*		
Reception	N/A		
Admitting	N/A		
Staff	Stairs		
Patient	N/A		
Volunteer	Stairs		
Visitors	Stairs		
Goods	Small service elevator		
Hallways, main			
Service	Unit hall		
Other	N/A		
Exit goods	Same		
Laundry	N/A		
Dead	N/A		
9. Parking	N/A		
Connections to other facilities	N/A		
Connection to neighborhood	N/A		
Street visibility	N/A		
Landscaping			
Front yard	Trees		
Back yard	Trees, shrubs		
10. Services			
Laundry	Utility room	1	120
Clean			
Dirty			
Janitorial			
Closet		1	20
Stores			
General stores	Off unit		
Offices	N/A		
Garbage	Off unit		
Garbage pickup	N/A		
Equipment storage	N/A		
Mail	N/A		
Miscellaneous	N/A		

Note: N/A = data not available.

BELLIN HOSPICE: PROXIMITY MATRIX

Variables	Variable Numbers													
	1.	2.	3.	4.	5.	6.	7.	8.	9.	10.	11.	12.	13.	14.
1. Patient	B													
2. Family	C	A												
3. Chapel/transition room	B	A	A											
4. Nature (outdoors)	D	D	D											
5. Nurses' station	C	C	B	D	E									
6. Inpatient services	E	E	E	D	E	E								
7. Kitchen	D	D	D	D	D	E	D							
8. Kitchenette	C	A	B	D	C	E	D							
9. Offices	B	B	A	D	B	E	D	B	A					
10. Main entry/facility	D	D	D	D	D	E	D	D	D					
11. Bed entry/unit	C	A	A	D	C	E	D	A	B	C				
12. Parking/staff	*	*	*	*	*	*	*	*	*	*	*			
13. Parking/visitors	*	*	*	*	*	*	*	*	*	*	*	*		
14. Janitorial	C	A	B	D	D	E	D	A	C	D	B	*	*	A

Key:
- A = within 16-foot radius (based on 8-foot corridors)
- B = within 32-foot radius
- C = related areas (see plan)
- D = distant
- E = scattered, disparate association
- blank = no relation
- * = no information available

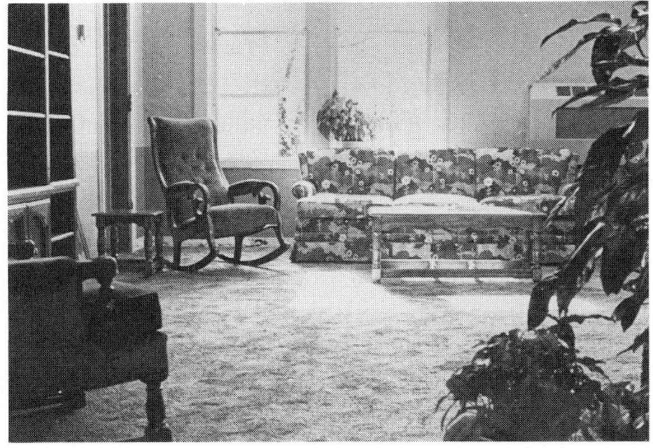

Bellin family lounge

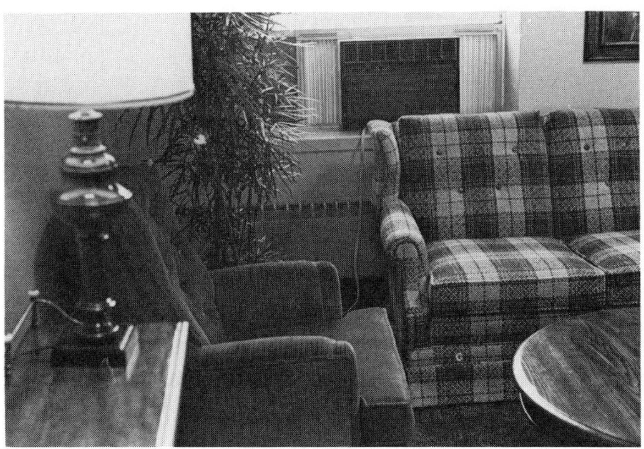

Detail of family lounge, Bellin Hospice

BELLIN HOSPICE: DESCRIPTIVE MATRIX (Environmental Factors)

| | *Patient (Bedrooms)* | | *Family (Lounge)* | |
	Intent	*Existing*	*Intent*	*Existing*
View				
Window	light	treetops	light	treetops
Doors	nonabandonment, privacy	hall, N.S., entry, and transition room	central, open	near entry, open to kitchenette
Each bed	window and doors	low sill windows, open doors, relights	N/A	N/A
Other: artwork	homelike, comforting	plants, nature scenes	homelike, comforting	plants, nature scenes
Window				
Treatment	N/A	N/A	N/A	N/A
Trim	homelike	wood	homelike	wood
Operation	existing	double-hung	existing	double-hung
Covering	light, adjustable, homelike	shades	light	none
Lighting				
Type	homelike	lots of natural light, fluorescent/incandescent	homelike	lots of natural light, fluorescent
Fixtures	flexible, homelike	overhead fluorescent lamps	flexible, homelike	overhead fluorescent
Handicap access				
Bed and wheelchair	recliners	roomy, large doorways, grouped furniture, low-pile carpet	recliners	roomy, grouped furniture
Dominant colors	homelike	earthtones, green plants, wicker browns	homelike, comforting	domestic floral prints, browns, green plants, pastels
Dominant materials	homelike, clean, natural	wood, paint, plastic laminate, metal, carpet, acoustical tile	homelike, warm, comforting	paint, wood, soft fabrics, pile carpet, acoustical tile
Furniture type	homelike, movable, flexible	hospital beds, residential chairs, tables, built-in closets	homelike, movable, private	sofas, rocker, tables, side chairs, picnic table, bookcase, all residential
Ceiling height/ treatment	existing, practical	approximately 8', acoustical tile	existing, practical	approximately 8', acoustical tile
Floor surfacing	homelike	low-pile carpet	homelike	pile carpet
Personalization	homelike	plants, places for display	homelike	plants, places for books, magazines
Organization	existing with modification	mixed use on double-loaded corridor	homelike	large room with kitchen. counter, near unit entry
Equipment	adaptable, comfortable, noninstitutional	HVAC, lights	homelike, comfortable	HVAC, lights, kitchen equipment
Signs	N/A	N/A	N/A	N/A

Transition Room

	Intent	*Existing*
View		
Window	light	treetops
Doors	private, convenient	hall, entry, offices, one patient room
Each bed	N/A	N/A
Other: artwork	nondenominational, homelike, comforting	nature scenes
Window		
Treatment	N/A	N/A
Trim	homelike	wallboard
Operation	existing	double-hung
Covering	light, adjustable, homelike	shade
Lighting		
Type	homelike, adjustable	natural light, fluorescent/incandescent
Fixtures	homelike, practical	overhead fluorescent/incandescent lamps
Handicap access		
Bed and wheelchair	bed, recliner	large door, grouped furniture
Dominant colors	homelike	plaid couch, earth-tones, pastels
Dominant materials	soft, warm, homelike, durable	paint, velour, twill, carpet, wood, brass, cane, plants
Furniture type	homelike, comfortable, nondenominational	soft couch, chair, coffee table, side cabinet, side chairs
Ceiling height/treatment	existing, practical	8' approximately, acoustical tile
Floor surfacing	homelike	carpet
Personalization	homelike, adaptable	plants, room for flowers
Organization	existing with modification	room off double-loaded hall near entry
Equipment	adaptable, comfortable, homelike	air conditioning, HV, lights
Signs	N/A	N/A

• CABRINI HOSPICE AT CABRINI HOSPITAL

227 East 19th Street
New York, New York 10003

Classification: Hospice

Sponsoring agencies: Cabrini Medical Center, Missionary Sisters of the Sacred Heart

Type: Skilled nursing facility in hospital (separate unit)

Area served: New York City and environs

Inpatient population: 15 beds; Catholic, Jewish, and Protestant. Mostly Jewish patients; 16 years and older

Established: Original unit in October 1980; this unit May 1982. Original unit was remodeled four-story Sisters' residence, with fifteen private one-bed rooms, moved to be closer to doctors and to provide larger rooms.

Scope of work involved: formerly skilled nursing facility, offices; remodel in progress
   Architect: inhouse planner

Cost of work: N/A
   Build: N/A
   Furnishings: N/A

Comprehensive intention of building selection and/or design: Homelike, secure, cheerful, and comfortable hospice environment

Location: City center, ward of large hospital (sixth floor for view, air)

Description:
   Double-loaded, L-shaped wing
   Community image: part of Cabrini Hospital
   Interior image: quiet, older ward, away from main activity
   Convenience: hard to find from hospital entry

Other: Not completely renovated at the time of visit
   Changes: Carpet, paneling over tile, cabinets in dayroom, blinds in rooms

Users:
   Outpatient staff: 2 home-care nurses
   Volunteers: N/A
   Inpatient staff: Five full-time equivalent—
     2 LPNs, 2 RNs, 1 director of nursing
   Average inpatient population: 12–15
   Average length of inpatient stay: 14–21 days
   Family/visitors per week: N/A

Services rendered: Inpatient care, home care, bereavement counseling

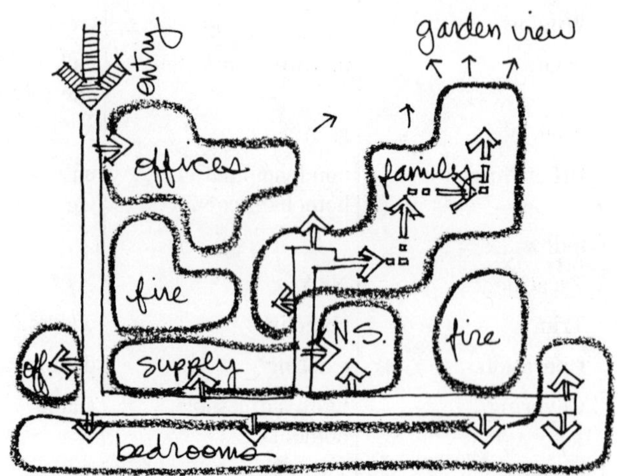

Parti drawing of Cabrini Hospice

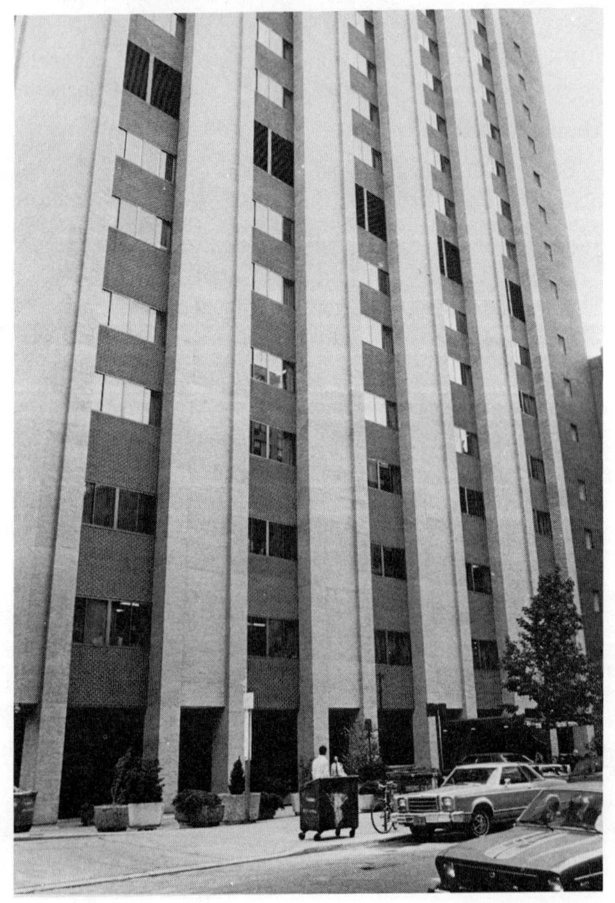

Entrance, Cabrini Hospice

CABRINI HOSPICE: ARCHITECTURAL COMPONENTS

Architectural Components	Notes	Wing/Total Number	Rough Dimensions or Size, Square Feet
1. Patient room	Single	5	8′ × 14′
	Double	4	11′ × 14′
	Other (double)	1	8′ × 14′
Bathrooms	Shared by 2 rooms	5	21
	Shower room	1	7′ × 7′
2. Family lounge	Sun room	1	12′ × 20′
Child area	None		
Eating area	See sun room		
Other	Active lounge	1	8′ × 18′
Family private room	None		
Family other	None		
Bathrooms	Off lounges	1	30
Conference	None		
3. Garden	Roof top, lower floor	1	1,200
Gardening area	In sun room		
Chapel	Off unit		
Transition room	In patient rooms		
Meditation room	None		
Chaplain office		1	72
4. Nurses' station		1	52
Medication room		1	20
Nurses' retreat	Off unit		
Staff rooms	None		
Bathrooms	W.C.	1	30
5. Daycare	None		
Childcare	Off-unit services		
Massage	Off-unit services		
Physical therapy	Off-unit services		
Occupational therapy	Off-unit services		
Library	None		
Music/reading	See sun room, lounge		
Barbershop	None		
Tavern	None		
Store	None		
Game room	None		
6. Kitchen facilities	N/A		
Storage			
Supplies	Off unit		
Preparation			
Cleaning			
Office			
Dietary staff			
Unit dining			
Other dining	See sun room, lounge		
Nutrition station		1	3′ × 8′
Kitchenette (coffee lounge)	See family active lounge		

CABRINI HOSPICE: ARCHITECTURAL COMPONENTS (*cont'd.*)

Architectural Components	Notes	Wing/Total Number	Rough Dimensions or Size, Square Feet
7. Offices		8 total	
Director/administrator		1	99
Nurse coordinator (D.N.)		1	80
Social work coordinator		1	48
Boardroom	None		
Conference room	None		
Volunteer coordinator		1	110
Business office	Admin. sec'y.	1	78
Files	Home care	1	112
Other	Medical director	1	80
8. Entry, front door	Hospital entry	1	
Reception	Unit entry		
Admitting	At unit		
Staff	Stairs, elevators		
Patient	Hospital emergency/elevators		
Volunteer	Elevators, hospital		
Visitors	Elevators, hospital		
Goods	Service elevators, hospice	2	4' × 6'
Other	Via hospital corridors		
Hallways, main	Hospital corridors		
Service	Hospice corridors		952
Other	Nurses' station, lounge hall		160
Exit goods	Service elevators, hospice		
Laundry	Service elevators, hospice		
Dead	To morgue (hospital)		
Miscellaneous	Fire stairs	2	144
9. Parking	N/A		
Connections to other facilities	N/A		
Connection to neighborhood	N/A		
Street visibility	N/A		
Landscaping	N/A		
Front yard			
Back yard			
10. Services			
Laundry			
Clean	Linen	1	42
Dirty	Linen	1	49
Janitorial			
Closet		1	21
Stores	General storage	1	30
General stores			
Offices	Off unit		
Garbage	Off unit		
Garbage pickup	N/A		
Equipment storage	See general storage		
Mail	N/A		
Miscellaneous	Storage, patients' items		10

CABRINI HOSPICE: PROXIMITY MATRIX

Variable Numbers

Variables	1.	2.	3.	4.	5.	6.	7.	8.	9.	10.	11.	12.	13.	14.
1. Patient	C													
2. Family	C													
3. Chapel	D	D												
4. Nature (view)	C	D	*											
5. Nurses' station	B	B	*											
6. Inpatient services	D	D	*	C	D									
7. Kitchen	*	*	*	*	*	*								
8. Kitchenette	C	A	*	C	A		*							
9. Offices	C	C	*	C	B	D	*	C						
10. Main entry/facility	D	D	C	D	D	D	*	D	D					
11. Bed entry/unit	C	D	*		C		*	D	C	D				
12. Parking/staff	D	D	D	D	D	D	*	D	D	D	D			
13. Parking/visitors	D	D	D	D	D		*	D	D	D	D	A		
14. Janitorial	B	C	*	D	A		*	B	C		C		B	

Key:

    A = within 16-foot radius (based on 8-foot corridors)
    B = within 32-foot radius
    C = related areas (see plan)
    D = distant
 blank = no relation
   * = off unit

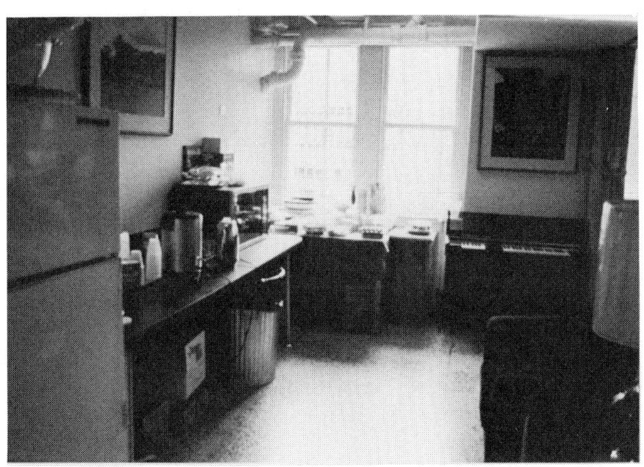

Kitchenette area of family lounge, Cabrini Hospice

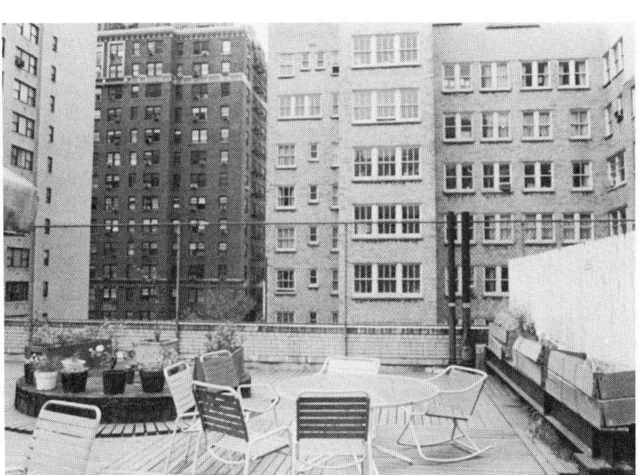

Rooftop garden

CABRINI HOSPICE: DESCRIPTIVE MATRIX (Environmental Factors)

	Patient (Bedrooms)		Family (Lounge)	
	Intent	*Existing*	*Intent*	*Existing*
View				
Window	bright, airy	south light, high (5th-6th floors)	open, nature	view rooftop garden, windows on 3 sides
Doors	nonabandonment, privacy	single-loaded bedrooms, near nurses' station, offices	private, cozy	cul-de-sac location
Each bed	homelike, nonabandonment	low beds, television, residential, furnishing, views	N/A	N/A
Other: artwork	plants, homelike, natural	windowsills, landscapes	homelike, intimate	windowsills, nature scenes
Window				
Treatment	existing	3 × 2 paning	existing	3 × 2 paning
Trim		wood		wood
Operation		operable, double-hung		operable, double-hung
Covering	adaptable, homelike	drapes	bright, airy	none, many large windows on 3 sides
Lighting				
Type	homelike, flexible	natural light, fluorescent/ incandescent	homelike, flexible	natural light, fluorescent/ incandescent
Fixtures	homelike, existing	lamps, overhead ceiling lights	existing, homelike	windows, residential lamps, ceiling lights
Handicap access				
Bed and wheelchair	chair and bed accessibility	wide doors, stable furniture, few pieces	wheelchair access	grouped furniture, stable furniture
Dominant colors	homelike, clean	pastels, including blues, yellows	homelike, warm, cheerful, earth tones	pastels, light beiges, browns
Dominant materials	homelike, cleanable	paint, linoleum, fabrics, metal, plastic laminate, wood	homelike	paint, plastic laminate, velour, wood, fabrics, linoleum
Furniture				
Type Colors	practical, homelike, browns, beiges	hospital beds, tables, residential table, television cart, recliner, built-in closet	homelike, comfortable, adaptable	residential couch, chairs, tables, lamps, organ
Ceiling height/ treatment	existing	approximately 8'6", paint	existing	high 9', paint
Floor surfacing	carpeting	linoleum	carpeting	linoleum
Personalization	homelike, adaptable	sills, tables for objects, pictures	homelike, comfortable	books on sills, plants, pictures
Organization	nonabandonment, modified existing	most on one side of double-loaded L corridor	homelike, comfortable, cheerful	2 rooms with activity areas, quiet areas
Equipment	practical, noninstitutional, diversions	oxygen/suction, no intercom, television, phones	homelike, noninstitutional, inexpensive	kitchenette with refrigerator, coffee pot, microwave, no television
Signs	practical, existing	room numbers	homelike	none

	Rooftop Garden		Nurses' Station	
	Intent	*Existing*	*Intent*	*Existing*
View				
Window	from garden (4th floor)	open to street on two sides, sky, hospital behind	internal	no windows
Doors	N/A	N/A	open	no doors
Each bed	to garden	hospice family rooms, offices, rehabilitation above (old wing)	open	very low counter
Other: artwork	N/A	N/A	N/A	N/A
Window				
Treatment	N/A	N/A	N/A	N/A
Trim	N/A	N/A	N/A	N/A
Operation	N/A	N/A	N/A	N/A
Covering	N/A	N/A	N/A	N/A
Lighting				
Type	day use only	no lights	existing	fluorescent
Fixtures	N/A	N/A	existing	overhead
Handicap access				
Bed and wheelchair	staff assists patient	recliner chairs, from hospice to elevator short corridor	visibility	desk-height counter, open plan
Dominant colors	seasonal, natural, homelike	yellow, brown, green, red, wood, bright colors	cheerful, homelike	pastel/light brown wallpaper
Dominant materials	natural, maintenance-free	plants, flowers, wood, metal, fabric, brick	practical, homelike	paint, linoleum, plastic laminate, acoustical tile, fabric
Furniture				
Type	residential, sheltering, weather-resistant	inexpensive patio (aluminum) furniture, wood planters, wood roof slats	open, homelike, office friendly, cluttered	long desk, office chair, medical cabinet, countertop curtain, carts
Ceiling height/ treatment	visibility, security	chain metal fence	existing	8' lowered with acoustical tile for HVAC, lights
Floor surfacing	maintenance-free	gravel	practical	linoleum
Personalization	volunteer-maintained	plants, furnished by contributions	casual, busy, friendly	pictures, bulletin board, personal objects
Organization	existing	large rooftop	central, friendly	L with low desk, meds and visibility
Equipment	practical, maintenance-free	hoses, storage shed	noninstitutional	medical cabinet, sink, no charts or office equipment visible
Signs	private facility	no signs	noninstitutional	no signs

Cabrini Hospice: General Notes

This is Cabrini Hospital's second hospice; the first was in a remodeled Sisters' residence nearby. The first hospice, a four-story building with fifteen single rooms, was unsatisfactory for several reasons. The bedrooms were too small and all of the same type, providing no variety. In addition, the unit was too far from the hospital; doctors seemed to find it inconvenient. However, it was a nice, residential atmosphere.

At the time of the survey, remodeling was still to take place. Tiles on corridor walls were to be replaced with paneling, cabinets were to be constructed in the dayroom, and carpeting and window blinds were to be added. The rooftop garden was also to be revitalized by hospice personnel and volunteers.

Overall, Cabrini Hospice was a pleasant, slightly cluttered, and very comfortable unit. Hospice personnel clearly worked with what they had and made do with much. The artwork was all first-rate, framed, and mounted everywhere. They needed a general meeting room, as the offices were too small for large meetings. It was difficult to find the hospice from the hospital entry; there were few signs. The absence of signs conveyed the feeling that a visitor must be an "insider" to find the hospice.

The organization of the unit contributed to the privacy, comfort, nonabandonment, and homelike qualities of the hospice. The L-shaped wing functioned as a U, with bedrooms and windows on the outside of the corridor, and nurses' station, offices, and family rooms in the compact center and other side of the corridor. This arrangement permitted a mixture of functions, promoted an atmosphere of nonabandonment, and left the family area as a cul-de-sac—farthest from the unit entry and, therefore, most private, yet still accessible. The family rooms viewed down to the rooftop garden. The high floor permitted more light and views into the hospice, which might otherwise have been difficult to obtain in the hospice's urban location. Religious services were held in the chapel and memorial services held in the tower's sixteenth-floor cafeteria. Religious symbols were visible in a few of the offices.

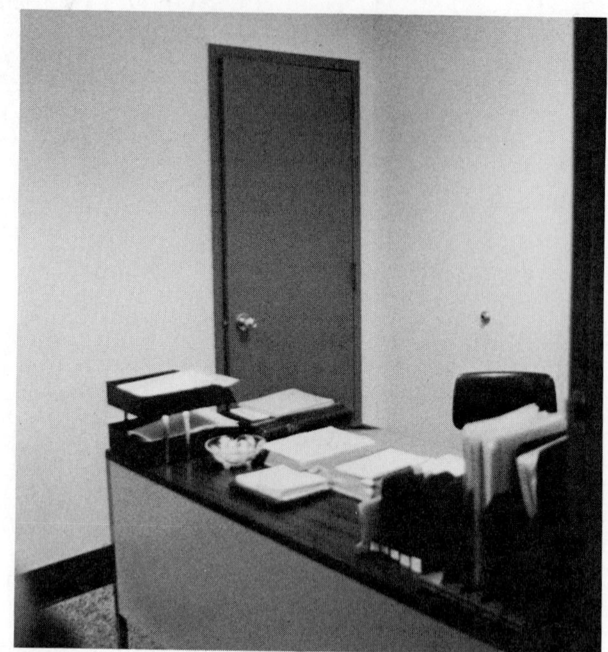

Hospice reception area

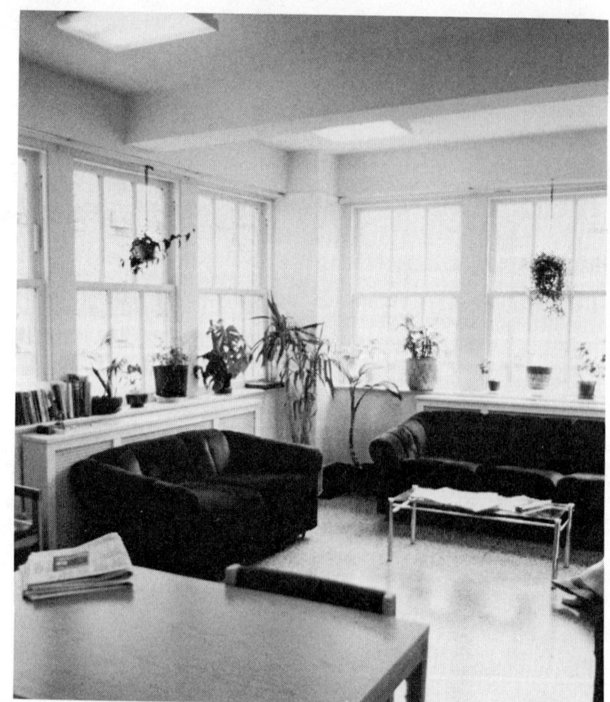

Sunroom

• CALVARY HOSPITAL

1740–70 Eastchester Road
Bronx, New York 10461

Classification: Pre-hospice/special hospital, acute care for the terminally ill

Sponsoring agencies: Department of Health and Hospitals, Catholic Charities of the Archdiocese of New York

Type: New inpatient facility (six-story)

Area served: New York City and metropolitan area

Inpatient population: 200 beds, approximately 2,000 patients per year

Established: This facility, 1978. Previous Calvary Hospital, on different site in the Bronx, had 111-bed population

Scope of work involved: 173,000 sq. ft. new construction

    Architect: Rogers, Burgun, Shahine & Deschler
            521 Fifth Avenue
            New York, NY 10175

Cost of work: 12 million
    Build: concrete frame, $69 per sq. ft.
    Furnishings: N/A

Comprehensive intention of building selection and/or design: Nonabandonment, modified intensive care

General intention: Shared amenities, single rooms

Location: Hospital area in Bronx, near train yards, factories, other facilities.

Description:
    Flat red-brick facade, with large plain windows, factory-like appearance from street.
    Community image: small six-story hospital.
    Interior image: modern, interior courtyard, spacious hospital, bright and clean.
    Convenience: parking, bus, subway, easy to reach and enter. Windy site.

Other: Calvary takes patients that cannot go to St. Rose's Home; has OR, radiology therapy, more active palliative care.
    Changes: Extensive changes planned. See General Notes.

Users:
    Outpatient staff: doctors, nurses
    Volunteers: 200
    Inpatient staff: 300 professionals/paraprofessionals

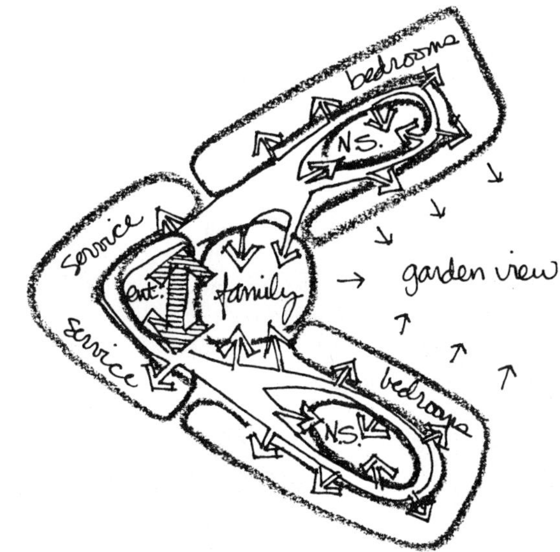

Parti drawing, Calvary Hospital

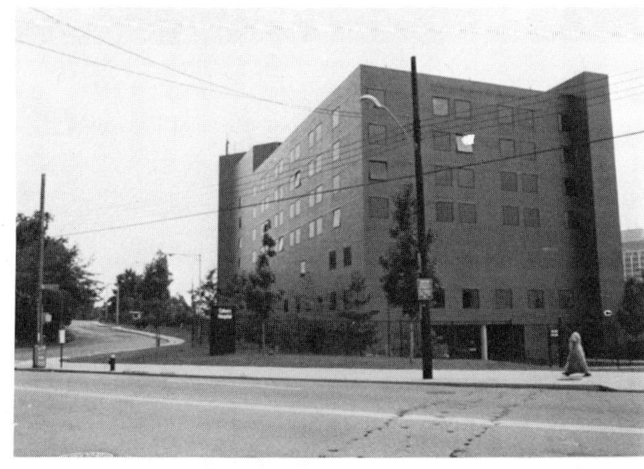

View of Calvary Hospital from street

    Outpatients served: 40 at one time
    Inpatient average population: 182
    Inpatient average length of stay: 60 days
    Family/visitors per week: Varies

Services rendered: Inpatient, outpatient, active palliative care, bereavement care, education and training, inpatient festivities, regular religious services, family sleeps in patient's room only in emergency.

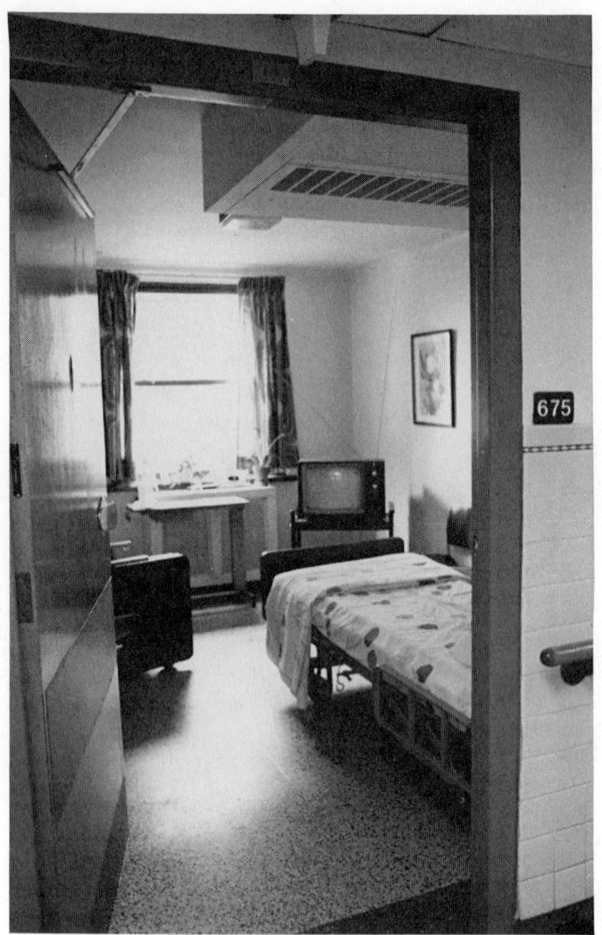

Patient room

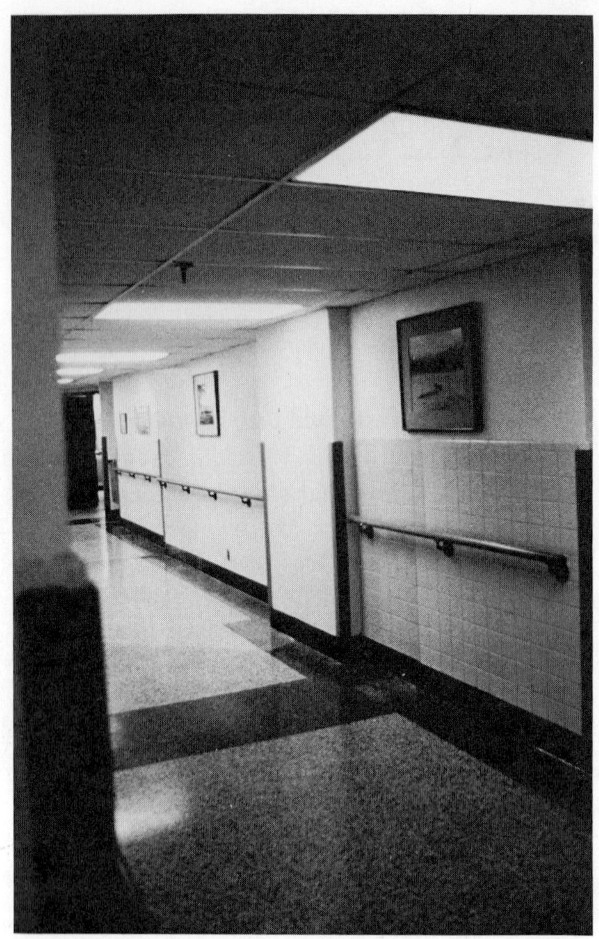

Hospice corridor

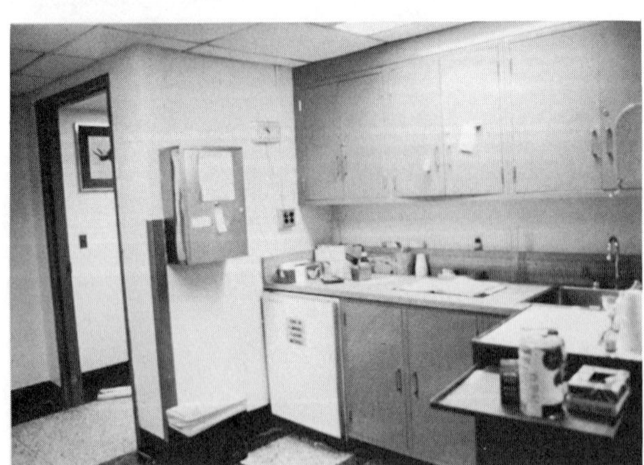

Nutrition station

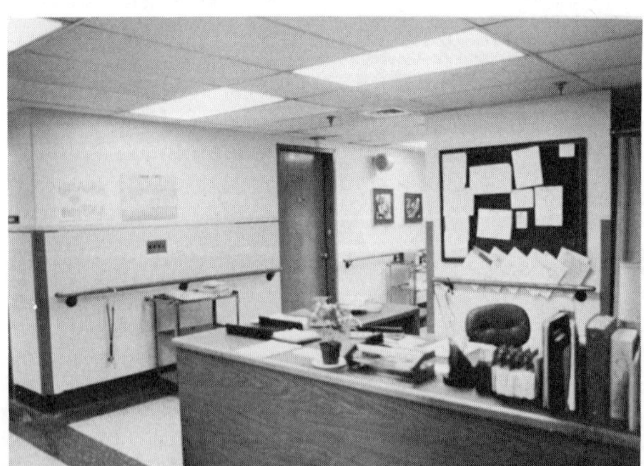

Nurses' station

CALVARY HOSPITAL: ARCHITECTURAL COMPONENTS

Architectural Components	Notes	Wing/Total Number	Rough Dimensions or Size, Square Feet
1. Patient room	Single	25/200	168
	Other (W.C.)	14/112	25
Bathrooms	Showers	1/8	110
	W.C. (m/f)	1/8	300
2. Family lounge	Dayroom	1/4	940 (usable)
Child area	N/A		
Eating area	Day/patient rooms		
Other	Games, television		
Family private room	N/A		
Family other	See coffee shop		
Bathrooms	W.C. (m/f)		
Conference	and ambulatory care	1	2,000
3. Garden	Patio, including landscaping	1	11,000
Gardening area	Dayrooms		
Chapel	See meditation room		
Transition room	Bereavement room	1	80
Meditation room	Chapel, 1st floor	1	760
Chaplain offices	1st floor	2	80
Terraces	2nd floor	2	1,975 (each)
Morgue/autopsy	Basement	1	900
4. Nurses' station		1/8	600
Medication room	Part of nurses' station		72
Nurses' retreat	On patient floors	1/8	80
Staff rooms	Lounge (basement)	1	250
Bathrooms	Staff lockers, m/f, basement	1	850
	Nurse lockers, m/f, patient floors	1/4	415
5. Daycare	See family lounge		
Childcare	See auditorium		
Massage	In patient rooms		
Physical therapy	1st floor		400
Occupational therapy	Recreational therapy	1	1,225
	Radiology, 2nd floor		1,500
	Laboratory, 2nd floor		1,750
	Surgical suite, 2nd floor		1,400
Other	Auditorium, 1st floor	1	1,900
6. Kitchen facilities	Total	1	4,100
Storage	N/A		
Supplies	Central, basement	1	3,500
Preparation	See total		
Cleaning	See total		
Office	None		
Dietary staff	None		
Unit dining	See family lounge, patient rooms		
Other dining	Cafeteria, basement	1	2,050
Nutrition station	At nurses' station	1/8	
	Pantry, patient floors	1/4	475
	Coffee shop, 1st floor	1	1,575

Architectural Components	Notes	Wing/Total Number	Rough Dimensions or Size, Square Feet
7. Offices			
Director/administrator			2,500
Nurse coordinator			2,375
Social work coordinators		2/8	300
Boardroom	See administration		
Conference room	N/A		
Volunteer coordinators		1	900
Business offices	1st floor		1,800
Files	Medical records		825
Other	Public relations		575
	Personnel		1,100
	Employee clinic		500
	On-call space, 2nd floor	2	150
8. Entry, front door	Divided: bed/pedestrian		1,650 (T)
Reception	1st/2nd floor	2	170/500
Admitting	1st floor, including offices		1,200
Staff	Main entry/staff entry		
Patient	Main entry		
Volunteer	Main entry		
Visitors	Main entry		
Goods	Service entry		
Other	Lobby, part of front door		1,050
Hallways, main	Above ground floors		
Service	Basement		
Exit goods	Service entry, basement		100
Laundry	Linen/trash exit, basement		550
Dead	Staff entry, basement		100
9. Parking	2 lots, 170 spaces		
Connections to other facilities	N/A		
Connection to neighborhood	N/A		
Street visibility	N/A		
Landscaping			
Front yard	Covered drive		
Back yard	Patio		
10. Services			
Laundry	Linen supply, basement	1	1,000
Clean	Boiled linen, basement	1	425
Dirty	Basement	1	400
Janitorial	and housekeeping, basement	1	1,000
Closet	Each floor		
General stores	See kitchen		
Offices	N/A		
Garbage	Incinerator	1	250
Garbage pickup	Trash collection	1	250
Equipment Storage	Each patient floor	1/4	50
Mail	Main entry, 1st floor	1	200
Plant maintenance	Basement		1,500
Pharmacy	Basement		1,600
Mechanical	Basement		6,600
Security	Basement		150
Central sterile supply	Basement		3,600

CALVARY HOSPITAL: PROXIMITY MATRIX

						Variable Numbers								
Variables	1.	2.	3.	4.	5.	6.	7.	8.	9.	10.	11.	12.	13.	14.
1. Patient	C													
2. Family (dayroom)	C	D												
3. Chapel/meditation room	C	D												
4. Nature (patio)	C	C	D											
5. Nurses' station	C	D	D	D										
6. Inpatient services	C	D	C	C	D									
7. Kitchen	D	D	D	D	D	D								
8. Kitchenette (pantry)	D	A	D	D	D	D	C							
9. Offices	C	D	A	C	D	C	D	D						
10. Main entry/facility	D	D	A	C	D	E	D	D	E					
11. Bed entry/unit	D	A	C	C	D	D	D	A	D	C				
12. All parking	C	D	C	D	D	E	C	D	E	C	C			
13. Linen/laundry	D	C	D		C	D	A	C						
14. Janitorial	C	C	C	C	C	C	A	C	C	C	C			C

Key: A = within 16-foot radius (based on 8-foot corridors)
B = within 32-foot radius
C = related areas (see plan)
D = distant
E = scattered, disparate association
blank = no relation

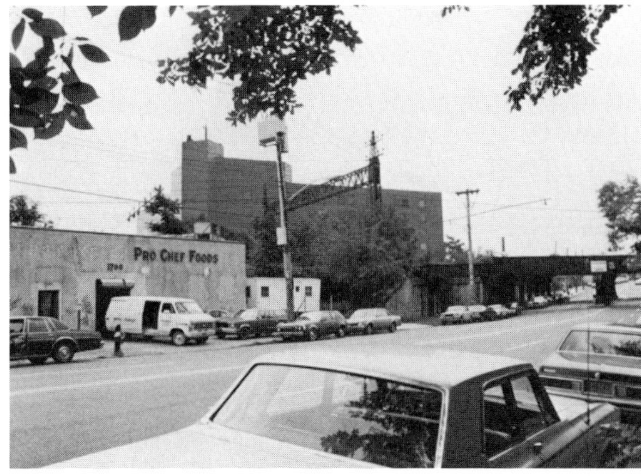

Back view of Calvary Hospital from street

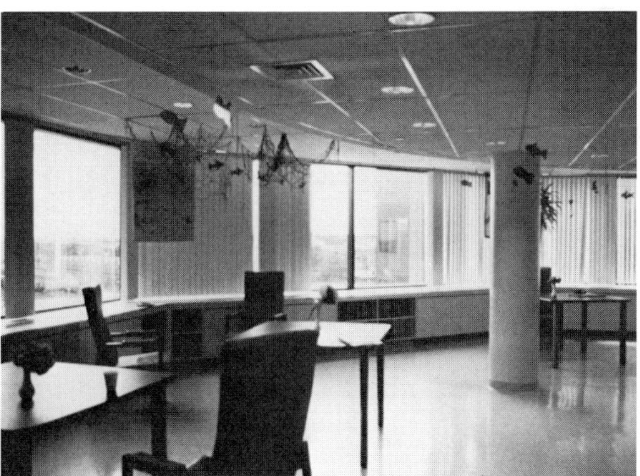

Dayroom

CALVARY HOSPITAL: DESCRIPTIVE MATRIX (Environmental Factors)

	Patient (Bedrooms)		Family (Dayroom)	
	Intent	*Existing*	*Intent*	*Existing*
View				
Window	light, turned inward/ high	large views, 36% view inward	light, turned inward	band of windows, overlooks patio
Doors	nonabandonment, privacy	single rooms, 68% view of nurses' station	open, welcoming, nonabandonment	open to hall both sides
Each bed	nonabandonment, nature, control	looks onto hall, window, built-ins, television	patio, activity, events	high view, books, television, hall, counter
Other: artwork	homelike, spiritual	nature pictures, plants, religious art	homelike, cheerful	patient art, prints, plants, colors
Window				
Treatment	energy-efficient	double pane (metal)	energy-efficient	double pane (metal)
Trim	modern	gypsum wall board	modern	gypsum wall board
Operation	homelike	operable	none	
Covering	light, clean	none, internal louvers for light control	bright, control	vertical blinds
Lighting				
Type	natural, flexible	large windows, incandescent/fluorescent	natural, warm task lighting	large windows, incandescent/fluorescent
Fixtures	choice, homelike	recessed wall fluorescent/incandescent lamps	choice, low gradient	ceiling fluorescent, incandescent lamps
Handicap access				
Bed and wheelchair	Lummox chair, bed	grouped furniture, built-ins	bed, Lummox chair, walker	grouped furniture, built-ins, large space, handrails
Dominant colors	clean, bright, variety	white, bright accent colors, browns	clean, bright, variety	white, bright accent colors, browns, greens
Dominant materials	clean, durable, cheerful	linoleum, paint, wood, plastic laminate, metal, fabrics	clean, durable, cheerful	linoleum, paint, glass, plastic laminate, woods, acoustical tile, fabrics
Furniture type	flexible, comfortable, noninstitutional	hospital bed, overbed table, Lummox chair, built-in closets, side tables, chair	flexible, homelike, cleanable	card tables, chairs, built-in counter, bookshelves, windowsill, lamps
Ceiling height/ treatment	homelike, meets building code	approximately 8', painted	windowhead	dropped acoustical ceiling with lights
Floor surfacing	durable, clean	linoleum	durable, clean	linoleum
Personalization	encouraged	windowsill, tables, built-ins, walls for display	encouraged	windowsill, shelves, walls for display

	Patient (Bedrooms)		Family (Dayroom)	
	Intent	*Existing*	*Intent*	*Existing*
Organization	nonabandonment, privacy	patient rooms encircle nurses' station on two wings, for four floors	nonabandonment, central, warm	between wings, axis with entry, patio, coffee shop
Equipment	comfortable, nonabandonment, choice	oxygen/suction, television, phone, louvers, temperature, lights	noninstitutional, comfortable, flexible	television, lights, radio, stereo, (pantry nearby) coffee shop
Signs	noninstitutional, minimal	small room number	noninstitutional, homelike	none, handmade signs

	Meditation Room		Nurses' Station	
	Intent	*Existing*	*Intent*	*Existing*
View				
Window	private, soft, glowing light	opaque stained-glass window	internal	no windows
Doors	private, accessible	large wood doors	nonabandonment, central	no doors
Each bed	view of speaker and outdoors	dais, large window	visibility	low countertops
Other: artwork	spiritual, comforting	religious symbols	warm colors	painted hallways
Services	accessible	televised	N/A	N/A
Window				
Treatment	spiritual	abstract in stained glass	N/A	N/A
Trim	modern	gypsum wall board	N/A	N/A
Operation	none	none	N/A	N/A
Covering	none	none	N/A	N/A
Lighting				
Type	indirect, soft, quiet	window, incandescent spot, fluorescent	flexible, economical	task area, indirect fluorescent
Fixtures	low-level, discreet	wallwashing lamps, recessed ceiling	low-level, flexible	ceiling cans, lamps, wallwash hall
Handicap access				
Bed and wheelchair	Lummox chair, walkers	large door, movable chairs, little furniture	beds, chairs, walkers, (outside nurses' station)	large open corridor, central nurses' station, surrounded
Dominant colors	warm, soft, quiet, peaceful	deep reds, browns, golds, light brown, green, white	light, clean, bright	white, light wood, accent colors, black, beige, metal
Dominant materials	warm, quiet, soft, natural, textured	carpet, paint, wood, glass, fabric, acoustical tile, plastic laminate	clean, smooth, modern	linoleum, wood, paint, plastic laminate, acoustical tile, metal

	Meditation Room		Nurses' Station	
	Intent	*Existing*	*Intent*	*Existing*
Furniture type	flexible, simple, durable, comforting	lectern, altar, chairs, carpeted dais	flexible, complete, modern, concealed	institutional clock, built-in cabinets, storage, telephones, monitors, medications
Ceiling height/ treatment	window head, typical, practical	8', acoustical tile	airy, practical, variety	10' over nurses' station, dropped over hall, paint/acoustical tile
Floor surfacing	quiet, warm, homelike	low-pile carpet	clean, durable	linoleum
Personalization	by celebrant	adapted for various services, flowers	some personalization	plants, signs by nurses, flowers
Organization	convenient, private	small room off 1st-floor entry	central, visible	large oval in center of patients' rooms
Equipment	flexible	lights, microphone, television	complete, concealed, practical	telephone, nutrition station, medications, countertop light, monitors, storage
Signs	noninstitutional, spiritual	small sign, religious symbols	noninstitutional, practical	handmade signs, sign of white nurses' uniform

	Kitchen Facilities (Coffee Shop)		Kitchen Facilities (Cafeteria)	
	Intent	*Existing*	*Intent*	*Existing*
View				
Window	light, open, nature	greenhouse to patio on South	light, no view	skylight to window well
Doors	controlled entry, exit	hall to entry, glass to patio	controlled entry, exit	hall to entry
Each bed	not applicable	not applicable	not applicable	not applicable
Other: artwork		gift shop visible through relights	colorful setting	painted, wall plants, mural
Window				
Treatment	lots of light	one side of room, large greenhouse	indirect lighting	dull window well
Trim	modern	no trim	modern	no trim
Operation	none	none	none	none
Covering	none	none	none	none
Lighting				
Type	natural, flexible	windows, incandescent/fluorescent	natural, low gradient	window well, incandescent
Fixtures	economical, low gradient	ceiling cans	economical	ceiling cans

| | Kitchen Facilities (Coffee Shop) | | Kitchen Facilities (Cafeteria) | |
	Intent	*Existing*	*Intent*	*Existing*
Handicap access				
Bed and wheelchair	Lummox chairs	large entry door	N/A	N/A
Dominant colors	light, warm, cheerful, clean	white, green, and beige; blond wood	clean, warm, simple	white, dark red, brown, orange
Dominant materials	clean, cheerful, home-like, durable	wood, paint, acoustical tile, glass, linoleum, plastic laminate	clean, warm, durable	paint, glass, plastic laminate, linoleum, metal, acoustical tile
Furniture type	homelike, comfortable, movable, practical	rustic chairs, plastic laminate tables, counter chairs, built-in counter	practical, movable	lunch tables, chairs, serving tables, line
Ceiling height/ treatment	typical, dropped	8′, acoustical tile	typical, practical	8′, dropped acoustical tile
Floor surfacing	practical, clean	linoleum	practical	linoleum
Personalization	minimal	plants	minimal	plants
Organization	central, bright, flexible	axis with entry and patio, south exposure door to patio	central console with kitchen	typical serving line
Equipment	restaurant equipment/self-serve	short-order restaurant, refrigerator, stove, cabinets, sinks, register, etc.	central console with kitchen	disorienting, dark basement room, near kitchen
Signs	restaurant	meal signboard, institutional clock	none	none

Calvary Hospital: Summary of Additional Needs

Nursing services: Specially trained nurses in cancer, psychiatry, and surgical procedures, enterostomal therapy. Needs offices.

Staff development: With nursing services provides training for the paraprofessional and professional personnel. Needs meeting space.

Outpatient services: Home care program to be started, with clinic in nutritional support, pastoral care, and social work, as well as enterostomal therapy and education. Needs office, examining room, conference room, secretary, storage.

Social services: Needs more office space and private conference room for private and group family support.

Pastoral care: Needs round-the-clock staff rooms, more office and conference space. Needs new, larger, safer chapel, with meeting space for bereavement counseling.

Kitchen and dietician offices: Larger kitchen, with more storage, food preparation, washing areas, work space. Needs offices for five clinical dieticians.

Ancillary services: Needs consolidation onto one floor. Needs department of physical therapy (now done on floors in halls) with office and equipment.

Recreation therapy: More room for family participation and patients. Offices for music therapy, ceramics, horticulture. Needs special-event space in a larger assembly room (current auditorium is too small for events; patient bed chairs cannot fit existing space). Also needs storage, library, game room.

Department of volunteers: Needs more office and education space, in conjunction with home-care division.

Educational programs: Needs group meeting space. Could double with recreation therapy auditorium.

Calvary Hospital: General Notes

Other problems with existing design include the following: inadequate parking facilities, inadequate on-call space, small, inconvenient service entry, uncontrolled windy conditions at terrace entry, no covered shelter on terrace, inadequate visibility from nurses' station to eight of the twenty-five patient rooms, overheated coffee shop, cracked brick on facade, small, inconveniently located staff lounge (in windowless basement), and overall a strict geometric column grid, which works effectively in wings but not in the central core. The coffee shop was designed for table service, not tray service, which it now has. All of the above are being addressed in a 12-million-dollar remodeling and new construction project, except visibility from the nurses' station and change of grid, which are impossible to remedy.

Overall, Calvary Hospital is simply too big for a pre-hospice and acute-care facility of this kind. Such a large bed contingent entails separation of functions and economies of scale out of place for personalized and individual care—the development of a close community of staff, nurses, and doctors becomes impossible to achieve. Calvary is a noble effort, however, as the demand for this kind of terminal care is high. The facility and patients are clean and attended to regularly. Corridors are shiny and long, but patient care areas are light and varied in colors. There is need for more family areas as the patient demographics change to a more wealthy and young population: there are, for instance, no overnight rooms for family within the environs of the hospital; private family conference space is hard to find within the hospital; and the group activities auditorium is not large enough to include all the patients, let alone their family members.

Innovations at Calvary include many positive elements, however: centralized nurse's station, which promotes nonabandonment of the patients; decentralized pantry for breakfast meals (often the only meal a cancer patient can eat); private rooms, selected for privacy, mix of ethnic and religious custom and behavior, and severity of debilitation; and close, centralized dayrooms, operable windows, and convenient access to the patio. Moreover, the patient bed entry (ambulance) and main pedestrian entry are combined, so that patients do not enter through a back door.

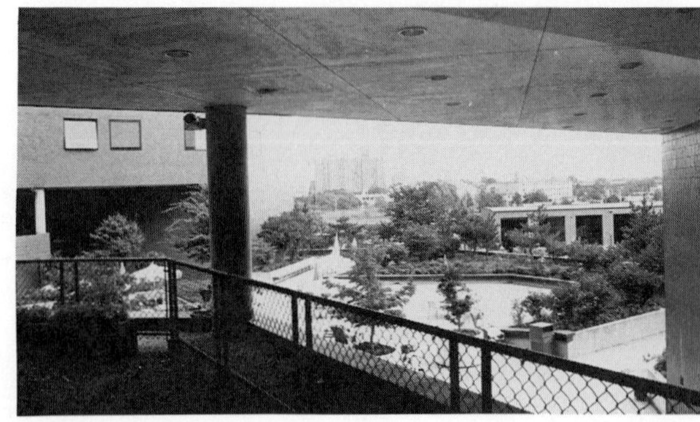

Garden patio

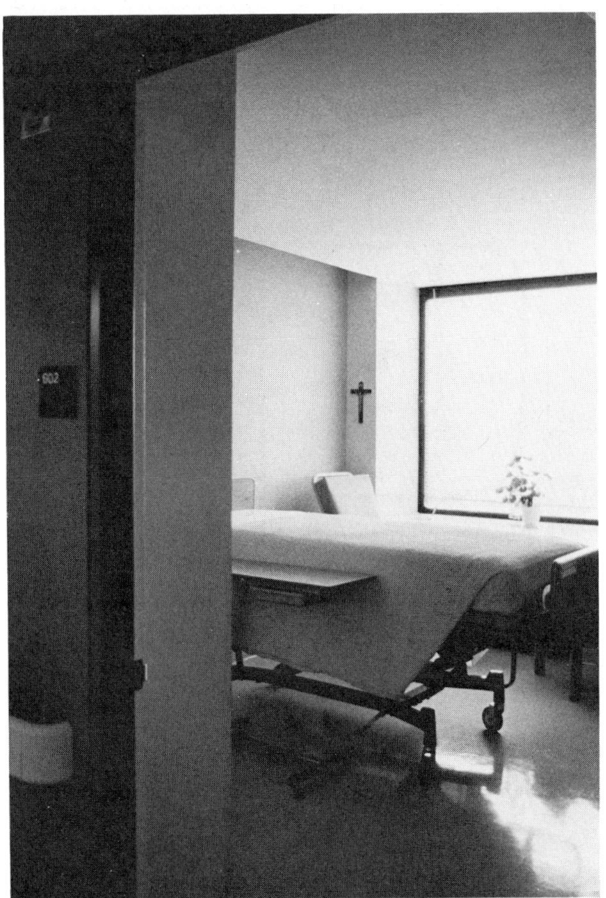

Patient room

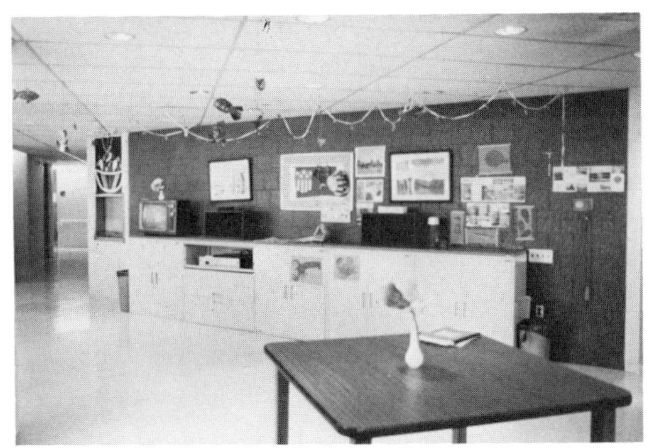

Dayroom

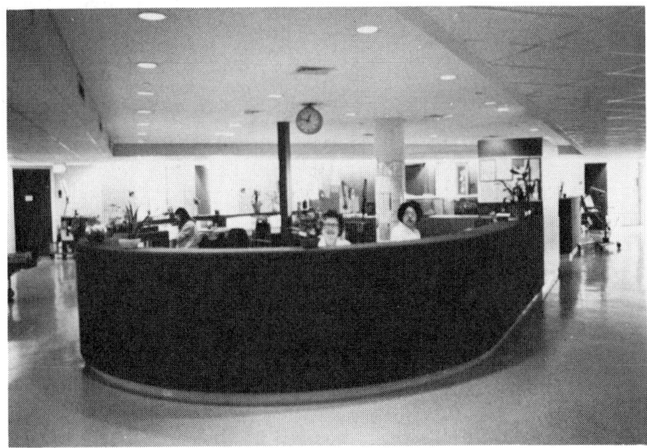

Nurses' station

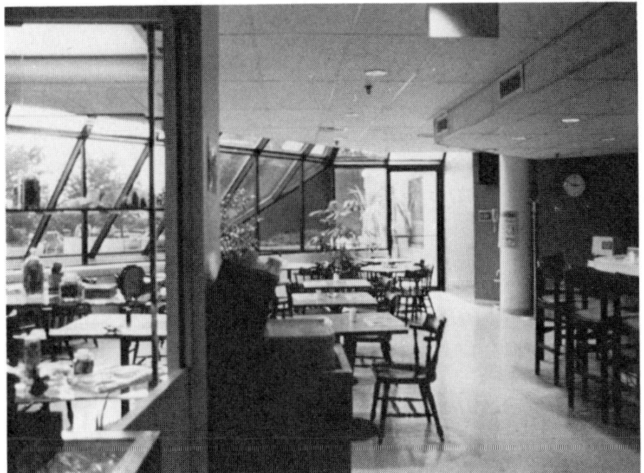

Coffee shop, Calvary Hospital

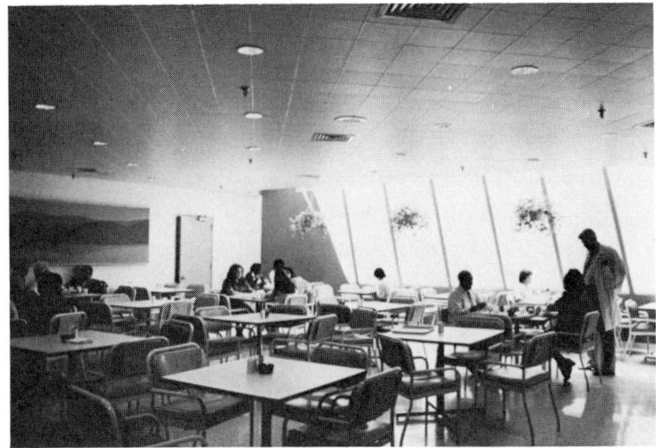

Staff cafeteria

• CLOVER HOSPICE

440 Minot Avenue
Auburn, Maine 04210

Classification: Hospice unit
Sponsoring agencies: Clover Living Center
Type: Separate ward (some shared areas)
Area served: Lewiston-Auburn vicinity
Inpatient population: 5 (French, Catholic, low-income)
Established: 1981–1982
Scope of work involved: New construction
    Architect: W. Gillis
              A. L. & H. Engineer Company
              Lewiston, Maine
Cost of work: $75,000 new
    Build: N/A
    Furnishings: N/A
Comprehensive intention of building selection and/or design: N/A
General intention: Intimate, distinct, noninstitutional, special facility
Location: Distinct unit in living center
Description:
    Community image: special part of living center
    Interior image: homelike, personal, nice, small
    Convenience: special entry
    Changes: sunroom to be built
Users:
    Outpatient staff: N/A
    Volunteers: N/A
    Inpatient staff: N/A
    Outpatients served: N/A
    Inpatient average population: N/A
    Inpatient average length of stay: N/A
    Family/visitors per week: N/A
Services rendered: Inpatient, daycare, family sleep in patient rooms.

Parti drawing, Clover Hospice

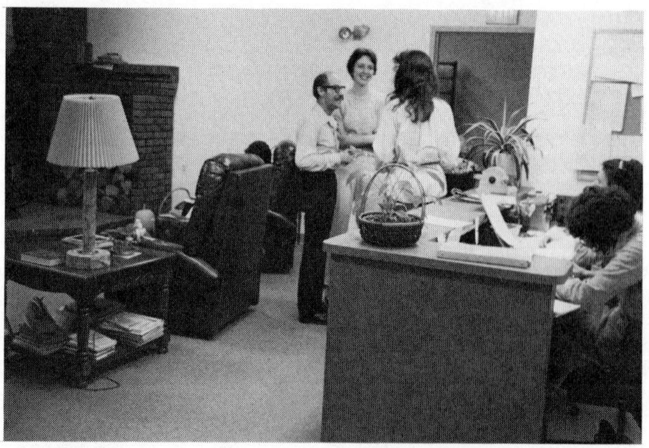

Family lounge and nurses' station, Clover Hospice

CLOVER HOSPICE: ARCHITECTURAL COMPONENTS

Architectural Components	Notes	Wing/Total Number	Rough Dimensions or Size, Square Feet
1. Patient room	Single	5	130 (approx.)
Bathrooms	W.C.	2/1	25/30
	Shower room	1	72
	Waiting area	1	360
2. Family lounge	Off unit		
Child area	None		
Eating area	Multipurpose	1	900
Other	None		
Family private room	Quiet room	1	190
Bathrooms	Off unit		
Conference	Off unit		
3. Garden	Children's playground	1	1,575
Gardening area	with landscaping		
Chapel			
Transition room			
Meditation room			
Chaplain office			
4. Nurses' station		1	40
Medication room		1	30
Nurses' retreat	Off unit		
Staff rooms	Off unit		
Bathrooms	Off unit		
5. Daycare	N/A		
Childcare	Off unit	1	
Massage	In patient rooms		
Physical therapy	Off unit		
Occupational therapy	See multipurpose		
Library	None		
Music/reading	None		
Barbershop	None		
Tavern	None		
Store	None		
Game room	None		
Other	N/A		
6. Kitchen facilities	Off unit		
Storage			
Supplies			
Preparation			
Cleaning			
Office			
Dietary staff			
Unit dining	In rooms		
Other dining			
Nutrition station	See multipurpose		

CLOVER HOSPICE: ARCHITECTURAL COMPONENTS (*cont'd.*)

Architectural Components	Notes	Wing/Total Number	Rough Dimensions or Size, Square Feet
7. Offices			
Director		1	98
Nurse coordinator		1	98
Social work coordinator	None		
Boardroom	None		
Conference room	None		
Volunteer coordinator	None		
Business office	Off unit		
Files	None		
Other	None		
8. Entry, front door	Hospice area	1	60
Reception	Hospice unit, see waiting		
Staff	Off unit		
Patient	Hospice area entry		
Volunteer	Hospice area entry		
Visitors	Hospice area entry		
Goods	Off unit		
Hallways, main	L-shaped corridor	1	8' × 84'
Service	Unit hall	1	8' × 30'
Other	ICF apt. units		
Exit goods	Off unit		
Laundry	Off unit		
Dead	Through hospice area entry		
9. Parking			
Connections to other facilities	For total facility		
Connection to neighborhood	N/A		
Street visibility	N/A		
Landscaping	N/A		
Front yard	N/A		
Back yard	N/A		
10. Services			
Laundry			
Clean	Linen	1	11
Dirty	Linen	1	28
Janitorial			
Closet	In waiting	1	8
Stores	Off unit		
General stores	Off unit		
Offices	Off unit		
Garbage	Off unit		
Garbage pickup	N/A		
Equipment storage	Off unit		
Mail	N/A		
Miscellaneous	N/A		

CLOVER HOSPICE: PROXIMITY MATRIX

| | Variable Numbers | | | | | | | | | | | | | |
Variables	1.	2.	3.	4.	5.	6.	7.	8.	9.	10.	11.	12.	13.	14.
1. Patient	A													
2. Family	B													
3. Chapel (none)														
4. Nature (garden)	C	B												
5. Nurses' station	A	A		B										
6. Inpatient services	E	E		C	E									
7. Kitchen	*	*		*	*	E								
8. Kitchenette	D	A		D	B	E	*							
9. Offices	D	C		B	D	E	*	D	A					
10. Main entry/facility	D	C		B	C	E	*	D	B					
11. Bed entry/unit	B	A		C	A	E	*	B	D	C				
12. All parking	D	D		C	D	E	*	D	C	B	D			
13. Laundry rooms	A	A		B	A	E	*	B	D	D	A		B	
14. Janitorial	B	A		D	B	E	*		D	D	B			

Key:
    A = within 16-foot radius (based on 8-foot corridors)
    B = within 32-foot radius
    C = related areas (see plan)
    D = distant
    E = scattered, disparate association
blank = no relation
    * = off unit

CLOVER HOSPICE: DESCRIPTIVE MATRIX (Environmental Factors)

Family (Waiting Room)

	Intent	*Existing*		
View				
Window	interior	no windows		
Doors	private	entry to unit		
Each bed	accessible, friendly, homelike	low nurses' station counter, residential finishes		
Other: artwork	homelike	seasonal pictures		
Window				
Treatment	N/A	N/A		
Trim	N/A	N/A		
Operation	N/A	N/A		
Covering	N/A	N/A		

Family (Waiting Room)

	Intent	Existing		
Lighting				
Type	homelike, practical	fluorescent and incandescent		
Fixtures	homelike, practical	overhead fluorescent/ incandescent lamps		
Handicap access				
Bed and wheelchair	space for bed, recliner, wheelchair, walker	large door, wall bars, grouped furniture, low-pile carpet, light		
Dominant colors	noninstitutional, clean, special	white, brown, brick red, wood, greens, black		
Dominant materials	noninstitutional, clean, special	paint, wood, stuffed "leather," brick, plastic laminate, carpet, tile		
Furniture type	homelike, clean, comfortable, unique	residential soft chairs, lamps, tables, wood stove, brick flue, woodpile, magazine rack		
Ceiling height/ treatment	homelike, practical	approx 8', acoustical tile		
Floor surfacing	homelike, lasting	institutional carpet		
Personalization	noninstitutional, flexible	bulletin board, plants, books		
Organization	welcoming, homelike	unit entry open to bedrooms, central area		
Equipment	homelike, noninstitutional, practical	wood stove, HVAC, emergency lights, clock, nurses' station		
Signs	practical	exit sign, clock, unit name		

• THE CONNECTICUT HOSPICE

61 Burban Drive
Branford, Connecticut 06405

Classification: Freestanding nonprofit hospice
Sponsoring agencies: The Connecticut Hospice Inc.,
Visiting Nurses' Association
Type: New construction
Area served: New Haven and environs plus five-
state area: New York, New Jersey, Massachusetts,
New Hampshire, Ohio
Inpatient population: 44 patients maximum
Established: 1980; home care program begun in
1976
Scope of work involved: New construction
    Architect: Lo-Yi Chan
              Prentice and Chan Ohlhausen
              500 Fifth Avenue
              New York, New York 10110
Cost of work: 2.9 million
    Build: N/A
    Furnishings: N/A
*Comprehensive intention of building selection
and/or design*: N/A
General intention: Warm, light, homelike, exper-
imental hospice
Location: Mixed residental and industrial area; Lion's
Park nearby, school across the street
Description: Modern, low-profile, brick exterior,
suburban-school image, familiar, approachable
    Community image: Small institution for the dying
    Interior image: contemporary, geometric, linear,
    "black and white," serene, clean
    Convenience: main door is for everyone; parking
    facilities inadequate
Other: Experimental, innovative design; transition
areas important
    Changes: Many additional items are needed: linen
    closet; audio-visual area; more office space; larger
    nurses' station; windows in grieving room; better
    overall heating system; better heating in the tub
    rooms; more parking facilities; and single-sex pa-
    tient rooms (rooms are now coed). Other problems:
    physical/occupational therapy is not used; bath-
    room doors swing the wrong way; the "scream
    room" is now a meditation room.

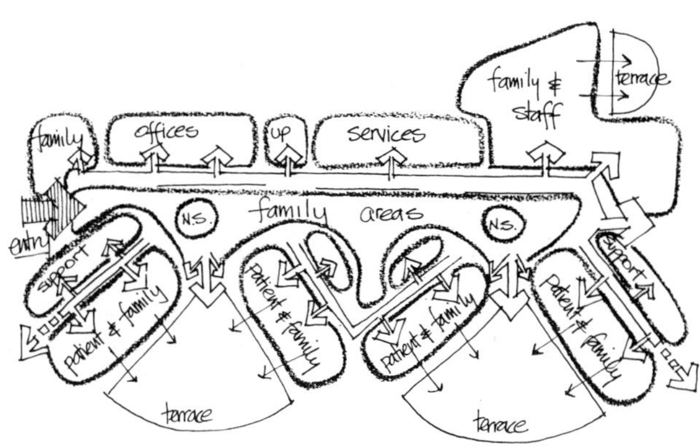

Parti drawing, Connecticut Hospice

Users (Based on 6-month statistics; 31 discharges,
215 deaths):
    Outpatient/inpatient staff: 125 average
    Volunteers: 250 average
    Outpatients served: 3-4 beds held open
    Average inpatient population: 39
    Average inpatient length of stay: 10-12 days; 18
    median
    Family/visitors per week: Varies
Services rendered: Home care, counseling, bereavement, inpatient care, 24-hour sleeping facilities for family, cots in patient rooms, education
and training, hospice promotion. Child pre-
school, Health Care Financing Administration
demonstration.

CONNECTICUT HOSPICE: ARCHITECTURAL COMPONENTS

Architectural Components	Notes	Wing/Total Number	Rough Dimensions or Size, Square Feet
1. Patient room	Single	4	251/383
	Other four/hall	10	609/741
Bathrooms	W.C.s	12/4	66/108
	Tub rooms		
	Shower room	4	104
2. Family lounge	Living rooms	2	1,048
Child area	See childcare		
Eating area	See family kitchens		
Other			
Family private room		1	414
Family other	Reading room	4	49
Bathrooms	Patient and m/f public	2	153 (each)
Conference	Patient	2	126 (each)
Lounge		1	115
3. Garden	Terraces	2	2,250
Gardening area	Greenhouses	4	450
Chapel		1	200
Transition room	Antechamber to viewing room	1	236/148
Meditation room	See scream room		
Chaplain office		1	153
4. Nurses' station		2	50
Medication room	Office area	2	183
Nurses' retreat	Staff lounge	1	688
Staff rooms	Lockers (m/f)		238/363
Bathrooms	m/f	2	142
Other	Inglenook	2	66
Scream room	Staff meditation	1	114
5. Daycare			
Childcare	Charlie Mills preschool	1	742
Massage	N/A		
Physical therapy	has W.C.	1	210/28
Occupational therapy	Preschool	1	140
Library	Reading room		
Music	Commons room	1	722
Barbershop	Hairdresser	1	153
Tavern	N/A		
Store	Gift shop	1	40
Game room	N/A		
6. Kitchen facilities		1	1,430
Storage	Garbage	1	210
Supplies	N/A		
Preparation	N/A		
Cleaning	N/A		
Office	N/A		
Dietary staff	N/A		

Architectural Components	Notes	Wing/Total Number	Rough Dimensions or Size, Square Feet
Unit dining	Staff/guest terrace	1	918/454
Other dining	Staff canteen		446
Nutrition station	N/A	2	102
Kitchenettes	Family kitchens		
7. Offices			
Director/executive		1	138
Nurse coordinator		1	138
Social work coordinator		1	218
Boardroom	2nd floor	1	370
Conference room	Ground floor	1	244
Volunteer coordinator		1	330
Business office		1	138
Files	Open office area	Hall	2,014
Other	General offices, 2nd floor		1,818
	Home-care offices		1,040 total
	Xerox room		100
8. Entry, front door	Vestibule	1	114
Reception		1	675
Admitting	Exam room (has W.C.)	1	144/24
Staff	Main entrance		
Patient	Main entrance		
Volunteer	Main entrance		
Visitors	Main entrance		
Goods	Service entry vestibule	1	81
Other	Daycare entry/exit	1	80
Hallways, main	Spine circulations, 2nd floor	Total	2,500
Service	Wing corridors	4	500
Other	Greenhouse gallery	4	416
Exit goods	Service entrance/garbage		
Laundry	Service entrance		
Dead	Hall to elevator to View Room to Elevator to service exit		
Miscellaneous	Service stairs/elevators	1/1	135/48
	Staff stairs	2	100
9. Parking		1	58
Connections to other facilities	N/A		
Connection to neighborhood	N/A		
Street visibility	N/A		
Landscaping			60', set back
Front yard	N/A		
Back yard	N/A		
Total site			5 acres
10. Services			
Laundry	Family laundry area		N/A
Clean	Laundry, linen room	1	170
Dirty	Laundry, linen room	1	175

CONNECTICUT HOSPICE: ARCHITECTURAL COMPONENTS (*cont'd.*)

Architectural Components	Notes	Wing/Total Number	Rough Dimensions or Size, Square Feet
Janitorial			
Closet	Ground floor	1	50
Stores	See general stores		
General stores	Total 2nd-floor storage		950
Offices	Ground-floor storage on wings	6	100
Garbage			
Garbage pickup			
Equipment storage	Hall alcoves	12	12
Mail	See reception		
Miscellaneous	Pharmacy	1	214
Preparation room		1	84
Wing linen supplies		6	100
Patient closets		8	36
Mechanical space/office		1/1	980

CONNECTICUT HOSPICE: PROXIMITY MATRIX

	Variable Numbers													
Variables	1.	2.	3.	4.	5.	6.	7.	8.	9.	10.	11.	12.	13.	14.
1. Patient (bedrooms)	E													
2. Family (living rooms)	C	E												
3. Chapel	C	C												
4. Nature (outdoors)	A	A	D	E										
5. Nurses' station	D	A	D	B	E									
6. Inpatient services	C	B	A	D	C									
7. Kitchen	D	C	C	A	C	B								
8. Kitchenette	C	A	D	B	A	C	C							
9. Offices	D	D	D	D	D	C	D	D						
10. Main entry/facility	C	C	C	A	C	C	D	C	C					
11. Bed entry/unit	D	A	D	D	B	C	C	B	D	C				
12. Parking/staff	D	C	C	A	C	D	D	D	C	C	C			
13. Parking/visitors	D	C	C	B	C	A	B	C	D	D	D	D		
14. Pharmacy	D	C	C	D	C	B	C	C	D	C	D	D	C	D

Key: A = within 16-foot radius (based on 8-foot corridors)

        B = within 32-foot radius

        C = related areas (see plan)

        D = distant

        E = scattered, disparate association

  blank = no relation

CONNECTICUT HOSPICE: DESCRIPTIVE MATRIX (Environmental Factors)

| | Patient (Bedrooms) | | Family (Living Rooms) | |
	Intent	*Existing*	*Intent*	*Existing*
View				
Window	light, nature, territorial	greenhouse gallery, terrace, park	nature, patient areas	12′ sliding doors to terrace
Doors	nonabandonment, privacy	low partitions, private corridor	open near patients, connect access	many entries, zoned for privacy
Each bed	community, privacy	large 4-bed wards, curtains, views, south light	homelike	8′ corridor openings, grouped furniture
Other: artwork	natural, varied	plants, footboard display, shelves	natural, varied, quality	plants, prints by local artists
Window				
Treatment	light, natural	greenhouse	light, access	doors, clerestory
Trim	greenhouse	metal, gypsum wall board	standard	metal, gypsum wall board
Operation	accessible	doors, grade, terrace	access	doors, grade, terrace
Covering	cheerful, natural	plants, separate from patient room	control, homelike	drapes, open clerestory
Lighting				
Type	homelike, cheerful	N/A	homelike, natural	incandescent, fluorescent, clerestory
Fixtures	homelike, flexible	N/A	low gradient	lamps, recessed down lights
Handicap access				
Bed and wheelchair	chair, walker	all at grade, 4′ doorways, large, open rooms, grouped furniture	bed, chair, walker	all at grade, 4′, 8′ doors, grouped furniture, open plan
Dominant colors	light, cheerful background, clean, serene	gray, brown, white, yellow, green, rust, blue, pink, reds	light, cheerful, clean, homelike	red, white, brown, green, rust
Dominant materials	homelike, clean, lasting, warm	carpet, paint, wood, slate, acoustical tile, glass, fabrics, bricks, aluminum	homelike, clean, lasting, warm	brick, paint, glass, wood, plastic laminate, acoustical tile, carpet
Furniture type	homelike, flexible, sturdy, comfortable	hospital beds, built-ins, rocking chairs, lounge chairs, clocks	homelike, clearn, adaptable, sturdy, contemporary	couches, fireplace, chairs, tables, lamps, bookcases, plants
Ceiling height/ treatment	practical	acoustical tile	N/A	N/A
Floor surfacing	homelike, lasting	carpet (salt-and-pepper pattern)	homelike	carpet, rugs
Personalization	encouraged	bulletin board, plants, furniture, shelves for display	allowed to some extent	plants, gifts, display areas

CONNECTICUT HOSPICE: DESCRIPTIVE MATRIX (Environmental Factors)

	Patient (Bedrooms)		Family (Living Rooms)	
	Intent	*Existing*	*Intent*	*Existing*
Organization	light, private, spacious, open	4 V-wing pavilions, single-loaded patient areas, service corridor, greenhouse	central, near patient area, out-of-doors	triangle between two patient wings off spine, nurses' station, kitchenette
Equipment	convenient, controllable, noninstitutional	television with headphones, phone (princess), oxygen, HVAC, curtains, afghans	convenient, noninstitutional	lights, HVAC, telephone, curtains
Signs	homelike	none	homelike	none

	Family (Family Room)		Chapel	
	Intent	*Existing*	*Intent*	*Existing*
View				
Window	private, local, entry, parking	entry, parking, private lawns	sacred, introspective	bubble skylight
Doors	private	one door, bend of L-shaped room	adaptable, private or open	opens into commons area for large service
Each bed	family only	not applicable	accessible	4' door, grouped furniture
Other: artwork	homelike, intricate	wall sketches	special, ecumenical, symbolic	tapestries on walls
Window				
Treatment	light	wall windows	light, symbolic	skylight
Trim	N/A	wood, gypsum wall board	N/A	N/A
Operation	N/A	N/A	N/A	N/A
Covering	homelike, energy-conserving	drapes	N/A	N/A
Lighting				
Type	homelike, natural	windows, incandescent, fluorescent	special	incandescent
Fixtures	homelike, low gradient	lamps, recessed down lights	adaptable, controllable	rheostatted lights
Handicap access				
Bed and wheelchair	walker	3' doorway, grouped furniture	bed, walker, chair	4' door (small)
Dominant colors	warm, homelike, contemporary, varied	brown, white, red, green, blue carpeting	warm, special, comfortable, contemporary	red, brown, bright accents, sky, white
Dominant materials	homelike, coordinated	brick, carpet, glass, wood, acoustical tile, fabrics	warm, special, coordinated, quiet	wood, brick, carpet, fabrics, plastic

CONNECTICUT HOSPICE: DESCRIPTIVE MATRIX (Environmental Factors)

	Family (Family Room)		*Chapel*	
	Intent	*Existing*	*Intent*	*Existing*
Furniture type	comfortable, home-like, lasting, contemporary	chairs, couches, tables, crib, hassock	ecumenical, adaptable, special, lasting	hand-carved round "altar," brushed bottom ladderback chairs
Ceiling height/ treatment	practical, fireproof	acoustical tile, 8′	special, symbolic	9′ skylight
Floor surfacing	warm, comfortable, homelike	carpet, medium pile	warm, quiet	carpet
Personalization	some	plants, books, home-made items	some	places for flowers, different services
Organization	private, isolated, but convenient	L-shaped room near building entry, zoned areas	symbolic, enclosing, adaptable	round, center of hospice, opens to commons area
Equipment	homelike, communication	television, telephone, lights, curtains, HVAC, clocks	special	hand-carved round "altar"
Signs	homelike	None	symbolic, special, sacred	N/A

	Viewing and Anterooms		*Nurses' Station*	
	Intent	*Existing*	*Intent*	*Existing*
View				
Window	none (internal)	no windows	indirect	through living room doors, clerestory
Doors	private, transition area	alcove, then linear progression	open, secure, with privacy	open counter, offices behind
Each bed	hidden	curtain over door from prep room	nonabandonment, visible	low counter, open
Other: display	shelves	behind-body for flowers, etc.	homelike, variety	pictures
Window				
Treatment	none	N/A	none	N/A
Trim	N/A	N/A	N/A	N/A
Operation	N/A	N/A	N/A	N/A
Covering	N/A	N/A	N/A	N/A
Lighting				
Type	soft	N/A	adaptable, practical	incandescent, fluorescent
Fixtures	low gradient	N/A	low gradient, task	lamps, recessed down lights
Handicap access				
Bed and wheelchair	chair, walker	elevator to 2nd floor, smaller doors, chambers	wheelchair height; no access behind counter	same

CONNECTICUT HOSPICE: DESCRIPTIVE MATRIX (Environmental Factors)

	Viewing and Anterooms		Nurses' Station	
	Intent	*Existing*	*Intent*	*Existing*
Dominant colors	background, simple	white, brown, rust	background, contemporary, coordinating	browns, gray, white, accent colors
Dominant materials	background, simple, quiet, warm	curtain, wood, acoustical tile, carpet, fabrics, gypsum wall board	background, matching, clean	carpet, acoustical tile, plastic laminate, fabric, wood, metal
Furniture type	comfortable, warm, contemporary	couch, tables, chairs, built-in shelf ledge	efficient, comfortable, contemporary	built-in cabinets, counter, desks, chairs, files
Ceiling height/ treatment	practical	8', acoustical tile	practical	8', acoustical tile
Floor surfacing	practical, homelike, quiet	carpet	practical, homelike, quiet	carpet
Personalization	some	shelf for flowers or other decoration	some	nurses' personal items
Organization	private, transitions, central	chambered private rooms, 2nd floor near elevator, service entrance	restricted, humanized, functional	small area off living rooms
Equipment	homelike, adaptable	lights, cold temperature	practical, adaptable	lights, files, telephones, etc.
Signs	homelike	N/A	homelike	N/A

	Nurses' Scream Room		Kitchen, Staff Canteen, Dining	
	Intent	*Existing*	*Intent*	*Existing*
View				
Window	introspective, natural	skylight over platform	light, nature, separate	separate back patio, trees, grass
Doors	private, secure	door off staff lounge stairs	haven, secure, separate	opposite end of spine, near preschool
Each bed	not applicable		not applicable	not applicable
Other: artwork	N/A	N/A	homelike, variety	pictures
Window				
Treatment	natural	skylight	light, open	wall windows
Trim	N/A	N/A	N/A	N/A
Operation	N/A	not operable	N/A	not operable
Covering	N/A	no covers	N/A	drapes
Lighting				
Type	adaptable, economical	fluorescent	adaptable, economical	fluorescent
Fixtures	practical, personal control	with rheostat ceiling	practical, personal control	recessed down lights

CONNECTICUT HOSPICE: DESCRIPTIVE MATRIX (Environmental Factors)

| | *Nurses' Scream Room* | | *Kitchen, Staff Canteen, Dining* | |
	Intent	*Existing*	*Intent*	*Existing*
Handicap access				
Bed and wheelchair	N/A	N/A	beds, chairs, walkers	large doors, open plan, grouped furniture
Dominant colors	serene, background, quiet	gray-mauve walls; floor, steps, black, brown	serene, clean, warm, homelike	red, blue, black, white, green, brown, gray
Dominant materials	soundproof, warm, cozy, simple	carpeted walls, floor, steps, metal, wood, Plexiglas	clean, economical, cozy, lasting	plastic laminate, linoleum, tile, brick, acoustical tile, wood, fabric
Furniture type	built-in, comfortable, simple	carpeted steps, bean bag chair resting on platform, below skylight	adaptable, clean, homelike, simple	captain's chairs, laminate-top tables, childrens' chairs, tables, plants
Ceiling height/ treatment	varied, special	approx. 8'–12', acoustical tile, skylight	practical	8', acoustical tile
Floor surfacing	quiet, comfortable	carpet	practical, clean, cheerful	linoleum tile
Personalization	none	none	some	plants, pictures
Organization	special, womblike, private	oval with platform open to sky, access from staff rooms	roomy, practical, open, angular	dining off serving canteen, near pre-school entrance
Equipment	N/A	N/A	practical, handy, clean	kitchen serving tables, etc.
Signs	special, symbolic	N/A	practical, adaptable	meal sign boards

• DEER'S HEAD CENTER HOSPICE

P.O. Box 2018
Salisbury, Maryland 21801

Classification: Hospice in skilled nursing facility of hospital

Sponsoring agencies: Deer's Head Center

Type: Remodeled interior

Area served: Nine counties within rural eastern shore of Maryland, primarily lower three counties

Inpatient population: 6 beds, black, white, middle- and lower-income population

Established: January 1980

Scope of work involved: Remodeled section
    Formerly: SNF, chronic patients
    Architect: Administration and volunteers

Cost of work: N/A
    Build: N/A
    Furnishings: Donations plus $1,200 new items

Comprehensive intention of building selection and/or design: Homelike, cheerful, private area of ward, comfortable

Location: 3rd floor, nursing facility

Description: Separate area of nursing facility. Has homelike touches, wallpaper, furnishings
    Community image: part of hospital
    Interior image: small-scale revisions, more comfortable
    Convenience: still part of larger general ward
    Changes: Adding pastel sheets, bedspreads, and complementing privacy curtains

Users:
    Outpatient staff: N/A
    Volunteers: N/A
    Inpatient staff: N/A
    Outpatients served: N/A
    Inpatient average population: N/A
    Inpatient average length of stay: N/A
    Family/visitors per week: N/A

Services rendered: Team, inpatient care, 24-hour visiting with family sleeping accommodations.

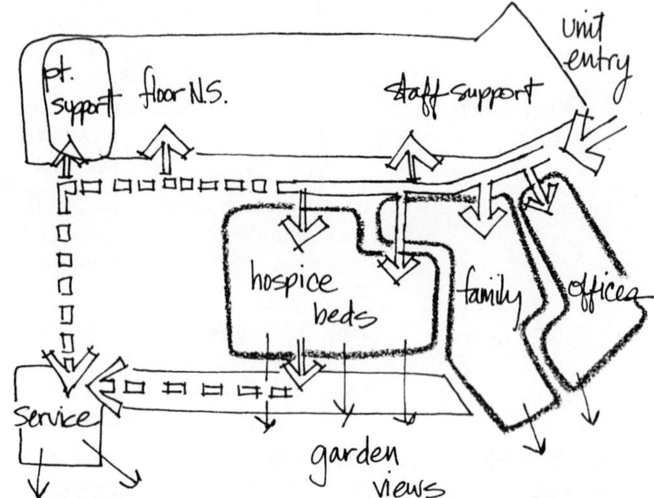

Parti drawing, Deer's Head Center Hospice

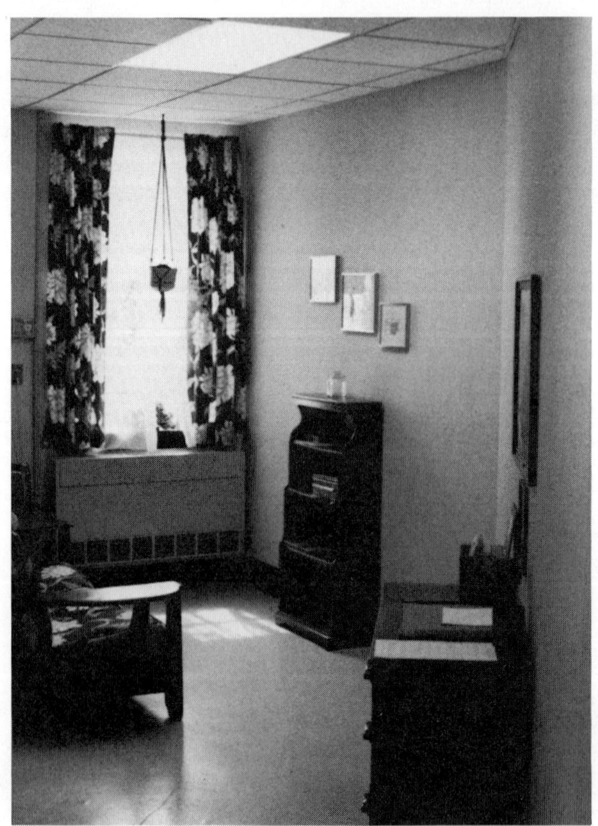

Hospice lounge

DEER'S HEAD CENTER HOSPICE: ARCHITECTURAL COMPONENTS

Architectural Components	Notes	Wing/Total Number	Rough Dimensions or Size, Square Feet
1. Patient room			
Single	(Were doubles)	2	10′–7″ × 16′–6″
Other	(Four bed)	1	22′ × 24′
Bathrooms	W.C.	1	6′ × 6′
	m/f toilets	1 ea./wing	240 (each)
2. Family lounge		1	200
Child area	None		
Eating area	None		
Other	See kitchenette		
Family private room	See lounge		
Family other	None		
Bathrooms	None		
3. Garden	Shared, 2 floors down		
Gardening area	N/A		
Chapel	Shared, off unit	1	
Transition room	None		
Meditation room	None		
Chaplain office	N/A		
Sunroom	Shared, on wing	1	38′ × 13′
4. Nurses' station	Shared	1	16′ × 24′
Medication room	Shared	1	8′ × 9′
Nurses' retreat	Shared, off unit		
Staff rooms	N/A		
Bathrooms	W.C., shared	1	25
5. Daycare	None		
Childcare	None		
Massage	In patient rooms		
Physical therapy	Off unit		
Occupational therapy	Off unit		
Library	None		
Music/reading	None		
Barbershop	None		
Tavern	None		
Store	None		
Game room	None		
Other	None		
6. Kitchen facilities	Off unit		
Storage	N/A		
Supplies	N/A		
Preparation	N/A		
Cleaning	N/A		
Office	N/A		
Dietary staff	N/A		
Unit dining	Shared	1	1,055
Other dining	None		

Architectural Components	Notes	Wing/Total Number	Rough Dimensions or Size, Square Feet
Nutrition station	See nurses' station		
Kitchenette closet	Lounge	1	8
7. Offices			
Director/doctor		1	11' × 17'
Nurse coordinator		1	9' × 16'
Social work coordinator	None		
Boardroom	None		
Conference room	None		
Volunteer coordinator	None		
Business office	None		
Files	None		
Other	None		
8. Entry, front door	Off unit		
Reception	N/A		
Admitting	N/A		
Staff	Elevators or stairs	1	6' × 8'
Patient	Elevators		
Volunteer	Elevators		
Visitors	Elevators		
Goods	Service elevator	1	6' × 8'
Other	Outdoor corridor, shared	1	
Hallways, main	3rd floor entry hall	1	1,112
Service	Shared, on wing	1	1,484
Other	Outdoor corridor, shared	1	128' × 8'
Exit goods	Service elevators		
Laundry	Service elevators		
Dead	Main elevators, morgue off unit		
Miscellaneous	Stair on wing	1	160
9. Parking	Main hospital parking		
Connections to other facilities	N/A		
Connection to neighborhood	N/A		
Street visibility	N/A		
Landscaping			
Front yard	Formal		
Back yard	Gardens		
10. Services			
Laundry	Off unit		
Clean	Shared	1	150
Dirty	Shared	1	161
Janitorial			
Closet	On wing, shared	2	50
Stores			
General stores	Off unit		
Offices			

DEER'S HEAD CENTER HOSPICE: PROXIMITY MATRIX

Variables	Variable Numbers													
	1.	2.	3.	4.	5.	6.	7.	8.	9.	10.	11.	12.	13.	14.
1. Patient	A													
2. Family	B	A												
3. Chapel	D	D												
4. Nature (sunroom)	C	D	*											
5. Nurses' station	C	C	*	C										
6. Inpatient services	D	D	*	D	D									
7. Kitchen (unit dining)	B	A	*	D	A	*								
8. Kitchenette	B	A	*	D	D	*	B							
9. Offices	C	A	*	D	C	*	B	B						
10. Main entry/facility	D	D	*	D	D	*	D	D	D					
11. Bed entry/unit	C	C	*	D	C	*	B	C	B	C				
12. Parking/staff	D	D	*	D	D	*	D	D	D	C	D			
13. Parking/visitors	D	D	*	D	D	*	D	D	D	C	D	C		
14. Janitorial	B	C	*	C	C	*	A	B	B		C			

Key:

- A = within 16-foot radius (based on 8-foot corridors)
- B = within 32-foot radius
- C = related areas (see plan)
- D = distant
- blank = no relation
- * = off unit

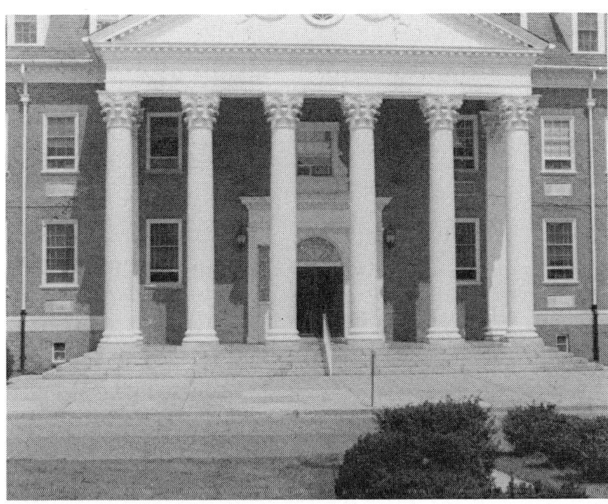

Entrance to Deer's Head Center

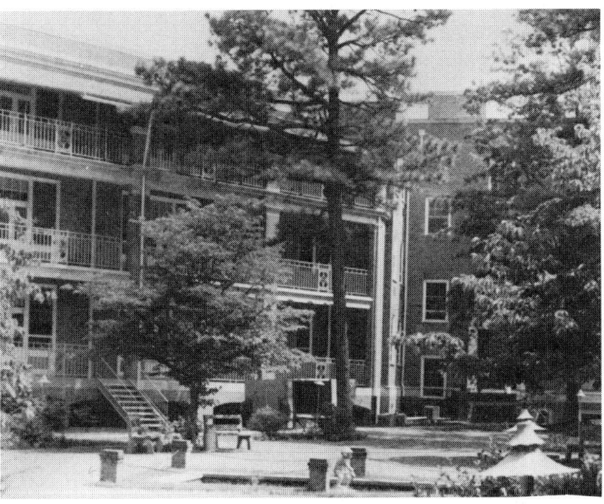

Garden

DEER'S HEAD CENTER HOSPICE: DESCRIPTIVE MATRIX
(Environmental Factors)

	Patient		Family	
	Intent	*Existing*	*Intent*	*Existing*
View				
Window	existing	to outdoor corridor, garden	homelike	garden view
Doors	nonabandonment	open, close to existing nurses' stations	homelike, private	privacy zoned room
Each bed	adaptability, homelike	curtains, roomy, residential dressers, mirrors, etc.	none	too small for bed access
Other: artwork	homelike, nature	prints, original artwork	homelike	prints
Window				
Treatment	residential	N/A	residential	N/A
Trim	existing	wood	existing	wood
Operation	existing	operable	existing	operable
Covering	residential	lace curtains and shades	residential, adaptable	drapes, curtains
Lighting				
Type	existing and task	fluorescent/incandescent	existing, task	fluorescent/incandescent
Fixtures	low-level, homelike	ceiling, wall, residential lamps	existing, homelike	ceiling, residential lamps
Handicap access				
Bed and wheelchair	existing, no modification	wide doors	existing	N/A
Dominant colors	soft colors	gold, green, blue, brown, white	soft colors	white, gold, dark green, dark brown
Dominant materials	existing, residential	paint, wallpaper, vinyl, wood, plastic laminate	existing, residential	paint, vinyl, tile, wood, residential-type fabrics
Furniture type	institutional and homelike residential	institutional beds and overbed tables, residential dressers, mirrors, chairs	residential comfort	desk, ashtrays, book shelves, lamps, old and soft chairs
Ceiling height/treatment	existing	approx. 8′6″, acoustical tile	existing	approx. 8′6″, acoustical tile
Floor surfacing	existing	vinyl	existing	vinyl
Personalization	homelike	dressers, wall space, plants	homelike	plants, pictures
Organization	existing area on double-loaded corridor	grouped hospice area, bigger patient space	existing private, adaptable	odd-shaped room, near beds, office on double-loaded corridor
Equipment	existing plus homelike	oxygen/suction, lights, HVAC, telephones, television	homelike, practical	sink and closet kitchenette, radio, telephone, lights
Signs	existing	overdoor call light number	N/A	N/A

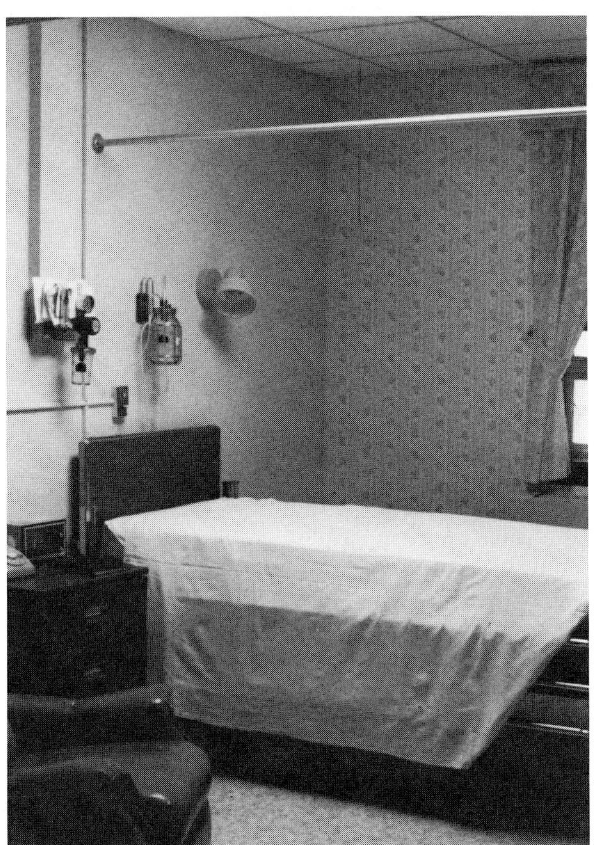

Patient room

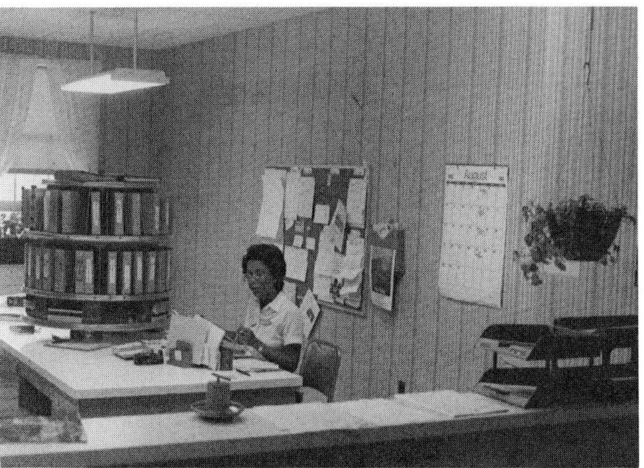

Nurses' station

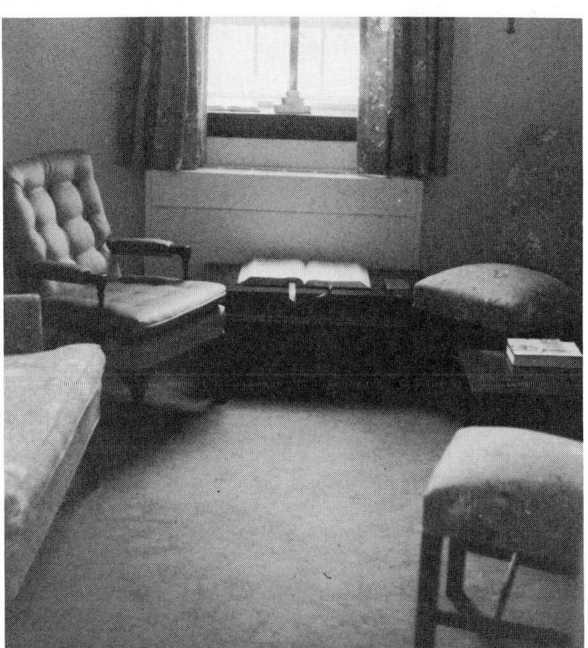

Chapel

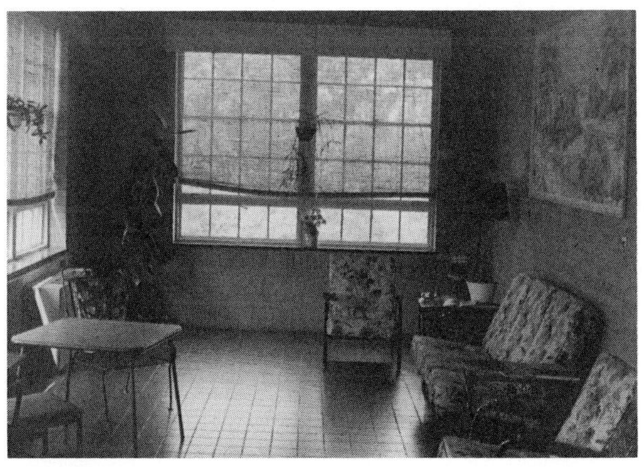

Sunporch

• HILLHAVEN*

Tucson, Arizona
(closed)

Classification: Freestanding hospice (National Cancer Institute demonstration hospice)

Sponsoring agencies: Hillhaven Foundation, Tacoma, Washington

Type: Revised, remodeled nursing home (skilled nursing facility)

Area served: Tucson and environs

Inpatient population: Maximum 39 beds

Established: 1977

Scope of work involved:
Formerly: nursing home
Architect: Inhouse

Cost of work: $186,000
Build: N/A
Furnishings: N/A

Comprehensive intention of building selection and/or design: N/A

General intention: patient and family emphasis, symbolic rooms and access to nature provided

Location: Urban area

Description: Remodeled skilled nursing facility
Community image: remodeled institution
Interior image: remodeled SNF with new rooms, nice finishes
Convenience: very convenient; ground-floor location with ramps

Other: Most satisfactory were chapel, outdoor areas, and kitchen
Changes: Recommended changes included the following: staff lounge and food preparation areas too small, patient rooms and nursing station cramped, badly organized. Floor plan separated patient rooms from social spaces; circular fireplace desired.

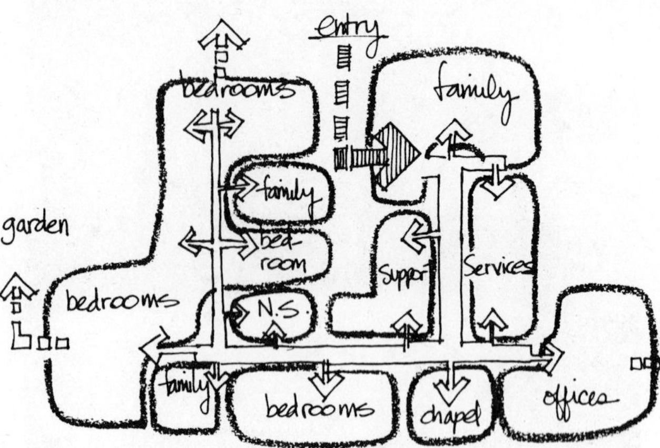

Parti drawing, Hillhaven Hospice

Users:
Outpatient staff: N/A
Volunteers: N/A
Inpatient staff: (FTE) N/A
Outpatients served: N/A
Inpatient average population: N/A
Inpatient average length of stay: N/A
Family/visitors per week: N/A

Services rendered: Inpatient, bereavement, counseling; family sleep in patient rooms or separate room.

* All data obtained from Dale Lupu and Deborah Monahan, *An Evaluation of a Hospice Inpatient Environment: Highlights of Results from a Post-occupancy Evaluation of Hillhaven Hospice*, 1980. See Bibliography.

HILLHAVEN: ARCHITECTURAL COMPONENTS

Architectural Components	Notes	Wing/Total Number	Rough Dimensions or Size, Square Feet
1. Patient room	Single with bath	1	190/59
	Double with W.C., closet	19	211/39
	Triple		
	Other		
Bathrooms	Showers	1	232
	Tub room	1	282
2. Family lounge	Activity room	1	880
Child area	Yes		
Eating area	Yes		
Other	N/A		
Family private room	East lounge, with W.C.	1	211/39
Family other			
Bathrooms	Public W.C. (m/f)	2	66
Conference	Medical director's office	1	213/39
3. Garden	Entrance patio	1	1,202
Gardening area	Rose garden patio	1	670
Chapel	with W.C.	1	213
Transition room	Viewing room with W.C.	1	213
Meditation room			
Chaplain office		1	211.5/39
Volunteer director	See chaplain's office		
4. Nurses' station		1	164
Medication room		1	42
Nurses' retreat	No windows	1	138
Staff rooms	N/A		
Bathrooms	W.C. in nurses' retreat	1	30
5. Daycare			
Childcare	Child area		
Massage	N/A		
Physical therapy	with W.C.	1	360/36
Occupational therapy/ craft room	N/A		
Library	Lounge with W.C.	1	211
Music/reading	Activity room	1	880
Barbershop	N/A		
Tavern	N/A		
Store	N/A		
Game room	Activity room		
Other	N/A		
6. Kitchen facilities	Total	1	406
Storage		1	91
Supplies	N/A		
Preparation	N/A		
Cleaning	N/A		
Office	N/A		
Dietary staff	N/A		

Architectural Components	Notes	Wing/Total Number	Rough Dimensions or Size, Square Feet
Other dining	Patient rooms, family lounge		
Nutrition station		1	47
7. Offices			
Director/administrator		1	211/39
Nurse coordinator		1	211/39
Social work coordinator		1	211/39
Boardroom			
Volunteer coordinator			
Business office		1	211/39
Files	Medical records	1	136
Other	Staff development	1	56
8. Entry, front door	Lobby	1	494
Reception	At lobby		
Admitting	N/A		
Staff	South exit, entrance lobby		
Patient	Entrance lobby		
Volunteer	Entrance lobby		
Visitors	Entrance lobby		
Goods	South exit, entrance lobby		
Other	N/A		
Hallways, main	All hallways 8′ wide		2,616
Service	N/A		
Other	N/A		
Exit goods	Entrance lobby		
Laundry	South exit		
Dead	South exit		
9. Parking	N/A		
Connections to other facilities	Skilled nursing facility		
Connection to neighborhood	N/A		
Street visibility	N/A		
Landscaping			
Front yard	N/A		
Back yard	N/A		
10. Services			
Laundry	Contracted		
Clean	Supply linen	1	143
Dirty	Supply linen	1	143
Janitorial	Housekeeping supplies	1	42
Closet	N/A		
Stores	N/A		
General stores		1	72
Offices	N/A		
Garbage	N/A		
Equipment storage	N/A		
Mail	N/A		
Miscellaneous	Locked storage	1	72

HILLHAVEN: PROXIMITY MATRIX

Variables	1.	2.	3.	4.	5.	6.	7.	8.	9.	10.	11.	12.	13.	14.
1. Patient (bedrooms)	C													
2. Family (activity room)	D													
3. Chapel	C	C												
4. Nature (outdoors)	C	A	C											
5. Nurses' station	C	D	C	C										
6. Inpatient services	D	B	B	D	D									
7. Kitchen	D	A	C	B	D	A								
8. Kitchenette	*	*	*	*	*	*	*							
9. Offices (director)	C	D	B	B	C	C	C	*						
10. Main entry/facility	D	A	C	A	D	B	A	*	D					
11. Bed entry/unit	*	*	*	*	*	*	*	*	*	*				
12. All parking	D	C	D	A	D	C	C	*	D	C	*			
13. Linen/laundry	C	D	C	D	A	C	C	*	C	D	*	D		
14. Janitorial	C	D	C	D	A	C	C	*	C	D	*	D	A	D

Key:

    A = within 16-foot radius (based on 8-foot corridors)
    B = within 32-foot radius
    C = related areas (see plan)
    D = distant
 blank = no relation
    * = no information available

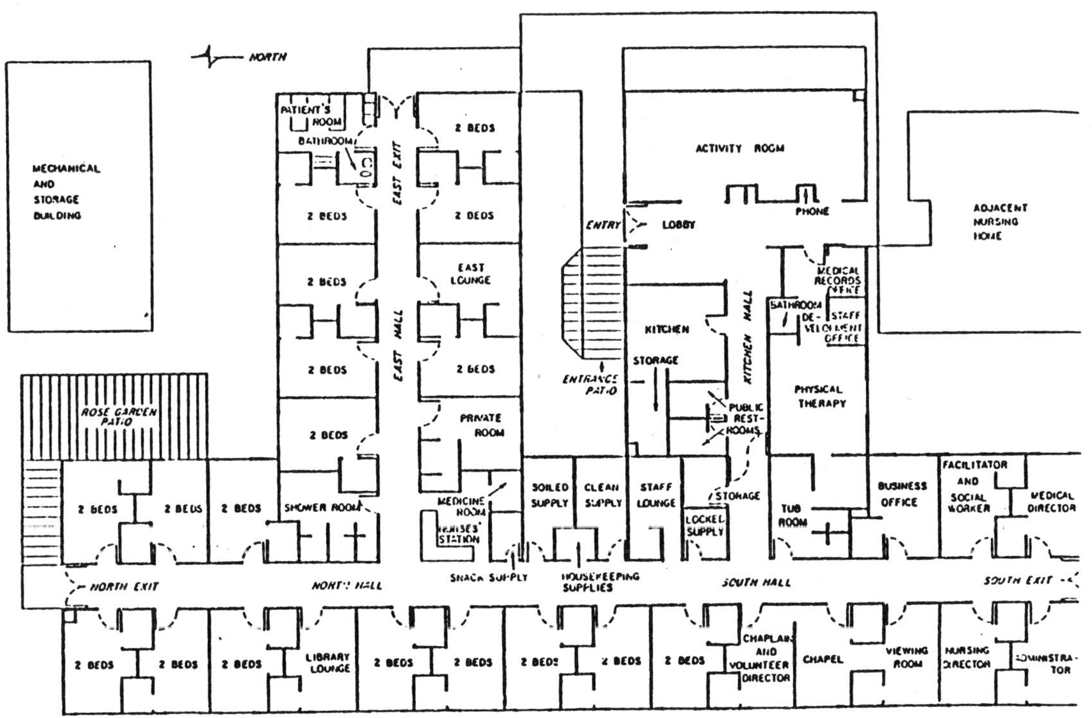

Schematic plan, Hillhaven Hospice

HILLHAVEN: DESCRIPTIVE MATRIX (Environmental Factors)

	General			
	Intent	*Existing*		
View				
Window	light, nature	ground-floor views		
Doors	nonabandonment, privacy	opposing doors on patient corridors		
Each bed	homelike, zoned	door, windows, personal items		
Other: artwork	variety, homelike	prints, sketches, nature, realism		
Window				
Treatment	control, homelike	N/A		
Trim	N/A	N/A		
Operation	N/A	N/A		
Covering	N/A	N/A		
Lighting				
Type	homelike	incandescent		
Fixtures	homelike	lamps, indirect sources		
Handicap access				
Bed and wheelchair	bed, chairs, walkers	wide doors, grouped furniture, sturdy furniture		
Dominant colors	homelike, comforting, clean	brown, blue, green, white, yellow, cream		
Dominant materials	homelike, warm, quiet, clean	carpet, wallpaper, wood, paint, fabrics, glass, acoustical tile		
Furniture type	homelike, comfortable, adaptable	residential furnishings, beds, tables, bookshelves, plants		
Ceiling height/ treatment	N/A	N/A		
Floor surfacing	homelike, clean	carpet, tile		
Personalization	encouraged	display area		
Organization	modified nursing facility	T ward with nurses' station at junction		
Equipment	homelike	television, telephones, minimized institutional safety		
Signs	homelike	noninstitutional		

• HOSPICE OF CINCINNATI, INC.

2710 Reading Road
Cincinnati, Ohio 45206

Classification: Freestanding; special hospital

Sponsoring agencies: Hospice of Cincinnati, Bethesda Hospital

Type: Remodeled two floors of nursing dormitory, second and third floors/basement and first used by hospital, building owned by Bethesda Hospital

Area served: Cincinnati and environs

Inpatient population: Currently, 18 maximum; room for 18 more in 4th-floor expansion

Established: 1981

Scope of work involved: Construction of new entry stair tower, remodeling of building included new HVAC, lights, plumbing, doors, and so on.

    Formerly: Nurses' residence

    Architect: William J. Rabon

            A. M. Kinney Assoc.

            2900 Vernon Place

            Cincinnati, Ohio 45219

Cost of work: N/A

    Build: N/A

    Furnishings: $55,000 plus donations

Comprehensive intention of building selection and/or design: N/A

General intention: Close to hospital, homelike, comfortable, pleasant-looking, functional

Location: Second, third, and fourth floors of remodeled nurses' dormitory, inner city, next to hospital

Description: Remodeled 1917 brick nurses' dormitory. Most existing walls remain; new entry stairs, elevator, mechanical systems

    Community image: part of hospital

    Interior image: remodeled L-shaped wards, new finishes, furniture

    Convenience: hampered by second-, third-story locations, hospital parking garage

Other: Initial design by Bethesda Hospital engineering staff

    Changes: Bigger nurses' station needed, as well as oxygen in walls, water closet for each room, better security, more storage, overnight accommodations for family, larger kitchen on patient floors, better patient meals, darker carpet (to hide stains), night-light system, elevator kill switch (hospice).

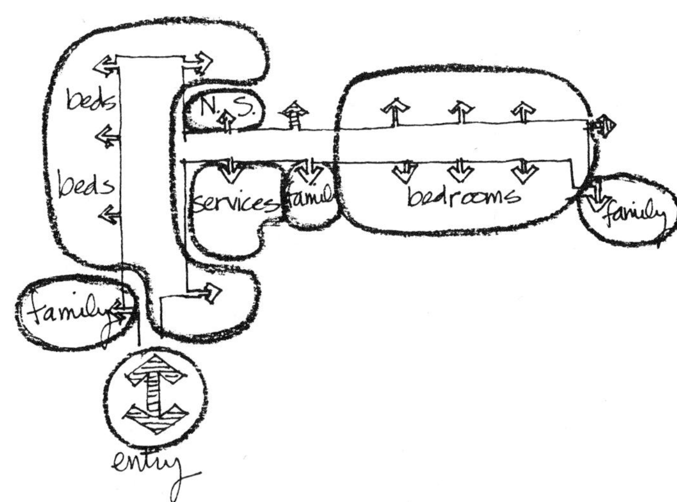

Parti drawing of patient floor, Hospice of Cincinnati

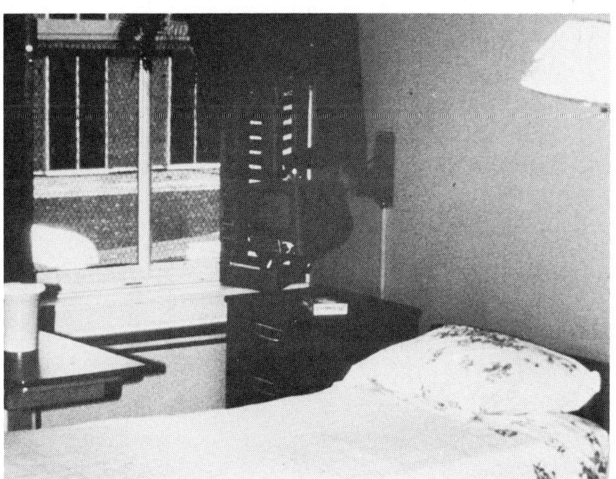

Patient room

Users:

    Outpatient staff: 4 home-care nurses

    Volunteers: 100

    Inpatient staff: 1 R.N. per every 3 patients

    Outpatients served: N/A

    Inpatient average population: 25 percent of care group

    Inpatient average length of stay: 8 days

    Family/visitors per week: Varies

Services rendered: Home care, inpatient care, social-services consultation. No family sleeping accommodations at this time, although ten cots will be added.

HOSPICE OF CINCINNATI: ARCHITECTURAL COMPONENTS

Architectural Components	*Notes*	*Wing/Total Number*	*Rough Dimensions or Size, Square Feet*
1. Patient room	Single	6	142/186
	Double	6	194/237
Bathrooms	Other: double with W.C.	1	54
	Patient bathrooms	2	125
2. Family lounge	2nd floor, with closet	1	165/9
Child area	Within family lounge		
Eating area	Within family lounge		
Other	Kitchen, 2nd floor		
	Family kitchenette, 3rd floor	1	124/10
Family other	Reading room, 3rd floor	1	157
Bathrooms	2nd floor, W.C. (m/f)	2	140
Conference	N/A		
3. Garden	Open, with cyclone fence		
Gardening area	See 3rd floor		
Chapel	None		
Transition room	Planned for 4th floor		
Meditation room		1	173.25
Chaplain office	See family lounge		
4. Nurses' station		1	86
Medication room	See nurses' station		
Nurses' retreat	N/A		
Staff rooms	Lounge, 2nd floor	1	158
Bathrooms	Staff, 3rd floor	1	36
	Staff, 2nd floor	1	140 (ave.)
5. Daycare	N/A		
Childcare	N/A		
Massage	N/A		
Physical therapy	N/A		
Occupational therapy	N/A		
Library	N/A		
Music/reading	See family lounge, 3rd floor		
Barbershop	N/A		
Tavern	N/A		
Store	N/A		
Game room	N/A		
Other	N/A		
6. Kitchen facilities	Provided by hospital		
Storage	N/A		
Supplies	N/A		
Preparation	N/A		
Unit dining	See patient rooms, family rooms		
Other dining	Staff dining room, 2nd floor	1	300
Nutrition station	Nurses' refrigerator, kitchen		
	for hospice staff, family	1	260

Architectural Components	Notes	Wing/Total Number	Rough Dimensions or Size, Square Feet
7. Offices			
Director/president	With closet	1	180/21
Nurse coordinator	With closet	1	164/12
Social work coordinator		1	143
Boardroom	See staff dining		
Conference room			
Volunteer coordinator	With closet	1	151/10
Business office	Home care and billing	1	620/150
Files	Secretary/bookkeeping	1	275
Other	Admitting (with closet)	1	135/10
Medical director	Exam room	1	135/10
Volunteer	Work room	1	200
8. Entry, front door	Stair tower, brick and concrete		
Reception	Waiting area, 2nd floor	1	300
Staff	Stair tower		
Patient	Stair tower		
Volunteer	Stair tower		
Visitors	Stair tower		
Goods	Hospice/hospital deliv. entrance		
Other	Fire stairs, with vestibule	2	190
Hallways, main	2nd-floor hallways		712 (6′ wide)
Service	3rd-floor hallways		957
Other	Stair and elevator tower	1	421
Exit goods	Hospice/hospital deliv. entrance		
Laundry	Hospital		
Dead	Service elevator to back court		
Miscellaneous	Elevator	1	6′ × 8′
	Service elevator	1	6′ × 8′

HOSPICE OF CINCINNATI: PROXIMITY MATRIX

| | Variable Numbers | | | | | | | | | | | | | |
Variables	1.	2.	3.	4.	5.	6.	7.	8.	9.	10.	11.	12.	13.	14.
1. Patient	C													
2. Family (2nd floor)	D	E												
3. Chapel (none)														
4. Nature (garden)	D	D												
5. Nurses' station	C	D		D										
6. Inpatient services	C	D		D	D									
7. Kitchen (hospital)	C	D		D	D	D								
8. Kitchenette (2nd floor)	D	A		D	D	D	D							
9. Offices (admitting)	D	B		D	D	D	D	A						
10. Main entry/facility	D	D		A	D	D	C	D	D					
11. Bed entry/unit (3rd floor)	C	D		D	C	D	D	D	D	C				
12. All parking	D	D		C	D	D	D	D	D	C	D			
13. Linen/laundry (3rd floor)	C	D		D	A	C	D	D	D	D	C			
14. Janitorial (2nd, 3rd floors)	C	C		D	C	D	D	B	A	D	C		A	D

Key:
- A = within 16-foot radius (based on 8-foot corridors)
- B = within 32-foot radius
- C = related areas (see plan)
- D = distant
- E = scattered, disparate association
- blank = no relation

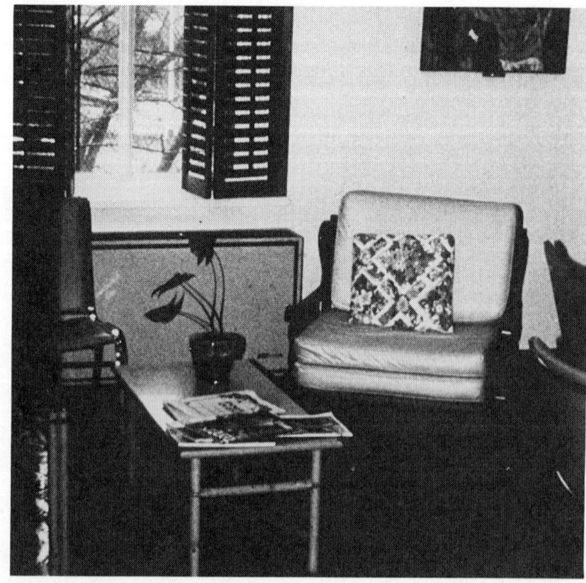

Family lounge area

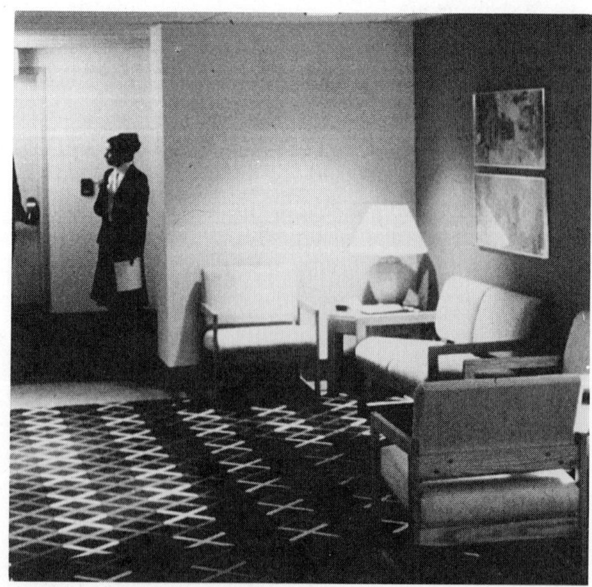

Reception area, located at hospice entrance

HOSPICE OF CINCINNATI: DESCRIPTIVE MATRIX (Environmental Factors)

	Patient (Bedrooms)		Family (2nd Floor)	
	Intent	*Existing*	*Intent*	*Existing*
View				
Window	light, homelike	high outside views from some/firewall	fire safety	no windows, wood shelves
Doors	nonabandonment, homelike	hallways, staggered room doors	connected, private	view to vending, hall end
Each bed	homelike, nonabandonment	furniture, television, telephone, (extra), hall/window		
Other: artwork	homelike	personalization encouraged	homelike	wall hangings
Window				
Treatment	obscuring, homelike		fire safety	wall blocked out
Trim	existing	wood trim	N/A	N/A
Operation	existing	operable	N/A	N/A
Covering	homelike, adjustable, obscuring	wooden window shutters, night light for firewall window	N/A	N/A
Lighting				
Type	homelike, practical	incandescent/ fluorescent	homelike, practical	incandescent
Fixtures	homelike, low gradient	fluorescent night, incandescent head swing, down light	homelike, low gradient	recessed down lights, lamps
Handicap access				
Bed and wheelchair	bed, chair, recliner, walker, crutches	large doors, hall bars, grouped furniture	bed, chair, recliner, walker	large doors, hall bars, grouped, movable furniture
Dominant colors	homelike, cheerful, contemporary	yellow, orange, beige, brown	homelike, cheerful, contemporary	brown, beige, yellow, orange
Dominant materials	homelike, clean, practical, warm	plastic laminate, paint, wood, ceramic, acoustical tile, carpet, fabric, metal	homelike, scrubbable, comfortable	fabrics, paint, wood, carpet, acoustical tile, toys, plastic laminate
Furniture type	practical, comfortable, homelike space-saving	hospital bed, table, wall cabinet, bed cabinet, rockers, lounge chair, curtains, bulletin boards	homelike, comfortable, scrubbable	couch, chairs, toy chest, bookcase, plants
Ceiling height/ treatment	practical	8′, acoustical tile	practical	8′, acoustical tile
Floor surfacing	homelike, warm	carpet	homelike	carpet
Personalization	encouraged	colored sheets, plants, pictures, furniture, bulletin boards	little	unused

HOSPICE OF CINCINNATI: DESCRIPTIVE MATRIX (Environmental Factors)

	Patient (Bedrooms)		*Family (2nd Floor)*	
	Intent	*Existing*	*Intent*	*Existing*
Organization	modified existing	double-loaded L-shaped corridor with many small patient rooms, nurses' station	modified existing	small room off patient floor, far from entry, action
Equipment	homelike, practical, convenient	lamps, call system, sink, night light, air conditioning, music	homelike, practical	lamps, closet, air conditioner
Signs	homelike	room numbers, bulletin boards, overdoor call lights	homelike	room numbers

	Family (Reading Room, Garden, Lounge)		*Nurses' Station*	
	Intent	*Existing*	*Intent*	*Existing*
View				
Window	light, airy, high views	high view, large windows, southern light	internal	no windows
Doors	open, but private	hall end, no door	open visibility	no doors but restricted visibility
Each bed	accessible	no door	visibility	4′ door, 3′ counter
Other: artwork	nature, cheerful	pictures, plants	restricted	small room
Window				
Treatment	gardenlike		N/A	N/A
Trim	existing	wood	N/A	N/A
Operation	existing	N/A	N/A	N/A
Covering	homelike	window shades	N/A	N/A
Lighting				
Type	homelike	incandescent	efficient	fluorescent
Fixtures	homelike, low gradient	recessed down lights	efficient, low gradient	recessed ceiling lamps
Handicap access				
Bed and wheelchair	chair, bed, lounge chair, walker, crutch	open, grouped furniture	counter is wheelchair height	same
Dominant colors	bright light, homelike, gardenlike	white, yellow, orange, green, brown, black	clean, coordinated	beige, brown, blue, white
Dominant materials	homelike, patio garden	wrought iron, plastic laminate, wood, paint, glass	clean, efficient, contemporary	plastic laminate, paint, acoustical tile, gypsum board, carpet
Furniture type	homelike, patio and garden furniture	wrought-iron tables, chairs, floor plants	space-efficient, contemporary, low-maintenance, clean	counters, cabinets, seating for 1 sink, refrigerator, intercom units

HOSPICE OF CINCINNATI: DESCRIPTIVE MATRIX (Environmental Factors)

	Family (Reading Room, Garden, Lounge)		Nurses' Station	
	Intent	*Existing*	*Intent*	*Existing*
Ceiling height/ treatment	practical	8', acoustical tile	practical	9', acoustical tile
Floor surfacing	homelike	carpet	homelike, coordinated	carpet
Personalization	encouraged	plants, pictures	limited	1-person enclosure, very cramped, files, cabinets
Organization	private, light location	hall end, south side, 3rd floor	central, visibility	at T crossing, small open room, poor visibility
Equipment	homelike, safety	fire exit sign	patient communication, nutrition station, practical	call system, refrigerator, sink, cabinets, medicine in locked cart, incom. unit
Signs	security, homelike	fire exit sign	central, open	location, hall signs, security camera

	Nurses (Staff Lounge)		Family (3rd-Floor Kitchen)	
	Intent	*Existing*	*Intent*	*Existing*
View				
Window	light, nature	southern light, big windows	light, nature	southern light, high views
Doors	private, convenient	hall end, double doors to dining	odor control, accessibility	4' door
Each bed	N/A	N/A	small, but accessible	family use
Other: artwork	minimal	staff contributed	cheerful, signs	plants, pictures
Window				
Treatment	homelike	N/A	homelike	N/A
Trim	existing	wood	existing	wood
Operation	existing	N/A	existing	operable
Covering	existing	none	homelike, adjustable	wood shutters
Lighting				
Type	homelike, warm	incandescent	homelike, efficient	fluorescent
Fixtures	homelike, low gradient	recessed down lights (ceiling)	low gradient	ceiling recessed louvered fixtures
Handicap access				
Bed and wheelchair	N/A	N/A	lounge chair, walker, wheelchair	large door, central to patient rooms
Dominant colors	clean, efficient coordinated	beige, brown, gray, black	clean, bright, coordinated	yellow, beige, brown, white
Dominant materials	clean, coordinated	metal, plastic laminate, carpet, acoustical tile	clean, homelike	metal, gypsum board, paint, wood, plastic laminate, linoleum

HOSPICE OF CINCINNATI: DESCRIPTIVE MATRIX (Environmental Factors)

	Nurses (Staff Lounge)		Family (3rd-Floor Kitchen)	
	Intent	*Existing*	*Intent*	*Existing*
Furniture type	practical, movable, economical	lockers, tables, chairs, pay phone	practical, movable, economical	countertop, refrigerator, hot water, ice machine, microwave, coffee machine
Ceiling height/ treatment	practical	8′, acoustical tile	practical, fire-safe	8′, suspended gypsum board
Floor surfacing	coordinated, homelike	carpet	practical	linoleum (vinyl)
Personalization	little	very underused	encouraged	much family use
Organization	private room near dining	alcove off unused area, dead end	alternate kitchen central to patient rooms	near nurses' station, patient rooms, W.C.s, action
Equipment	practical, clean	lockers, pay phone, lights, air conditioning	kitchen equipment, practical	lights, air conditioning, closet, call duty
Signs	homelike	hall signs, homemade signs	homelike	hall signs

	Kitchenette (Staff Dining)		Kitchenette (2nd Floor)	
	Intent	*Existing*	*Intent*	*Existing*
View				
Window	light, bright, views	southern light, 2 windows, views	light, bright views	southern light, 2 windows, views
Doors	privacy, connections	kitchen, hall, employee lounge	odor control, privacy	hall door
Each bed	minimal	hall doorways	minimal	hall doorways
Other: artwork	homelike, cheerful	plants, pictures	homelike, cheerful	plants, pictures
Window				
Treatment	existing	N/A	existing	N/A
Trim	existing	N/A	existing	wood
Operation	existing	operable	existing	operable
Covering	homelike, adaptable	wood shutters, latticework	homelike, adaptable	wood shutters
Lighting				
Type	homelike, cheerful	natural, incandescent	homelike, practical	natural, fluorescent
Fixtures	homelike, individually controlled	recessed down lights with dimmer	task, general	under cabinet fluorescent and recessed ceiling lights
Handicap access				
Bed and wheelchair	chair, walker accessibility	doors accessible	minimal chair, walker	narrow doors for beds, not on patient bed floors

	Kitchenette (Staff Dining)		Kitchenette (2nd Floor)	
	Intent	*Existing*	*Intent*	*Existing*
Dominant colors	cheerful, homelike coordinated	bright yellow, white, green, brown, beige, florals	homelike, cheerful, clean	pastel, yellow, green, beige, brown, rainbow
Dominant materials	homelike, adaptable, scrubbable	carpet, plastic laminate, wood, wallpaper, plaster, paint, acoustical tile	homelike, warm, clean, cheerful	acoustical tile, vinyl, plastic laminate, oak, metal, paint, wallpaper
Furniture type	adaptable, scrubbable, homelike, comfortable	5 tables with 4 chairs each, lights, telephone	homelike, useful, scrubbable, comfortable	cabinets, counters, table, chairs, refrigerator, microwave, stove, dishwasher, garbage disposal
Ceiling height/ treatment	practical	8′ acoustical tile	practical	8′ acoustical tile
Floor surfacing	homelike, coordinated	carpet	homelike, cleanable	linoleum (vinyl)
Personalization	some	used as dining, also as boardroom and conference room	encouraged	plants, food, etc.
Organization	central, near complementary uses	large room off corridor near offices, kitchen, family room	central, near complement uses	spacious room, off dining, nurses' station, volunteer, staff spaces
Equipment	dining room, efficient, noninstitutional	air conditioning, telephone, lights with dimmer, call duty	cooking, noninstitutional	furniture, utensils, exhaust fan, call duty, air conditioning
Signs	homelike	hall sign	homelike	hall sign

	Offices (Home Care)		Offices (Volunteer Work Room)	
	Intent	*Existing*	*Intent*	*Existing*
View				
Window	fire safety, light, views	5 boarded up, 2 view to west, entry	light, bright, low views	southern exposure, local views
Doors	entry, visibility, view	open to entry hall w/relight window	privacy	hall doorway
Each bed	limited	hall views	none	not applicable
Other: artwork	encouraged	pictures, plants	encouraged	pictures, plants
Territorial	personal spaces	carousel cubicles	N/A	N/A
Window				
Treatment	existing, fire safety	N/A	existing, homelike	N/A
Trim	see above	wood, gypsum board	existing	wood
Operation	see above	5 modified, 2 existing	existing	operable
Covering	fire safety, homelike, adaptable	bookshelves, wood shutters	homelike, adaptable	wood shutters

HOSPICE OF CINCINNATI: DESCRIPTIVE MATRIX (Environmental Factors)

	Offices (Home Care)		Offices (Volunteer Work Room)	
	Intent	*Existing*	*Intent*	*Existing*
Lighting				
Type	practical, economical	fluorescent and task incandescent	homelike, practical	fluorescent, task incandescent
Fixtures	practical, low gradient	recessed overhead desk lamps	practical, low gradient	recessed overhead desk lamps
Handicap access				
Bed and wheelchair	limited	3′ door entry	limited	3′ door entry
Dominant colors	homelike, cheerful warm, coordinated	yellow, orange, beige, brown, green, blue, white	homelike, donated, cheerful	pastel, yellow, white, brown, beige, green
Dominant materials	homelike, warm, quiet, privacy	fabrics, acoustical tile, carpet, paint, wood, paper, metal	homelike, practical, comfortable	paint, wood, fabric, glass, acoustical tile, carpet, plastic laminate
Furniture type	office; comfort, privacy	carousel cubicals, desk, chairs, bookcases, charts, cabinets, fireplace, shelves	homelike, adaptable, donated, comfortable	desk, couches, bookshelves, tables, soft chairs, mirror, sink
Ceiling height/treatment	practical	8′ acoustical tile	practical	8′ acoustical tile
Floor surfacing	homelike, warm, welcoming	carpet	homelike, warm, coordinated	carpet
Personalization	encouraged	staff items, plants, pictures, books, furniture	encouraged	donated furniture, art, plants, books
Organization	convenient, private, but open	large divided room near offices, entry, W.C., billing	convenient, private	near offices, away from patient floor, near W.C., volunteer director
Equipment	practical, comfortable	air conditioning, lights, typewriters, radio, telephones	practical, noninstitutional	air conditioning, lights, radio
Signs	location, noninstitutional, homelike	central location, hall sign, residential imagery	noninstitutional	hall sign, homemade signs

	Offices (Admitting)		Circulation (Halls)	
	Intent	*Existing*	*Intent*	*Existing*
View				
Window	fire safety	window now a bookcase	modified, existing	double-loaded corridors with light through rooms
Doors	privacy	3′ door	homelike but double-loaded	new wood doors

HOSPICE OF CINCINNATI: DESCRIPTIVE MATRIX (Environmental Factors)

	Offices (Admitting)		Circulation (Halls)	
	Intent	*Existing*	*Intent*	*Existing*
Each bed	limited	through door	light, airy, cheerful	pictures, light colors, residential lights
Other: artwork	homelike, variety	wall hangings, ceiling mobiles	homelike, cheerful	pictures
Window				
Treatment	N/A	N/A	through rooms	N/A
Trim	N/A	N/A	N/A	N/A
Operation	N/A	N/A	N/A	N/A
Covering	N/A	N/A	N/A	N/A
Lighting				
Type	homelike, efficient	fluorescent, built-in	light, airy, noninstitutional	fluorescent/ incandescent
Fixtures	efficient, low gradient	recessed ceiling fixtures, baffle	indirect, recessed	fluorescent wall wash, indirect ceiling, down lights
Handicap access				
Bed and wheelchair	chair, lounge chair, walker	3′ door, grouped furniture, wall bars	bed, chair, lounge chair, walker	wall bars, 6′ minimum width, elevator patient rooms, near elevators
Dominant colors	homelike, cheerful, coordinated	orange, beige, brown, green	serene, contemporary, homelike	beige, brown, blue off-white
Dominant materials	homelike, comfortable, scrubbable	carpet, acoustical tile, wood, paint, magazines, glass	contemporary, homelike, quiet, clean	carpet, mosaics, wood, acoustical tile paint, metal
Furniture type	homelike, comfortable, scrubbable	4 soft chairs, coffee table, bookcases, side tables	none	no conversation nooks, alcoves for patient/family except 2nd floor reception
Ceiling height/ treatment	practical	8′ acoustical tile	maximum possible, practical	7′-8″ acoustical tile
Floor surfacing	homelike, welcoming	carpet	homelike, warm, quiet	carpet
Personalization	encouraged	artwork, signs, plants, magazines	limited, some	no room for furniture, pictures, plants
Organization	homelike room near complementary facilities	small room off double-loaded corridor, near exam, kitchen, W.C.	modified existing	double-loaded corridor
Equipment	comfortable, communication	telephone, air conditioning, lights, music (tapes)	safety, handicapped	call lights, wall bars, fire equipment sign
Signs	noninstitutional	hall room sign	minimize institutional	fire exit signs, room signs, sprinkler head direct

Hospice of Cincinnati: General Notes

The Hospice of Cincinnati was originally programmed by Bethesda Hospital Facilities for the hospice tenant, as an economical plan. The existing walls were to remain, and this eventually turned out to restrict the design. The architect feels that in remodels of this type, it is probably no less expensive to tear out the walls and rebuild from scratch. This, of course, would provide for a more homelike and flexible design.

Hospice of Cincinnati has separated uses on floors, with offices on one floor and patient rooms on another. However, family uses were placed on the staff floor and this has not worked out. Instead, there has been duplication of function with family rooms and kitchen on both the patient and staff floors; the family rooms on the staff floors were just too far away from the hospice patients. These third-floor family rooms are afterthoughts and do not provide the spaciousness or detail of the second-floor rooms.

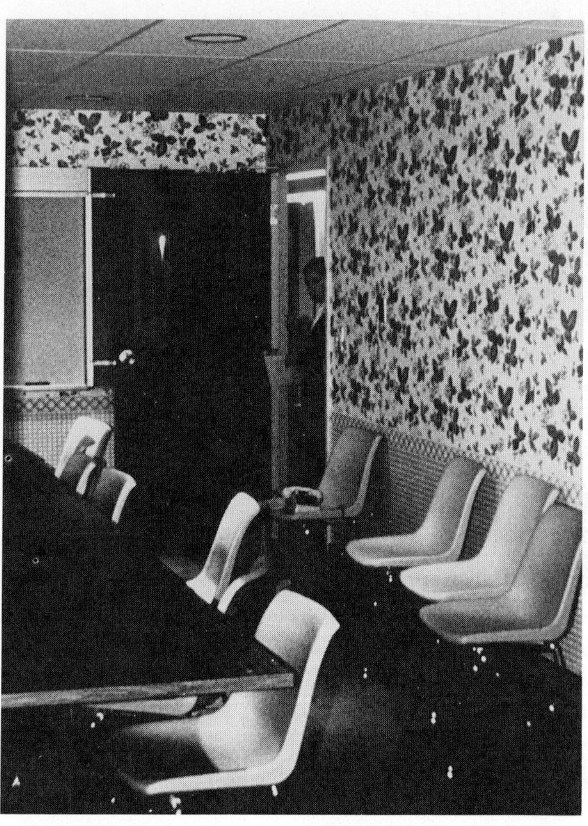

Office space

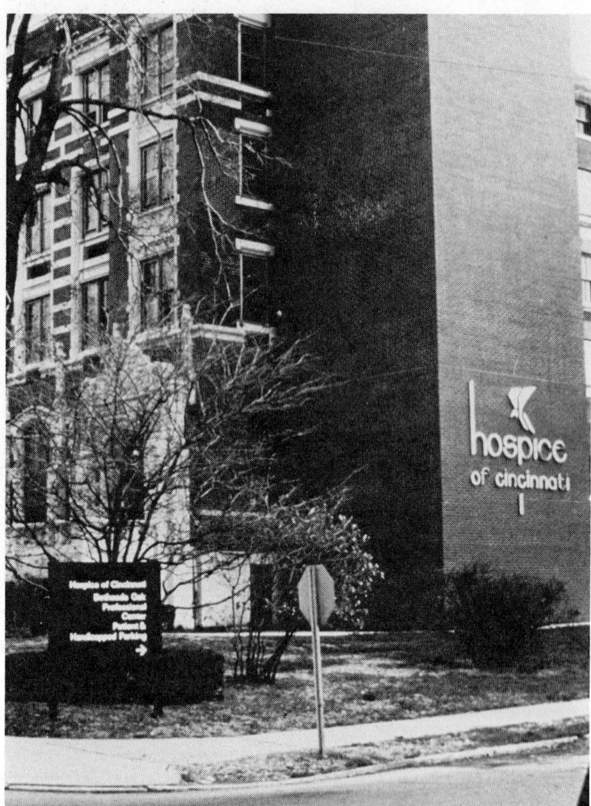

View of hospice from street

• HOSPICE OF THE GOOD SHEPHERD, INC.

Waban, Massachusetts 02168

Classification: Proposed facility, freestanding hospice, special hospital

Sponsoring agencies: Hospice of the Good Shepherd

Type: Remodeled school

Area served: Boston suburban environs; serves 5 to 7 area hospices

Hospice facility address:
465 Lowell Ave.
Newtonville, Massachusetts 02160

Inpatient population: 15-bed hospice, 17 apartments, physician's suite

Established: Hospice established 1978; original school built 1951, addition in 1959.

Scope of work involved: Widened access, landscaping, new access, new kitchen and food service, new deck, apartments, hospice facilities, sunroom, new windows, repaired facades.

Formerly: Claflin Elementary School
Architect: Steffian-Bradley Assoc., Inc.
      66 Canal Street
      Boston, Massachusetts 02114

Cost of work: 2.8 million
Build: See above
Furnishings: Additional $448,000 (hospice)

Comprehensive intention of building selection and/or design: N/A

General intention: Homelike, comfortable, light, airy, residential scale, character

Location: Five-acre grounds, mature trees, existing playing areas, in residential neighborhood of same age

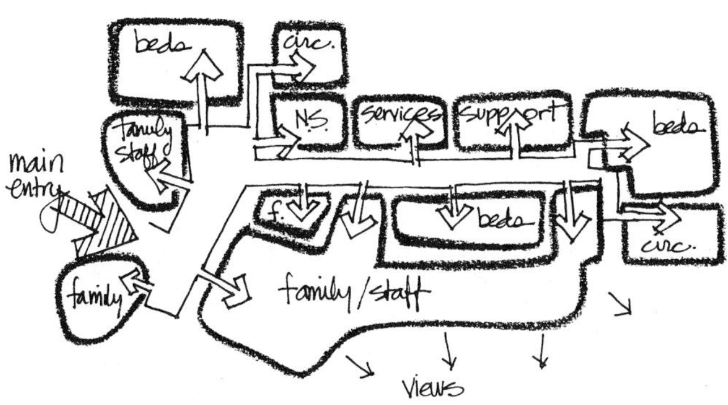

Parti drawing of the first floor, Hospice of the Good Shepherd

Description: Remodeled modern brick school
Community image: remodeled school with apartments
Interior image: open, bright, woodsy, clean, friendly, with variety, subtlety
Convenience: hilltop site with carpool/van access

Other: Fundraising effort, continuing (as of 1984)

Users:
Outpatient staff: N/A
Volunteers: N/A
Inpatient staff: (FTE) N/A
Outpatients served: N/A
Inpatient average population: N/A
Inpatient average length of stay: N/A
Family/visitors per week: N/A

Services rendered: Home care, inpatient care, bereavement counseling, education, 24-hour family visiting, family sleeping facilities

HOSPICE OF THE GOOD SHEPHERD: ARCHITECTURAL COMPONENTS

Architectural Components	Notes	Wing/Total Number	Rough Dimensions or Size, Square Feet
1. Patient room			
	Single with W.C.	2	177/40 (ave.)
	Single with bath	1	195/50
	Four with bath	2	557/57 (ave.)
Other	Four with bath	1	675/52
Bathrooms	Tub rooms	3	36
2. Family lounge	Living room	1	830
Child area	See living room		
Eating area	See dining		
Other	See sun room		
Family private room	With W.C.	1	220/45
Family other	Room and parlor	1	130/108
Bathrooms	Public restrooms	2	55
Conference/social work	See also entry lobby	1	120
3. Garden	See landscape/sun porch	1	640
Gardening area	Garden sun room	1	768
Chapel	None		
Transition room	N/A		
Meditation room	N/A		
Chaplain office	N/A		
4. Nurses' station		1	8′ × 25′
Medication room	Utility storage	1	100
Nurses' retreat	Staff lounge	1	220
Staff rooms	Lockers	1	96
Bathrooms	Public restroom, ground floor	2	40/60
5. Daycare	See living room		
Childcare	Multipurpose room	1	168
Massage	In patient rooms		
Physical therapy		1	80
Occupational therapy/ craft room	See unit dining		
Library	See boardroom		
Music/reading	See family rooms		
Barbershop	N/A		
Tavern	N/A		
Store	N/A		
Game room	See sun room		
Other	N/A		
6. Kitchen facilities	Ground floor	Total	1,368
Storage		1	230
Supplies	Refrigerator/freezer	1	240
Preparation		1	497
Cleaning		1	175
Office		1	226
Dietary staff	N/A		

HOSPICE OF THE GOOD SHEPHERD: ARCHITECTURAL COMPONENTS

Architectural Components	Notes	Wing/Total Number	Rough Dimensions or Size, Square Feet
Unit dining	1st floor (entertainment)	1	350
Other dining	Staff lounge, patient rooms		
Nutrition station	See nurses' station		
7. Offices			
Administrative reception		1	240
Director/executive		1	360
Nurse coordinator		1	56
Social work coordinator		1	110
Boardroom		1	600
Conference room		1	308
Volunteer coordinator		1	72
Business office	Fiscal manager	1	168
Volunteer/education		1	360
Facility manager		1	176
Home-care office		1	120
Files	Secretary	1	240
Assistant administrator		1	280
Administrative support	Copying/sorting	1	205/426
Administrative support	Home care	1	209
Home-care team rooms		2	465/228
Home-care work room		1	448
Bathrooms		2	56
8. Entry, front door	Main entry	1	96
Reception		1	80
Administration	Stairway	1	164
Staff	See main entry, home-care entry		
Patient	See main entry		
Volunteer	See main entry		
Visitors	Lobby, waiting area	1	276
Goods	Service area, receiving	1	143
Other	Conference room entry	1	154
Hallways, main	1st, 2nd floors		2,368
Service	Kitchen/service		664
Other	Home care corridors		350
Loading dock		1	540
Exit goods	See service goods/receiving		
Laundry	See service goods/receiving		
Dead	See service goods/receiving		
Miscellaneous	Elevator	1	6' × 8'
	Stairs	2	253
9. Parking	Front yard	47 spaces	
Connections to other facilities	N/A		
Connection to neighborhood	N/A		
Street visibility	N/A		
Landscaping			
Front yard	Existing trees, shrubs		
Back yard	Existing trees, shrubs		

Architectural Components	Notes	Wing/Total Number	Rough Dimensions or Size, Square Feet
10. Services			
Laundry	Contracted		
Clean linen	Closets	1/2	40/15
Dirty linen		1	40
Janitorial		1	110
Closet		1	44
Stores	N/A		
General stores	Miscellaneous storage	1	80
Offices	Storage	1	30
Garbage	Trash room	1	342
Garbage pickup	Dumpster at loading dock		
Equipment storage		1	90
Mail	See reception		
Miscellaneous	Mechanical/electrical		784/110
	Audio/visual storage	1	56

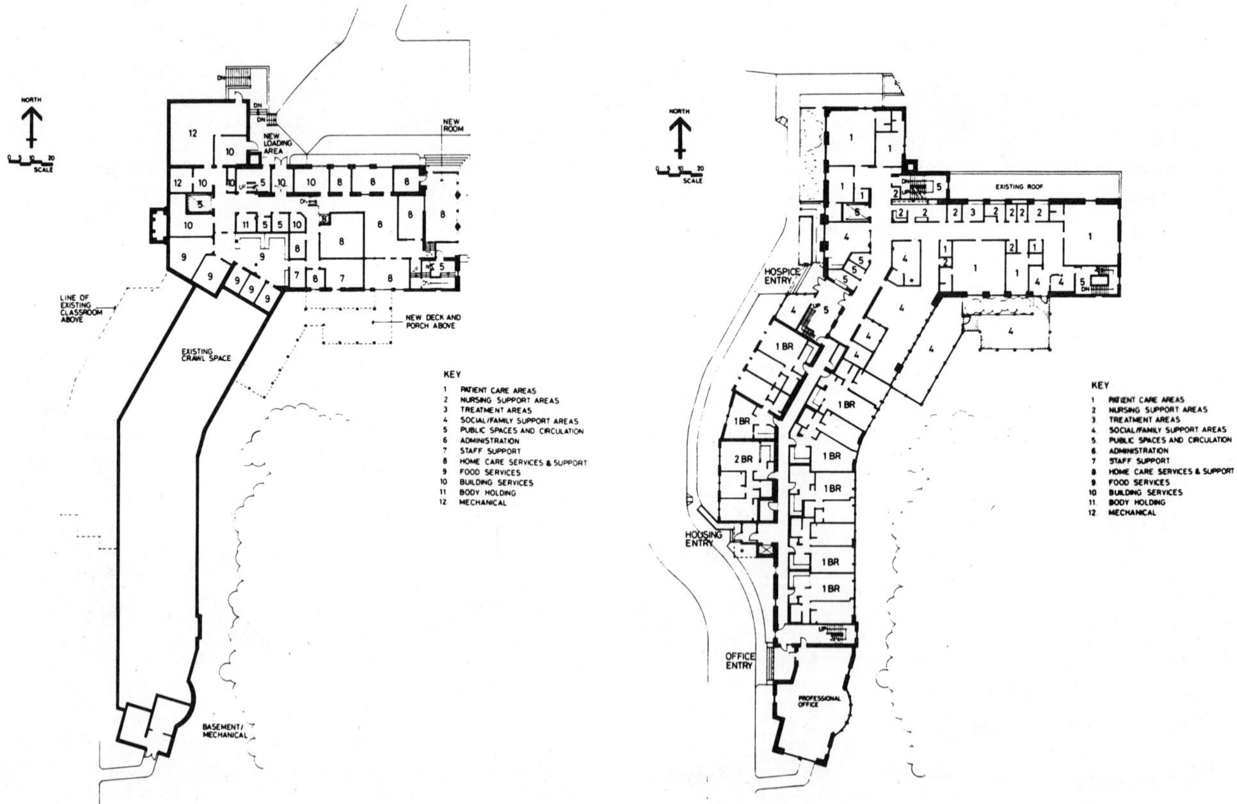

Plan, ground floor of hospice   *Plan, first floor of hospice*

HOSPICE OF THE GOOD SHEPHERD: PROXIMITY MATRIX

Variables	*Variable Numbers*													
	1.	*2.*	*3.*	*4.*	*5.*	*6.*	*7.*	*8.*	*9.*	*10.*	*11.*	*12.*	*13.*	*14.*
1. Patient														
2. Family	B													
3. Chapel	*	*												
4. Nature (sunroom, deck)	C	A	*											
5. Nurses' station	C	A	*	C										
6. Inpatient services	C	C	*	C	B									
7. Kitchen	D	D	*	D	C	D								
8. Kitchenette	C	A	*	C	B	C	C							
9. Offices (admin.)	D	C	*	D	C	D	D	C						
10. Main entry/facility	C	A	*	C	C	C	D	B	C					
11. Bed entry/unit	D	D	*	D	C	D	A	D	D	D				
12. All parking	C	C	*	C	D	D	D	C	D	B	D			
13. Linen/laundry	B	C	*		C	A	D	C	D	D	C	D		
14. Janitorial	D	D	*	D	C	D	B	C	D	D	A	D	D	

Key:

    A = within 16-foot radius (based on 8-foot corridors)

    B = within 32-foot radius

    C = related areas (see plan)

    D = distant

  blank = no relation

     * = no information available

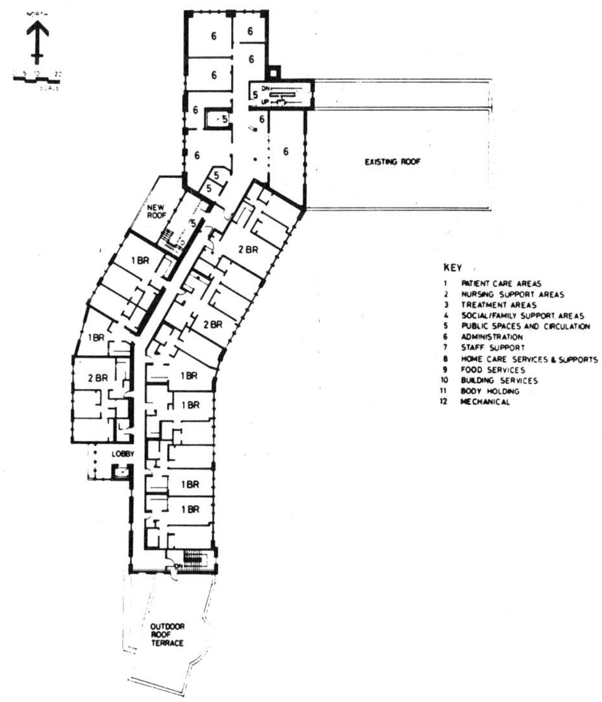

Plan, second floor of hospice

General				
	Intent	*Existing*		
View				
Window	light, nature, activity	trees, grass, play areas, entries		
Doors	nonabandonment, privacy, flexibility	wood, handicap access, alcoves		
Each bed	territorial, homelike	near and distant views		
Other: artwork	homelike, variety	changing professional art		
Window				
Treatment	energy-efficient, light, choice	new double-glazed		
Trim	homelike	wood		
Operation	homelike	operable		
Covering	homelike, choice	curtains, blinds, shutters		
Lighting				
Type	homelike	incandescent		
Fixtures	homelike, adaptable	lamps, wall washers, indirect sources		
Handicap access				
Bed and wheelchair	bed, lounge chair, walker	wall rails (wood), large doorways, grouped furniture		
Dominant colors	homelike, variety light, decorative	to be selected		
Dominant materials	homelike, warm, comfortable, clean, natural	wood, fabrics, carpet paint, wallpaper, texture		
Furniture type	homelike, comfortable, adaptable	hospital beds, residential furniture, lamps, tables, chairs		
Ceiling height/ treatment	varied, homelike	no acoustical tile		
Floor surfacing	warm, homelike, quiet	carpet, tile		
Personalization	encouraged	display areas, signboards, plants		
Organization	one floor of patient/ family use	T-shaped patient/ family layout with services, offices		
Equipment	homelike, friendly, nonabandonment	oxygen in walls, individual heat, lights, television, life-safety equipment		
Signs	homelike, friendly	N/A		

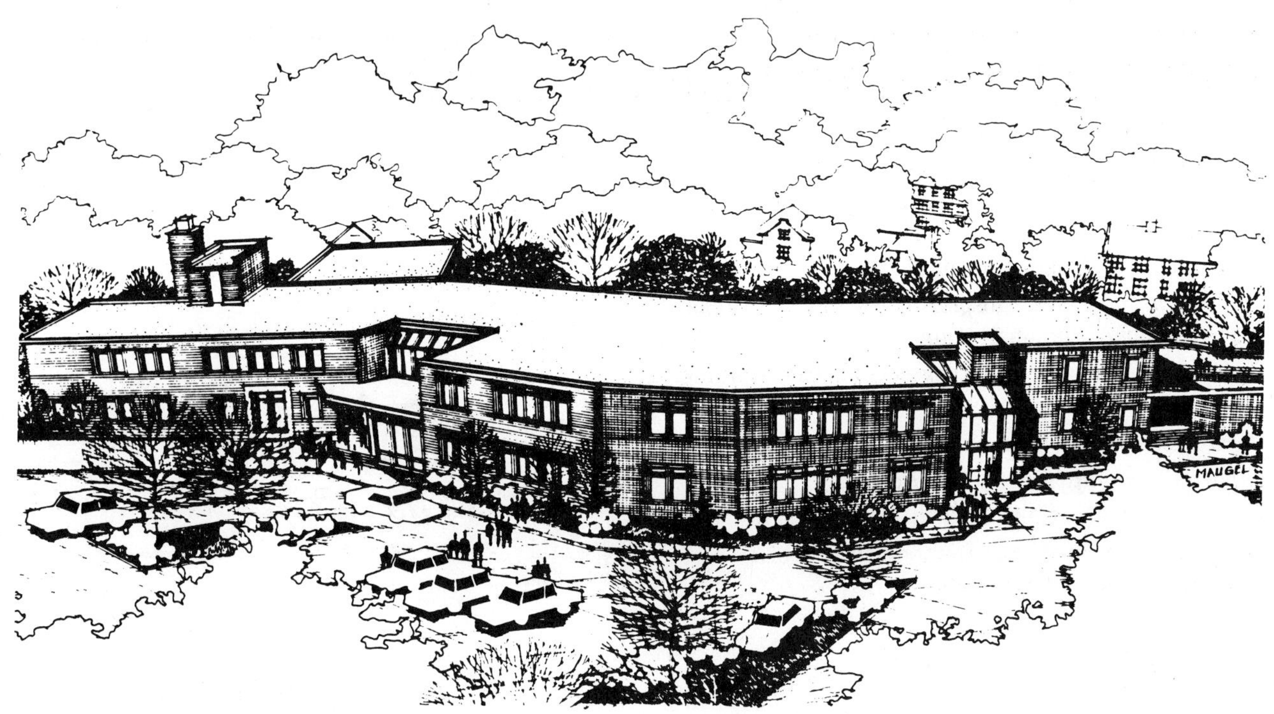

View of main entry, Hospice of the Good Shepherd

• HOSPICE OF NORTHERN VIRGINIA

4715 North 15th Street
Arlington, Virginia 22205

Classification: Special hospital

Sponsoring agencies: Hospice of Northern Virginia; part of HCFA demonstration

Type: Remodeled elementary school, freestanding hospice facility

Area served: Northern Virginia, Arlington

Inpatient population: Maximum 15

Established: Inpatient 1982; home care 1978

Scope of work involved: Remodeled school
   Formerly: Woodlawn School
   Architect: Engineer on board of directors

Cost of work: 1 million
   Build: N/A
   Furnishings: N/A

Comprehensive intention of building selection and/or design: N/A

General intention: Homelike decor coordinated with building's architecture.

Location: On landscaped, parklike grounds in quiet, residential area

Description: 1941 Georgian brick elementary school, relandscaped
   Community image: remodeled school
   Interior image: spacious, warm, gracious family and patient areas, modern and cheerful offices
   Convenience: ground-floor entry
   Changes: additional storage space needed; storage area in basement should be remodeled. Better nurses' lounge needed.

Users:
   Kitchen staff: 6
   Outpatient staff: 12
   Volunteers: 150+
   Inpatient staff: FTE 11.3 nurses, 7.5 aides, bereavement and education staff: 5
   Inpatient average population: Not yet known
   Inpatient average length of stay: N/A
   Family/visitors per week: Varies
   Administration and staff: 10

Services rendered: Home care, counseling, inpatient care, bereavement, family sleeping facilities (patient rooms, counseling room, or family lounge)

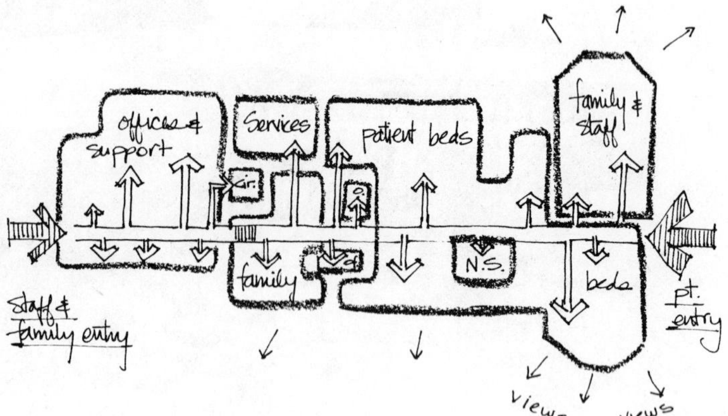

Parti drawing, Hospice of Northern Virginia

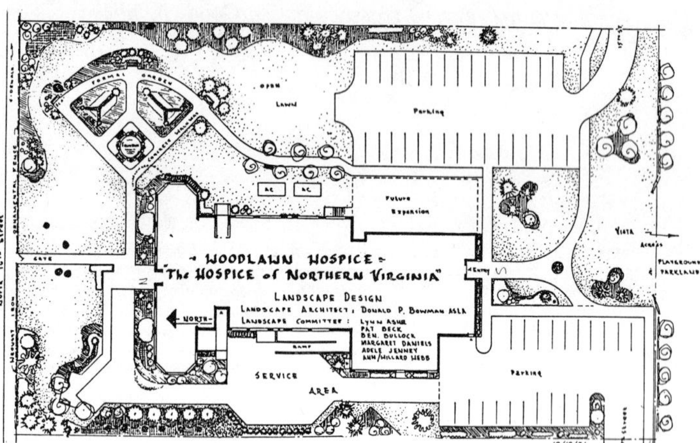

Landscape design

HOSPICE OF NORTHERN VIRGINIA: ARCHITECTURAL COMPONENTS

Architectural Components	Notes	Wing/Total Number	Rough Dimensions or Size, Square Feet
1. Patient room	Single with W.C.	1	156/25
	Single with W.C.	1	160/42
	Single	1	183
	Four-bed with W.C.	1	580/25
	Four-bed with W.C.	1	624/42
	Four-bed with W.C.	1	616/30
Patient bath/shower		1	120
2. Family lounge		1	725
Child area			
Eating area	See family lounge		
Other	Game area		
Family private room	Counseling	1	88
Family other	See kitchen, laundry		
Bathrooms	Handicap (m/f)	2	80
3. Garden	Landscaped grounds		
Gardening area	Plants in rooms		
Chapel	See meditation room		
Transition room	See meditation room		
Meditation room		1	240
Chaplain office	Bereavement counseling	1	70
4. Nurses' station		1	120
Medication room		1	35
Nurses' retreat	See multipurpose room		
Staff rooms	Lockers (basement)		
Bathrooms	W.C. in nurses' station	1	20
5. Daycare	See family lounge		
Childcare	See family lounge		
Massage	See nurses' lounge		
Physical therapy	Nurses' lounge	1	225
Occupational therapy	See nurses' lounge		
Library	See office/conference room		
Music/reading	See family lounge		
Barbershop	None		
Tavern	None		
Store	None		
Game room	See family lounge		
Other	None		
6. Kitchen Facilities			600 total
Storage	Freezer area		95
Supplies	Basement		
Preparation			361
Cleaning			144
Office	See facility manager		
Dietary staff	with W.C., shower	1	48
Unit dining	See patient rooms/lounge		
Other dining	Staff dining	1	510
Kitchenette		1	7' × 11'

HOSPICE OF NORTHERN VIRGINIA: ARCHITECTURAL COMPONENTS

Architectural Components	Notes	Wing/Total Number	Rough Dimensions or Size, Square Feet
7. Offices			
Director/executive		1	132
Director of Nursing		1	100
Nurse coordinator		1	126
Social work coordinator			
Boardroom	See conference room		
Conference room	Library	1	400
Volunteer coordinator		1	80
Business office		1	400
Files	Facilities manager	1	60
Other	Volunteer work room	1	204
Medical director	Inpatient counseling	1	80
8. Entry, front door	North entrance	1	40
Reception room		1	288
Admitting	See nurses' station		
Staff entrance	South entrance	1	40
Patient	North entrance		
Volunteer	South entrance		
Visitors	South entrance		
Goods	Service entrance (west)		
Other	N/A		
Hallways, main	Upper corridor		
Service	Lower corridor		
Other	Basement rooms		
Exit Goods	Trash out kitchen door		
Laundry	Basement (family also permitted to use)		
Dead	North entrance		
Miscellaneous	Stairs	3	4' × 10'
	Elevator	1	6' × 8'
9. Parking	2 lots east/west	55 spaces	
Connections to other facilities	N/A		
Connection to neighborhood	N/A		
Street visibility	N/A		
Landscaping			
Front yard	N/A		
Back yard	N/A		
10. Services			
Laundry	Basement	1	102
Janitorial			
Closet		2	
Stores	Basement		
General stores	Basement	1	864
Offices			
Garbage	Trash out kitchen door		
Garbage pickup	Service entrance		
Equipment storage	Offices/basement		
Mail	Reception area		
Miscellaneous	N/A		

HOSPICE OF NORTHERN VIRGINIA: PROXIMITY MATRIX

	Variable Numbers													
Variables	*1.*	*2.*	*3.*	*4.*	*5.*	*6.*	*7.*	*8.*	*9.*	*10.*	*11.*	*12.*	*13.*	*14.*
1. Patient	B													
2. Family	C													
3. Meditation room	C	C												
4. Nature (gardens)	C	A	D											
5. Nurses' station	B	B	C	C										
6. Inpatient services	C	D	B	D	C									
7. Kitchen	D	D	D	C	D	D								
8. Kitchenette (family)	C	A	C	C	A	C	D							
9. Offices (reception)	D	D	D	D	D	C	A	D						
10. Main entry/facility	D	D	D	A	D	D	A	D	A					
11. Bed entry/unit	C	A	D	A	B	C	D	A	D	D				
12. All parking	D	D	D	A	D	D	C	D	C	C	D			
13. Linen/laundry	C	D	C	D	C	A	D	D	D	D	D	D		
14. Janitorial	B	B	D	D	A	C	A	A	B	A	B	D	D	

Key: A = within 16-foot radius (based on 8-foot corridors)
B = within 32-foot radius
C = related areas (see plan)
D = distant
blank = no relation

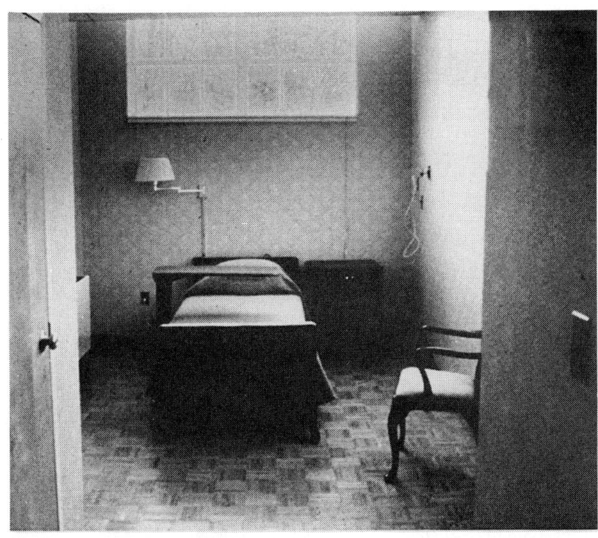

Single-bed patient room

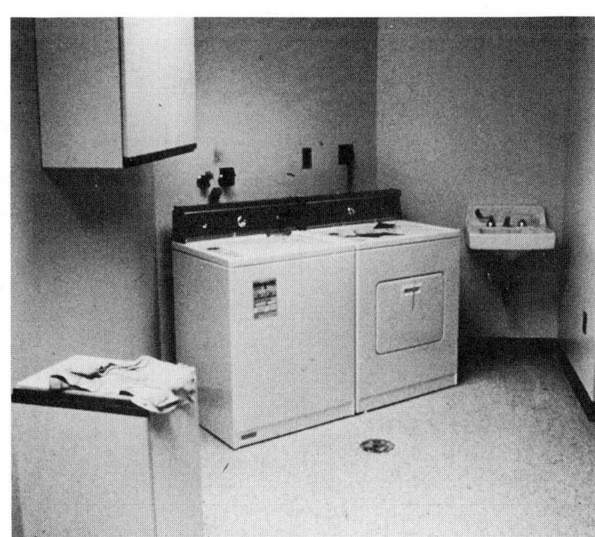

Laundry facilities

HOSPICE OF NORTHERN VIRGINIA: DESCRIPTIVE MATRIX
(Environmental Factors)

	Patient (Rooms)		Family (Lounge)	
	Intent	*Existing*	*Intent*	*Existing*
View				
Window	bright, natural	large windows to landscaped garden	bright, nature entry views	large window to garden, entry
Doors	nonabandonment, privacy	view nurses' station, hall	privacy, entry views	smaller door near patient rooms, entry
Each bed	nonabandonment, privacy, choice	multibed rooms with private curtain, zoned, single rooms also available	N/A	N/A
Other: artwork	variety, choice, quality	changing art displays	variety, comfort	artist-supplied pictures
Window				
Treatment	homelike	N/A	homelike	N/A
Trim	homelike	wood (painted)	homelike	N/A
Operation	homelike	operable	homelike	N/A
Covering	homelike, adjustable	curtains, venetian blinds	homelike, adjustable	N/A
Lighting				
Type	homelike, flexible	natural, incandescent	homelike, flexible	incandescent, natural
Fixtures	homelike	N/A	homelike	residential lamps
Handicap access				
Bed and wheelchair	bed, wheelchair, walker, patient lounge chair	halls have single bars, large doors, grouped table and chairs, parquet	bed, wheelchairs, walker, lounge chairs	large doors, grouped furniture, sturdy furniture, parquet floors
Dominant colors	warm, homelike, coordinated with architecture	green, coral, cream, mahogany, wood, florals	homelike, warm, coordinated	green, coral, cream, mahogany, wood, plants
Dominant materials	homelike, warm, durable, coordinated	wallpaper, paint, wood, fabrics, plaid, parquet	homelike, warm, coordinated	paint, wood, fabric, parquet, brick
Furniture type	homelike, flexible, coordinated, dignified	Queen Anne chairs, nightstand tables, chests, hospital beds, bed curtain, built-ins	homelike, warm, elegant, coordinated, comfortable	fireplace, piano, sofa beds, lamps, Georgian tables, desk, chairs
Ceiling height/treatment	varies, homelike	7'-6" to 9'	homelike	N/A
Floor surfacing	homelike, durable	parquet floors	homelike, durable	parquet floors
Personalization	encouraged	varied layout, walls, tables for display, storage	some	movable layout, plants, books, display

HOSPICE OF NORTHERN VIRGINIA: DESCRIPTIVE MATRIX (*cont'd.*)
(Environmental Factors)

| | Patient (Rooms) | | Family (Lounge) | |
	Intent	Existing	Intent	Existing
Organization	homelike, varied, convenient	range of room population size, shape, and location. Near north entry	homelike, welcoming, comfortable	large, open room, near patient entry, patient beds, family, kitchen, nurses' station
Equipment	homelike, noninstitutional, flexible	lights, telephones, television, central air, piped oxygen	homelike, comfortable, cheerful	dining area, lights, HVAC, toys, music
Signs	homelike	no intercom	homelike	no intercom

| | Nature (Gardens) | | Sacred (Meditation Room) | |
	Intent	Existing	Intent	Existing
View				
Window	East	formal garden, grass, parking	quiet, nature, airy, bright	east view, lawn, benches
Doors	West	service area, parking, shrubs	private, peaceful	door off hall, near office, library
Other	North	formal entry, gate from garden, grass	accessible, simple	large doorway, grouped furniture
	South	parking, south entry, vista across playground, park	N/A	N/A
Window				
Treatment	N/A	N/A	2 windows, homelike	5′ × 8′-8″ windows, 3 × 3 sill
Trim	N/A	N/A	homelike	wood
Operation	N/A	N/A	homelike	operable
Covering	N/A	N/A	homelike, adjustable	miniblinds
Lighting				
Type	daylight only	no lamps	special, sacred	incandescent, on dimmer
Fixtures	N/A	N/A	homelike, low gradient	12″ incandescent ceiling globes
Handicap access				
Bed and wheelchair	bed, wheelchair, patient lounge chair	ramp access, concrete paths	bed, wheelchair, patient lounge chair	large doorway, grouped furniture, sturdy furniture
Dominant colors	variety	hedges, evergreens, seasonal flowers, fountain	calm, serene, homelike, coordinated	green beige/ochre, dark woods

	Nature (Gardens)		Sacred (Meditation Room)	
	Intent	*Existing*	*Intent*	*Existing*
Dominant materials	homelike, variety, dignified	wrought-iron fence, ornamentals, evergreens, deciduous trees	homelike, comfortable, serene	wood, paint, carpeting, glass fixtures
Furniture type	variety, comfort	stopping places with conversation nooks, benches	homelike, comfortable, adaptable	"colonial" chairs, tables, couch, built-in cabinets
Ceiling height/ treatment	N/A	N/A	quiet, homelike	7'-9" (12')/hung acoustical tile
Floor surfacing	variety, handicap access	concrete, grass	homelike, quiet, soft	carpet
Personalization	encouraged	flowers, gardening	some	places for plants and flowers, neutral design
Organization	mixed, varied	English landscape, with formal garden, fenced environs	quiet, serene, adaptable, comfortable	L-shaped room off main hall, away from patient rooms
Equipment	maintenance equipment	mower, pruning equipment, paint, hoses, sprinklers (or on contract)	homelike, adaptable	places for religious articles, fan-coil, lights
Signs	simple, homelike	north entry, patient doors well-marked	homelike	N/A

	Kitchen (Family Kitchen)		Circulation (Halls)	
	Intent	*Existing*	*Intent*	*Existing*
View				
Window	none	none	variety, homelike	glimpses through rooms, doors
Doors	visible, controlled door	central to entry, nurses' station, door	homelike, spacious	variety of doors, nooks, room types
Each bed	homelike, central	located near patient pathways	homelike, variety	painted out wall bars, 2 levels
Other: artwork	homelike, clean	built-in modern with coordinated cabinets	homelike, variety	pictures, plants, light colors, wood
Window				
Treatment	none		none	
Trim				
Operation				
Covering				

HOSPICE OF NORTHERN VIRGINIA: DESCRIPTIVE MATRIX (*cont'd.*)
(Environmental Factors)

	Kitchen (Family Kitchen)		Circulation (Halls)	
	Intent	*Existing*	*Intent*	*Existing*
Lighting				
Type	homelike, practical	fluorescent	homelike, cheerful	
Fixtures	homelike, low gradient	ceiling	homelike, low gradient	
Handicap access				
Bed and wheelchair	none	none	beds, wheelchairs, patient lounge chairs, walkers	wide corridors, elevator, wall bars, door levers, stopping places
Dominant colors	coordinated, clean	cream, coral, green, wood	warm, cheerful, airy, light	cream, coral, green, wood
Dominant materials	cleanable, homelike, new	plastic laminate, enamel, glass, metal	homelike, warm	plastic laminate, paint, fabric, glass, acoustical tile
Furniture type	built-in, cleanable	countertop, cabinets above, refrigerator, sink, stove, ice machine with basket	homelike, practical, comfortable, accessible	lounge chairs, lamps, nurses' station with 44″ counter, 30″ desk, wall bar, elevator
Ceiling height/ treatment	homelike, practical	7'-11″ acoustical tile	homelike, practical	7'-11″ acoustical tile
Floor surfacing	homelike	parquet	homelike	parquet
Personalization	homelike	N/A	homelike	art, personal effects, plants, etc., at nurses' station
Organization	central, convenient welcoming, near activity	near patient entry, patient rooms, lounge, nurses' stations, for convenience	central, varied	double-loaded hall, 2 different entries, horizontal and vertical relief
Equipment	homelike, convenient, clean	coffee pot, toaster, microwave, blender. see Furniture	security, fire safety, general safety	signs, lighting, wall bars, nurses' station cart alcoves
Signs	noninstitutional	homemade instructions	noninstitutional, minimal	unobtrusive

General Notes

The Hospice of Northern Virginia has added considerably to the hospice definition of "homelike" with its selection of an older school for inpatient remodeling. The school has a recognized place in the neighborhood, an identifiable Georgian style, and is situated on parklike grounds near a playground for children. The internal remodeling has taken advantage of the site in several ways. The facility has two entries: the north entry, a formal front door at grade for patients, near the living room, kitchen, and nurses' station; and the south entry, used by family and staff, near a reception and office area for greeting and security. These entrances are part of a double-loaded corridor that runs through the building and provides connection of the areas. Although the corridor is double-loaded, considerable variety is afforded within the corridor by changes in grade and use as well as width and ceiling height differences. In effect, these two entrances serve to separate the residential and administrative functions of the hospice. There is considerable duplication of function in the two parts of the building, such as in greeting, meeting space, and dining, for example, but this duplication emphasizes the homelike nature of the hospice as well as the distinct nature of the two sections of the facility.

The hospice takes advantage of its building and site in other ways as well. The ground access provided by the school is perfect for a connection to the natural landscape. In addition, the distinct architectural style of the building is suitable for a matched interior style; the traditional, formal Queen Anne furniture and room treatments that were adopted increase the homelike quality of the hospice.

One other issue is addressed in this remodeling. Although many spaces have distinct functions, there is considerable ambiguity with offices, conference rooms, and so on, allowing for changes over time. This flexibility is especially important in a free-standing facility.

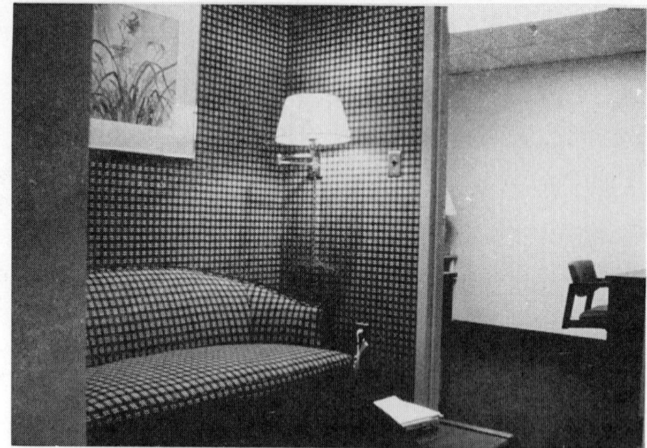

Anteroom

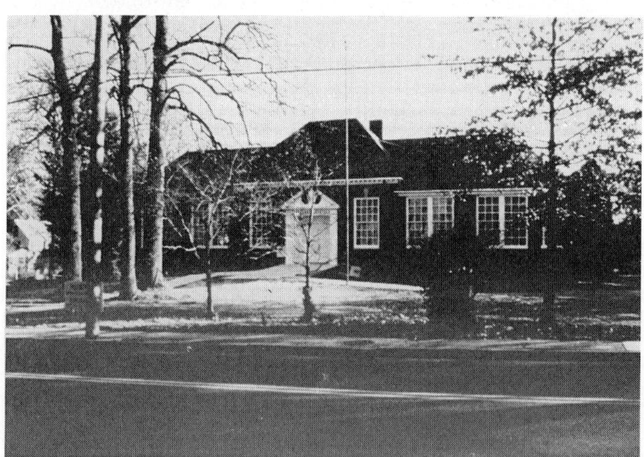

Front entrance of hospice

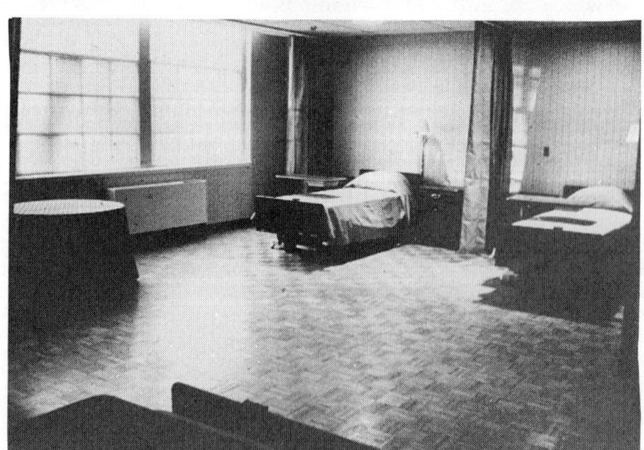

Four-bed patient room

• KAISER PERMANENTE HOSPICE PROGRAM

12500 South Hoxie Avenue
Norwalk, California 90650

Classification: Hospice in convalescent hospital
Sponsoring agencies: Kaiser Permanente System (HMO)
Type: Remodeling of existing space, separate hospice wings
Area served: Norwalk and vicinity
Inpatient population: 17 beds; patients 80% white, 20% black, primarily Christian
Established: 1978
Scope of work involved: N/A
    Formerly: acute ward in hospital
    Architect: Carolyn Brink
            Kaiser, Sunset and Vermont
Cost of work: $150,000
    Build: N/A
    Furnishings: N/A
Comprehensive intention of building selection and/or design: N/A
General intention: Homelike environment, soft, pleasant, special, well-lit
Location: Cross wards, ground floor of hospital
Description:
    Community image: part of hospital
    Interior image: homelike, modern light
    Convenience: good; special entry, ground-floor unit
    Changes: Need some private rooms for staff, families, and visitors, and more storage space
Users:
    Outpatient staff: N/A
    Volunteers: N/A
    Inpatient staff: (FTE) N/A
    Outpatients served: N/A
    Inpatient average population: N/A
    Inpatient average length of stay: N/A
    Family/visitors per week: N/A
Services rendered: Home and inpatient care, bereavement counseling, family sleeping facilities

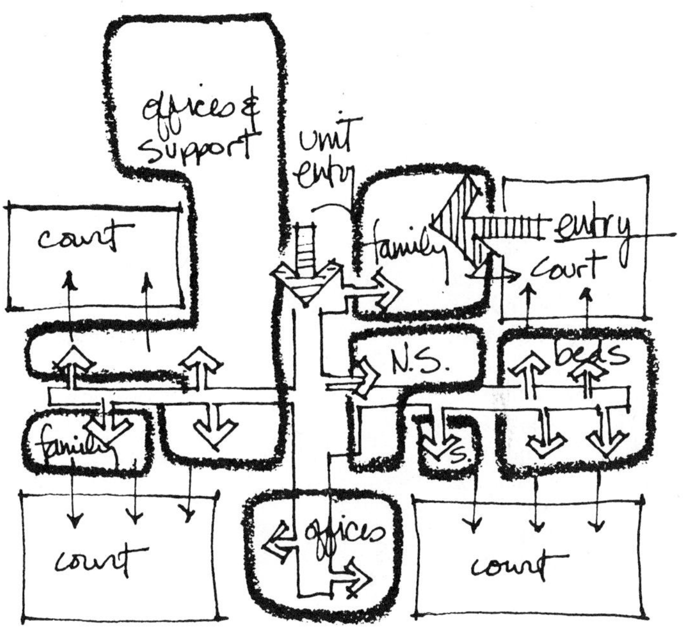

Parti drawing, Kaiser Permanente Hospice

KAISER PERMANENTE HOSPICE: ARCHITECTURAL COMPONENTS

Architectural Components	Notes	Wing/Total Number	Rough Dimensions or Size, Square Feet
1. Patient room	Single with W.C.	1	133/27
	Double	8	154
	Double	4	220
Bathrooms		1	240
	W.C. for doubles (shared)	4	26
2. Family lounge	Dayroom	1	22′ × 24′
Child area	Dayroom		
Eating area	Dayroom		
Other	See kitchenette		
Family private room	Guestroom with W.C.	1	154/26
Family other	Laundry (shared by staff)	1	77
Bathrooms	guest/staff bath	1	240
3. Garden	Patio gardens	8	8′ × 8′ (min.)
Gardening area	Dayroom garden		
Chapel		1	220
Transition room	Viewing, with W.C.	1	220/26
Meditation room	See chapel		
Chaplain office	With W.C.	1	220/26
4. Nurses' station		1	354
Medication room		1	56
Nurses' retreat	Staff lounge	1	168
Staff rooms	N/A		
Bathrooms	Women's	1	220
	Men's	1	220
5. Daycare	See dayroom		
Childcare	N/A		
Massage	N/A		
Physical therapy	Exam room	1	72
Occupational therapy	N/A		
Library	N/A		
Music/reading	See dayroom		
Barbershop	N/A		
Tavern	N/A		
Store	N/A		
Game room	N/A		
Other	N/A		
6. Kitchen facilities	Within larger hospital kitchen; undifferentiated space	1	920
Storage	N/A		
Supplies	N/A		
Preparation	N/A		
Cleaning	N/A		
Office	N/A		
Dietary staff	N/A		

KAISER PERMANENTE HOSPICE: ARCHITECTURAL COMPONENTS (*cont'd.*)

Architectural Components	Notes	Wing/Total Number	Rough Dimensions or Size, Square Feet
Unit dining	In patient rooms, dayroom		
Other dining	N/A		
Nutrition station		1	12′ × 9′
Kitchenette	In dayroom	1	6′ × 12′
7. Offices			
Director	With W.C.	1	143/21
Nurse coordinator		1	100
Social work coordinator	With 1 W.C.	1	154/26
Boardroom	Home care, with W.C.	1	240/26
Conference room	Staff	1	120
Volunteer coordinator			
Business office	Administration	1	190
Files	With W.C.	2	95
Other	Exam	1	72
	Waiting and reception	2	133/27
8. Entry, front door		1	14′ × 22′
Reception	See files		
Admitting	Main or parking entry		
Staff entrance	Main or parking entry		
Patient	Main or parking entry		
Volunteer	Main entry		
Visitors	Service entry		
Goods	Patient wing entry		
Other	Hospice unit halls	4	2,166
Hallways, main	N/A		
Service	N/A		
Other	Service		
Exit goods	Utility on unit		
Laundry	Hospice entry		
Dead			
9. Parking			
Connections to other facilities			
Connection to neighborhood	N/A		
Street visibility	N/A		
Landscaping	N/A		
Front yard	Gardens		
Back yard	Gardens		
10. Services			
Laundry	Utility room	1	192
Janitorial		1	17.5
General stores	Storage (small window)	1	220
Garbage service	N/A		
Equipment storage	See storage		
Mail	Nurses' station		

KAISER PERMANENTE HOSPICE: PROXIMITY MATRIX

Variables	Variable Numbers													
	1.	2.	3.	4.	5.	6.	7.	8.	9.	10.	11.	12.	13.	14.
1. Patient (bedrooms)	B													
2. Family (dayroom)	C													
3. Chapel	D	D												
4. Nature (outdoors)	A	A	A											
5. Nurses' station	C	A	C	C										
6. Inpatient services	D	C	D	B	C									
7. Kitchen	C	A	D	C	C	D								
8. Kitchenette	C	A	D	A	B	C	C							
9. Offices (admin.)	D	C	D	A	B	A	D	C						
10. Main entry/facility	D	A	D	A	C	D	B	A	C					
11. Bed entry/unit	C	A	C	C	A	C	B	B	C	C				
12. All parking	D	C	D	A	D	D	C	C	D	C	C			
13. Linen/laundry	C	B	C	C	A	B	D	C	B	D	B	D		
14. Janitorial	C	C	C	C	B	C	D	C	C	D	B	D	B	

Key:
A = within 16-foot radius (based on 8-foot corridors)
B = within 32-foot radius
C = related areas (see plan)
D = distant
blank = no relation

KAISER PERMANENTE HOSPICE: DESCRIPTIVE MATRIX
(Environmental Factors)

	Overall			
	Intent	*Existing*	*Intent*	*Existing*
View				
Window	light, direct access to nature	patios off most rooms		
Doors	existing open doors; privacy maintained	existing double-loaded corridor		
Each bed	privacy	special privacy drapes, cubicles		
Other: artwork	homelike	plants each room		
Window				
Treatment	existing windows	no change		
Trim	existing	no change		
Operation	existing	patio doors		
Covering	N/A	drapes		
Lighting				
Type	N/A	N/A		
Fixtures	homelike	residential lamps added		
Handicap access				
Bed and wheelchair	beds, recliner, wheel-chair, walker	most areas handicap size		
Dominant colors	homelike, comforting	soft colors, browns		
Dominant materials	homelike	all carpeted, fabrics, paints		
Furniture type	homelike	residential-type furni-ture added wherever possible		
Ceiling height/ treatment	N/A	N/A		
Floor surfacing	homelike	carpet		
Personalization	homelike	personal belongings encouraged		
Organization	existing near special hospice entry and kitchen	crosswards with dou-ble-loaded corridors; each wing has sepa-rate function		
Equipment	life-safety, hospital equipment	HVAC, lights, kitchen, laundry, no intercom		
Signs	N/A	N/A		

General Notes

Kaiser Permanente Norwalk has most of the home-like elements commonly found in hospices that are remodeled: residential furniture and finishes, family spaces, a variety of bedroom sizes and populations, more room per patient, and the location of the unit near activity (entry and kitchen). The difficulty of providing hospice patients with homelike, appetizing, cooked-to-order meals also seems to be addressed in the design of the hospice: the hospice is located near the hospital's kitchen and has a nutrition station on the hospice ward as well.

Kaiser Permanente also has a strong connection with nature; the hospice is located on the ground floor and most rooms have an adjoining outdoor patio. In addition to the chapel and viewing rooms, there are many staff support spaces, including staff lounges, sleep areas, and large offices. Compared with other medium-size remodeled facilities, it is generous in staff area allocation and provides a minimum of family space, although the areas provided are not small.

Perhaps the greatest criticism of Kaiser Permanente Norwalk comes from its rather typical cross-ward design, which does little to diminish the institutional organization of the plan. The placement of the nurses' station in the center of the crossing certainly emphasizes its importance in controlling the activity of the unit. Moreover, there is a wide separation of uses at Norwalk: bedrooms are located on one wing; administration on another; special hospice functions in the wing opposite the patient bedrooms; and the entry, kitchen, and dayroom placed on the fourth, truncated wing. A breakdown of these functions would stimulate more activity and more privacy, as well as deemphasize the institutional nature of the organization.

• LUTHERAN HOSPITAL PATHWAY HOSPICE

501 Tenth Avenue
Moline, Illinois 61265

Classification: Hospice in hospital

Sponsoring agencies: Lutheran Hospital, contracting home health agencies

Type: Inhouse remodeling of seventh-floor nurses' residence, full floor

Area served: Moline and environs

Inpatient population: 10 maximum

Established: 1981

Scope of work involved:
  Formerly: nurses' residence
  Architect: inhouse

Cost of work: $70,000–$80,000
  Build: N/A
  Furnishings: N/A

Comprehensive intention of building selection and/or design: N/A

General intention: Warm, homelike, flexible, light, bright

Location: Seventh (top) story of former nurses' residence, connected by bridge to hospital (acute ward)

Description: Light, warm, friendly, homelike patient floor
  Community image: part of hospital
  Interior image: special part of hospital
  Convenience: seventh floor
  Changes: More space and a connection to the outdoors are needed

Users:
  Outpatient staff: N/A
  Volunteers: N/A
  Inpatient staff: (FTE) N/A
  Outpatients served: N/A
  Inpatient average population: N/A
  Inpatient average length of stay: N/A
  Family/visitors per week: N/A

Services rendered: Inpatient and home care, bereavement, family sleeping in patient rooms. ". . . the patient care goals on the unit are to alleviate loneliness, pain, and other distressing symptoms, to integrate the family into the plan of care, and to make it possible for people to remain involved in life as long as possible" (staff notes derived from survey questionnaire).

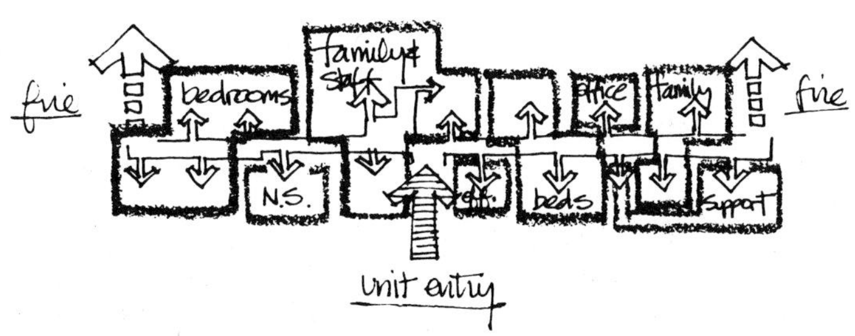

Parti drawing, Lutheran Pathway Hospice

LUTHERAN HOSPITAL PATHWAY HOSPICE: ARCHITECTURAL COMPONENTS

Architectural Components	Notes	Wing/Total Number	Rough Dimensions or Size, Square Feet
1. Patient room			
	Single	8	15′ × 20′
	Single	2	15′ × 20′
Bathrooms	W.C.	6	4′ × 4′
	Unit shower room	1	9′ × 9′
2. Family lounge		1	20′ × 30′
Child area	See family lounge		
Eating area	See family lounge		
Other	See kitchenette		
Family private room		1	155
Family other	Washer/dryer	1	8′ × 8′
Bathrooms	Handicap-accessible	1	8′ × 8′
Conference		1	10′ × 15′
3. Garden			
Gardening area	Outside 7th floor	1	10′ × 30′
Chapel	Off unit		
Transition room	None		
Meditation room	None		
Chaplain office	Off unit		
4. Nurses' station		1	20′ × 20′
Medication room	See nurses' station		
Nurses' retreat	Off unit		
Staff rooms	None		
Bathrooms	See family handicap		
Conference room	(Shared with family)		
5. Daycare	See family lounge		
Childcare	See family lounge		
Massage	In patient rooms		
Physical therapy	N/A		
Occupational therapy	N/A		
Library	None		
Music/reading	See lounge		
Barbershop	Off unit		
Tavern	None		
Store	None		
Game room	None		
Other	None		
6. Kitchen facilities	Off unit		
Unit dining	Patient rooms		
Other dining	Kitchenette		
Nutrition station	See nurses' station		
Kitchenette		1	10′ × 20′

Architectural Components	Notes	Wing/Total Number	Rough Dimensions or Size, Square Feet
7. Offices			
Director/head nurse		1	14' × 20'
Nurse coordinator			
Social work coordinator			
Boardroom			
Conference room			
Volunteer coordinator			
Business office			
Files	Hospice office	1	14' × 20'
Other	None		
8. Entry, front door	Pavilion	1	
Reception	N/A		
Admitting	N/A		
Staff	Hospital causeway		
Patient	Hospital causeway		
Volunteer	N/A		
Visitors	Hospital or pavilion		
Goods	Basement or causeway		
Other	N/A		
Hallways, main	Entry unit		
Service	Patient wings	1	8' × 185'
Other	Elevator	1	6' × 8'
Exit goods	See entry		
Laundry			
Dead	Exit via loading dock		
Miscellaneous	Stairs	3	10' × 20'
9. Parking	Hospital parking		
Connections to other facilities	N/A		
Connection to neighborhood	N/A		
Street visibility	N/A		
Landscaping			
Front yard	N/A		
Back yard	N/A		
10. Services			
Laundry	Off unit		
Clean linen		1	14' × 20'
Dirty linen		1	14' × 20'
Janitorial			
Closet		1	3' × 4'
Stores	N/A		
General stores	Off unit		
Offices	N/A		
Garbage service	Off unit		
Garbage pickup	N/A		
Equipment storage	N/A		
Mail	N/A		
Miscellaneous	N/A		

LUTHERAN HOSPITAL PATHWAY HOSPICE: PROXIMITY MATRIX

Variables														
Variable Numbers	1.	2.	3.	4.	5.	6.	7.	8.	9.	10.	11.	12.	13.	14.
1. Patient	C													
2. Family (lounge)	C													
3. Chapel	*	*												
4. Nature (patio)	C	A	*											
5. Nurses' station	C	A	*	B										
6. Inpatient services	*	*	*	*										
7. Kitchen	D	D	*	D	D	*								
8. Kitchenette	C	A	*	A	C	*	D							
9. Offices	C	B	*	C	C	*	D	B	A					
10. Main entry/facility	D	D	*	D	D	*	D	D	D					
11. Bed entry/unit	C	A	*	B	A	*	D	A	B	C				
12. All parking	D	D	*	D	D	*	C	D	D	C	D			
13. Linen/laundry	D	D	*	D	D	*	D	C	B	D	C	D		
14. Janitorial	C	A	*	B	A	*	D	B	C	D	A	D	D	

Key:
    A = within 16-foot radius (based on 8-foot corridors)
    B = within 32-foot radius
    C = related areas (see plan)
    D = distant
 blank = no relation
    * = off unit

LUTHERAN HOSPITAL PATHWAY HOSPICE: DESCRIPTIVE MATRIX
(Environmental Factors)

	Patient (Bedrooms)		*Family (Lounge)*	
	Intent	*Existing*	*Intent*	*Existing*
View				
Window	light, homelike, airy, warm	large windows, drapes, high view	open, homelike	open to patio, drapes high view
Doors	nonabandonment, privacy	8 rooms connected like doubles	welcoming, homelike	open to entry, next to kitchen
Each bed	homelike, accessibility	display of personal items, clock	welcoming, homelike	open to hall, viewing outdoors
Other: artwork	homelike	nature pictures	homelike, comforting	forest pathway mural
Window				
Treatment	homelike	N/A	homelike	N/A
Trim	existing	N/A	N/A	N/A
Operation	N/A	N/A	accessible	sliding doors
Covering	homelike	draperies	homelike	draperies
Lighting				
Type	homelike, flexible	natural light and incandescent only	homelike, choice	natural light and incandescent
Fixtures	homelike, flexible	residential lamps, no fluorescent	homelike	residential lamps, 4 overhead globes
Handicap access				
Bed and wheelchair	bed, recliner, walker	large doors, grouped furniture, built-ins	bed, recliner, walker	open to hall, grouped furniture
Dominant colors	warm, homelike, secure, varied	off-white, yellow and green, brown	welcoming, homelike	off-white, green, yellow, brown, blue
Dominant materials	homelike, durable	paint, fabrics, tile floor, wood, plastic laminate	homelike, comfortable, clean	paint, fabrics, tile, wood, toys, murals, plastic laminates
Furniture type	homelike, noninstitutional, practical	hospital bed, overbed table, recliner/rocker, sofa bed, desk, closet, bookshelves	homelike, comfortable, welcoming, flexible	sofa, side chairs, rocking chairs, table with checkers, lamps, toy box
Ceiling height/ treatment	existing, homelike	approx. 8', painted	existing, homelike	approx. 8', painted
Floor surfacing	homelike, durable	light-color tile	homelike, durable	light-color tile
Personalization	encouraged	lots of display space, bulletin board, plants	some	plants, books, donations
Organization	modified existing	8 double-loaded patient rooms; 2 rooms separate from these	modified existing	central to entry, nurses' station, and unit, open with patio
Equipment	homelike, practical	stretcher, bathing, HVAC, lights, telephone, television, storage	homelike, noninstitutional	phone, lamps, HVAC, drapes
Signs	homelike	bulletin boards, homelike clock	homelike	

• MERCY HOSPITAL HOSPICE

1000 North Village
Rockville Centre, New York 11570

Classification: Inhouse hospice

Sponsoring agencies: Mercy Hospital, Sisters of Mercy

Type: Remodel

Area served: Long Island, including Nassau, Queens, and part of Suffolk County.

Inpatient population: 18 maximum; mixed ethnic and religious population

Established: This unit opened May 1981. Demonstration unit on medical/surgical ward opened September 1978

Scope of work involved:
 Formerly: Women's pavilion (maternity)
 Architect: Weidersum Associates
  1455 Veteran's Highway
  Hauppauge, New York 11788

Cost of work: N/A
 Build: N/A
 Furnishings: N/A

Comprehensive intention of building selection and/or design: N/A

General intention: Hospice care in warm, soft environment, peaceful, homelike

Location: Behind hospital in park grounds and parking lots

Description: Small brick pavilion, double-loaded corridors
 Community image: part of hospital
 Interior image: clean, bright, quiet ward with friendly community spaces
 Convenience: by car, easy; by foot or through main hospital, difficult

Other: Remodel dictated by care providers.
 Changes: Connection to outdoors "icing on the cake" with sun protection and ramp.

Users:
 Outpatient staff: none
 Volunteers: 29 total (3-hour shifts)
 Inpatient staff: 20
 Outpatients served: none
 Inpatient average population: 15
 Inpatient average length of stay: 15 days
 Family/visitors per week: Varies

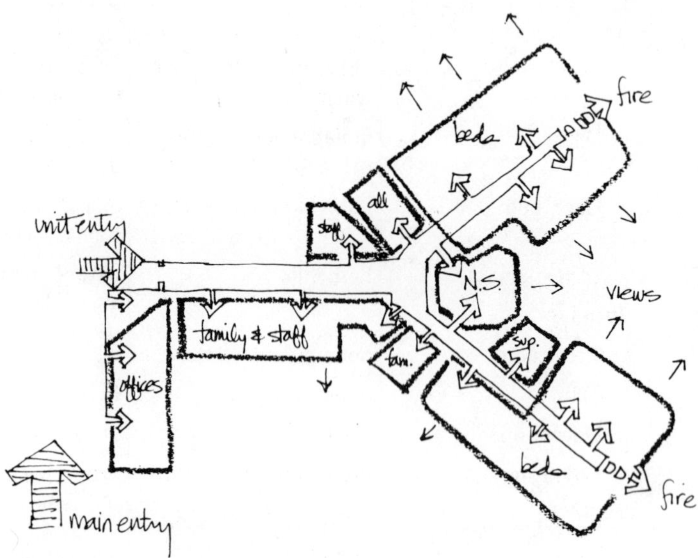

Parti drawing, Mercy Hospital Hospice

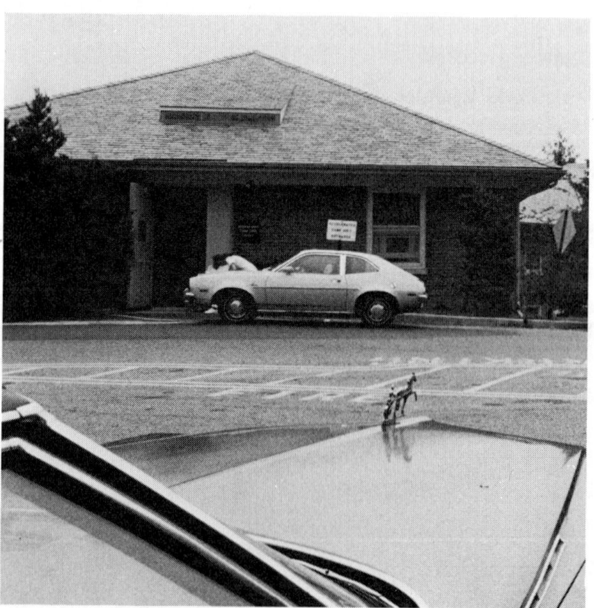

Bed entry to hospice

Services rendered: Inpatient, bereavement, home care (contract with three visiting nurse services through the hospital family), sleeping allowed in patient rooms

MERCY HOSPITAL HOSPICE: ARCHITECTURAL COMPONENTS

Architectural Components	Notes	Wing/Total Number	Rough Dimensions or Size, Square Feet
1. Patient room			
Single		2	156
Double	(Varies)	8	247/319
Bathrooms	Toilet	10	30
	Bath	1	72
	Showers	1	30
2. Family lounge	Multipurpose	1	731
Child area	None		
Other	See kitchenette		
Family private room		1	148.5
Family other	Laundry room	1	27
Bathrooms	Shared	2	25 (each)
Conference	See office		
3. Garden			
Gardening area	Plants in rooms		
Chapel	Can convert to multipurpose room	1	238
Transition room	None		
Meditation room	None		
Chaplain office	Off unit		
4. Nurses' station	Custom woodwork	1	130
Medication room		1	63
Nurses' retreat	None		
Staff rooms	With lockers (pink)	1	112
Bathrooms	Staff	1	30
5. Daycare	See family lounge		
Childcare	N/A		
Massage	N/A		
Physical therapy	Off unit		
Occupational therapy/ craft room	N/A		
Library	N/A		
Music/reading	N/A		
Barbershop	Off unit		
Tavern	None		
Store	None		
Game room	None		
Other	None		
6. Kitchen facilities	Off unit		
Unit dining	In bedrooms		
Other dining	See kitchenette		
Nutrition station			
Kitchenette	In multipurpose room	1	348.5
7. Offices			
Director		1	140
Nurse coordinator		1	70

Architectural Components	Notes	Wing/Total Number	Rough Dimensions or Size, Square Feet
Social work coordinator	None		
Boardroom	None		
Conference room		1	165
Volunteer coordinator	None		
Business office		1	135
Files	None		
Other	Office W.C.	1	17
	Entry W.C.	1	20
8. Entry, front door	Pavilion entry		
Reception	N/A		
Admitting	See offices, nurses' station		
Staff	Stairs, hallway		
Patient	Through Accelerated Care to entry hall of unit		
Volunteer	Entry hall of unit		
Visitors	Entry hall of unit		
Goods	Underground from hospital		
Hallways, main	Entry of unit		611
Service	Underground		
Other	Entry hall of unit		7' × 61'
Exit goods	Underground to hospital		
Laundry	Underground to hospital		
Dead	Through hallways to morgue		
Miscellaneous	Wing hallways	2	7' × 78'
9. Parking	Visitor lots	2	Large
Connections to other facilities	N/A		
Connection to neighborhood	N/A		
Street visibility	N/A		
Landscaping			
Front yard	N/A		
Back yard	N/A		
10. Services	Soiled linen room	1	64
Laundry	See family laundry room		
Clean	Workroom	1	42
Dirty	Workroom	1	81
Janitorial			
Closet	On unit	1	18
Stores	N/A		
General stores	Off unit		
Office	N/A		
Garbage	Off unit		
Garbage pickup	N/A		
Equipment storage	Stretchers	1	72
Mail	N/A		
Miscellaneous	Office storage area	1	14
General storage	Office	1	39
Unit storage		1	13.5
Closet		1	18

MERCY HOSPITAL HOSPICE: PROXIMITY MATRIX

| | Variable Numbers | | | | | | | | | | | | | |
Variables	1.	2.	3.	4.	5.	6.	7.	8.	9.	10.	11.	12.	13.	14.
1. Patient (bedrooms)	C													
2. Family (lounge)	C													
3. Chapel	D	A												
4. Nature (outdoors)	D	D	D											
5. Nurses' station	C	B	C	D										
6. Inpatient services	*	*	*	*										
7. Kitchen	D	D	D	D	D									
8. Kitchenette	C	A	B	D	A	*	*							
9. Offices (admin.)	D	D	C	D	D	*	*	D						
10. Main entry/facility	D	D	D	A	D	*	*	D	B					
11. Bed entry/unit	D	C	A	D	C	*	*	C	B	C				
12. All parking	D	D	D	A	D		C	D	C	B	D			
13. Linen/laundry	C	B	D	D	A	*	*	B	D	D	D	D		
14. Janitorial	C	B	C	D	B	*	*	C	D	D	D	D	B	

Key:
A = within 16-foot radius (based on 8-foot corridors)
B = within 32-foot radius
C = related areas (see plan)
D = distant
blank = no relation
* = off unit

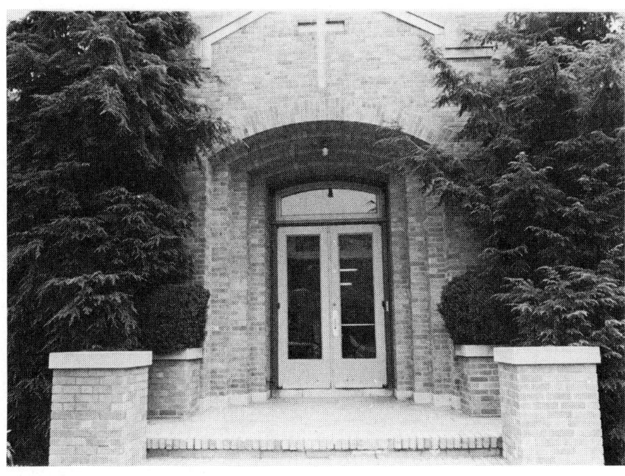

Front entrance, Mercy Hospital

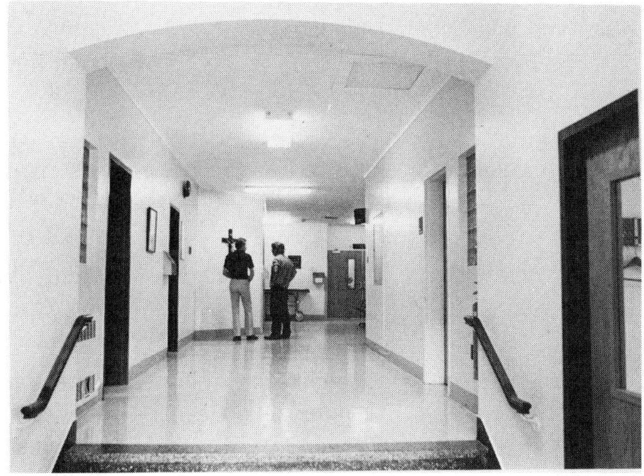

Entry hall

MERCY HOSPITAL HOSPICE: DESCRIPTIVE MATRIX (Environmental Factors)

	Patient (Bedrooms)		*Family (Lounge)*	
	Intent	*Existing*	*Intent*	*Existing*
View				
Window	residential, natural	3/4 of parking lot, hospital, lawn, trees	homelike, natural	same as patient rooms
Doors	homelike, nonabandonment	staggered doors on long, straight hall	flexible	chapel and multipurpose bed doors
Each bed	homelike, semiprivate	custom room divider, hall/window	not applicable	not applicable
Other: artwork	homelike, personal	landscapes, personal items	homelike, peaceful	landscapes
Privacy	flexible	bed curtain, divider	choice	small or large rooms
Window				
Treatment	choice, homelike	new sash windows	choice, homelike	new sash windows
Trim	homelike	new wood trim	homelike	new wood trim
Operation	choice	operable by patient	choice	operable
Covering	homelike, choice	blinds, curtains	homelike, choice	blinds, curtains
Lighting				
Type	flexible, homelike	flatwall module, remote fluorescent/incandescent	practical, homelike	fluorescent
Fixtures	flexible, choice	arm task light, recessed down lights	practical, distribution	overhead only rheostats
Handicap access				
Bed and wheelchair	openness	double doors that can open for bed access	openness	large rooms with gathered furniture groupings, solid furniture
Dominant colors	warm, secure, peaceful, clean	pastels, white, beige, dark woods (plastic laminate)	homelike, warm	pastels, earth colors, brown, dark wood
Dominant materials	homelike, clean	paint, plastic laminate, floral sheets, curtains	homelike, clean	paint, twills, wood, carpet, linoleum
Furniture type	homelike, flexible, comfortable, cleanable	institutional bed, over-bed table, recliner, custom room divider	homelike, comfortable, cleanable	neocolonial, dark woods, veneer tables, built-in kitchen cabinets
Ceiling height/treatment	homelike	8' 6" acoustical tile	homelike	8' 6" acoustical tile
Floor surfacing	homelike, clean	sheet linoleum, ceramic tile baths	homelike	carpet, some linoleum in kitchen
Personalization	in-view security	closet, bedstand, divider, bulletin board, shelves	donations	pictures, plants

MERCY HOSPITAL HOSPICE: DESCRIPTIVE MATRIX (Environmental Factors)

	Patient (Bedrooms)		Family (Lounge)	
	Intent	*Existing*	*Intent*	*Existing*
Organization	homelike as possible, given existing Y shape	hall walls load-bearing, rooms uniform and standard	homelike, flexible, welcoming	ex-nursery, expandable size. On single-loaded corridor
Equipment	flexible, comfortable, homelike	patient beds, tables, divider, residential clock, panel: oxygen/suction, HVAC	homelike, comfortable, peaceful	oxygen/suction, HVAC, telephone, kitchenette
Signs	homelike, minimal	over-door lights	homelike, minimal	small door plates

	Chapel		Nurses' Station	
	Intent	*Existing*	*Intent*	*Existing*
View				
Window	introspective quality, light	abstract stained glass	interior orientation	only offices have windows
Doors	welcoming	open, located at entry hall	open, welcoming	triangular nurses' station
Each bed	accessible	wide door through multipurpose (family) room	N/A	N/A
Other: artwork	nondenominational	abstract window	welcoming, natural	religious statue, donated prints
Privacy	flexible	accordian doors	visual	various work stations
Window				
Treatment	spiritual	stained glass	N/A	N/A
Trim	homelike	wood	N/A	N/A
Operation	N/A	N/A	N/A	N/A
Covering	translucent	abstract nature scene		N/A
Lighting				
Type	flexible, spiritual	fluorescent, incandescent	focal point and general lighting	fluorescent
Fixtures	central	ceiling wall lights	N/A	custom ceiling
Handicap access				
Bed and wheelchair	open, easy access	folding doors from multipurpose into chapel for beds, recliners	visual access	low nurses' station, desk, 3′ 8″ high
Dominant colors	peaceful, earth tones, spiritual	green, gold, dark wood, blue, pastels	friendly, calm	pastel pink, wood grain, off-white
Dominant materials	peaceful, quite	paint, glass, carpet, wood	friendly, central	paint, wood grain linoleum, light louvers

MERCY HOSPITAL HOSPICE: DESCRIPTIVE MATRIX (Environmental Factors)

	Chapel		*Nurses' Station*	
	Intent	*Existing*	*Intent*	*Existing*
Furniture type	comfortable, warm, multipurpose	altar, chairs, cabinet, dark wood	inviting, practical, modern, efficient	custom nurses' station desk, wood veneer, 3′ 8″ high
Ceiling height/ treatment	standard, modern	8′ 6″ acoustical tile	focal point, modern	at 8′ 2″ fixture, dropped lighting
Floor surfacing	quiet, homelike	carpet	clean, convenient	light, acoustical tile, linoleum rolls
Personalization	some	flowers, religious articles, "abstract" design	some	place for flowers, wall pictures
Organization	convenient, expandable	small room off entry and entry hall, multipurpose room	center of unit	intersection of Y arms, views entry hallway
Equipment	minimal	HVAC, lights, closet, altar, oxygen/suction	minimize clutter	call-light panel, telephone, typewriter, charts (built-in)
Signs	minimal	door only	minimal	none

	Hallways		*Outdoor Connections*	
	Intent	*Existing*	*Intent*	*Existing*
View				
Window	unimportant	only at end of ward halls, exits	N/A	N/A
Doors	firesafe with visibility	firedoors with wire-glass porthole	N/A	N/A
Each bed	N/A	N/A	use existing on grade entry	patient bed entry at outpatient care
Other: artwork	comforting, spiritual	crucifix in entry	existing	some religious symbols outside
Windows				
Treatment	N/A	N/A	new, to match existing	new, complements existing style
Trim	N/A	N/A	existing	remains
Operation	N/A	N/A	operable	new
Covering	N/A	N/A	existing	no exterior coverings, mostly evergreens
Lighting				
Type	bright, practical	fluorescent	use existing	parking lot lights, main entry lights
Fixtures	N/A	overhead in grid	N/A	incandescent fixture over east door

MERCY HOSPITAL HOSPICE: DESCRIPTIVE MATRIX (Environmental Factors)

	Hallways		*Outdoor Connections*	
	Intent	*Existing*	*Intent*	*Existing*
Handicap access				
Bed and wheelchair	some; main entry hall has stairs, no access	support bars for wall protection and physical help in some areas	use existing	main entry not modified for handicap access
Dominant colors	warm, friendly, clean	pastel, shiny light floor, white ceiling	on-site existing	green trees, grass, asphalt, brown, brick, white
Dominant materials	warm, friendly, clean	paint on stucco, linoleum, acoustical tile, wood, glass, metal	existing	grass, asphalt, cars, brick, wood trim, concrete
Furniture type	entry seating	couch, armchairs, leatherlike stretchers	existing	no lawn furniture or park seating
Ceiling height/ treatment	welcoming, modern	discrete lowering, acoustical tile		
Floor surfacing	clean, convenient	linoleum		
Personalization	view of personalized spaces	entry offices have visual relight connection, details	none	none
Organization	as existing	entry: double-loaded entry hall: single-loaded halls: double-loaded	existing pavilion siting	pavilion 140′ back of hospital; no physical connection
Equipment	minimum	fire safety, sprinklers, lights	existing	N/A
Signs	minimal	none at entry, small wall signs at unit (hard to find)	minimum additional signs	hospital to hospice, no signs; drive-in, one sign

General Notes

Constraints on remodeling were caused, in part, by the load-bearing corridor walls. Special doorways, with doors of two different sizes, were constructed to provide bed or walking access. Design emphasis was placed on privacy and individual control; patient rooms were supplied with room dividers, storage and display facilities for personal possessions, and cot closets. Patient rooms were also provided with operable windows (insulated, double-hung), piped-in music, and thermostat controls. It was troublesome to install the wall modules (equipped with oxygen, suction, HVAC, and light switches), because the many unions represented could not coordinate efforts in this work. The fire stairs at the end of the corridor were fitted with wire glass enclosures, as determined by state law.

A different organizational program at remodeling would have made Mercy more homelike. The nurses' station, at the end of the long corridor, is too prominent, does not look welcoming, and yet does not provide visibility from patient rooms. Except for the expandable family areas, the design offers little flexibility for changes over time.

Small changes could be made, however, to the existing design. Better signs should be posted in the connection of the hospital to the main hospice entry, although it would be even more helpful if an improved connection route were devised. At this point, the connection to the hospice seems to lead through the laundry room of the hospital. Indoors, patient rooms could be decorated differently from one another to provide greater distinction; corridors could be made more varied and residential through the use of such decorative finishes as vinyl wallpaper, carpeting, and more homelike furniture and lighting. Throughout, lighting is too standardized; rheostat incandescent lights, for example, are used only in the chapel.

It is also recommended that the main entry be modified for bed and wheelchair accessibility. Outdoors, traffic should be slowed in the parking lots and connections to the hospital delineated with crosswalks, changed pavings, and so on. Providing some landscaped exterior areas especially for the patients would be nice, although the hospice's preliminary proposal to add ramps proved too expensive.

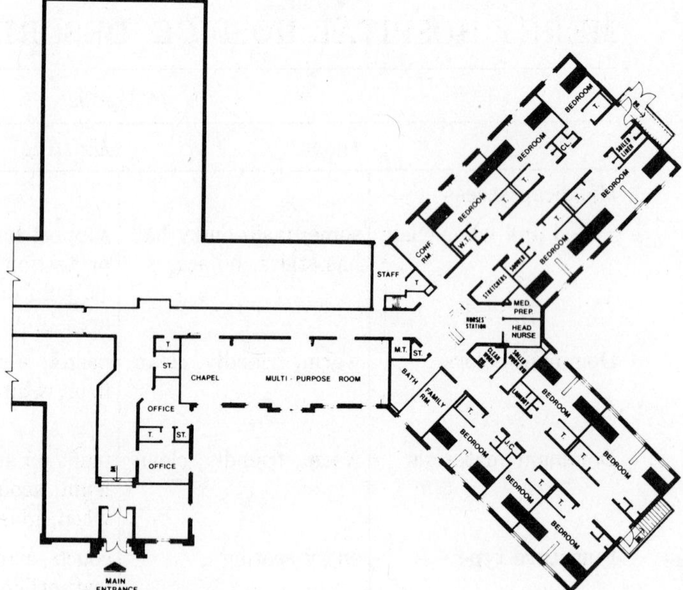

Plan of Mercy Hospice

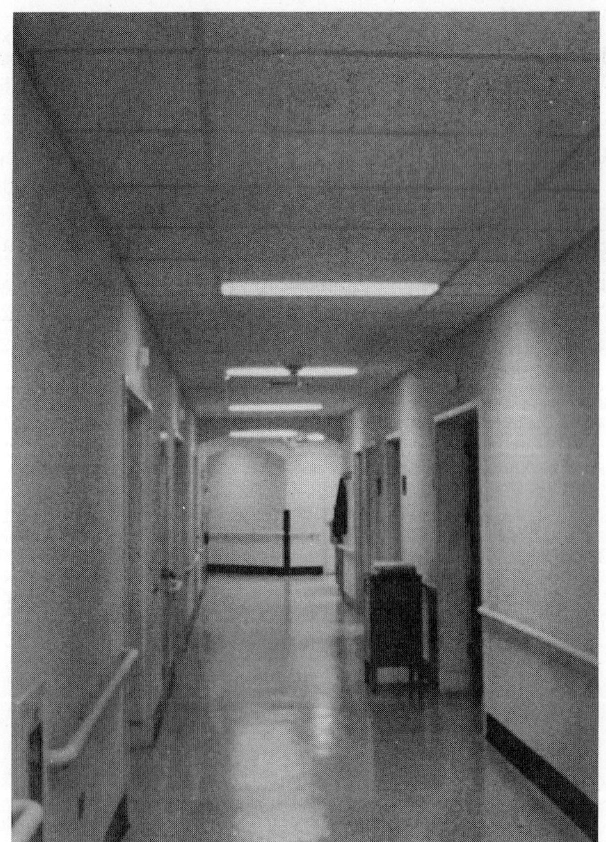

Corridor

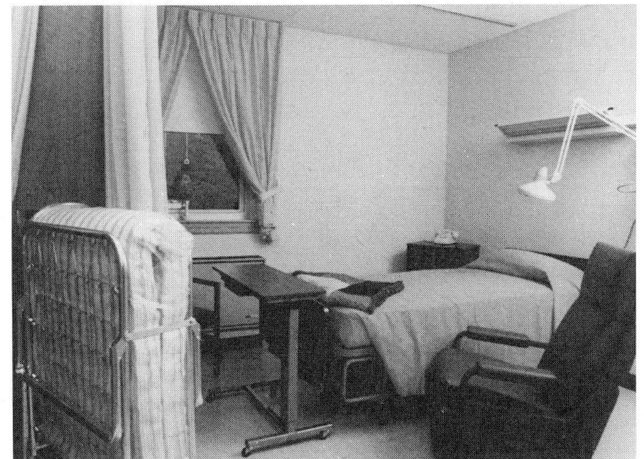

Patient room

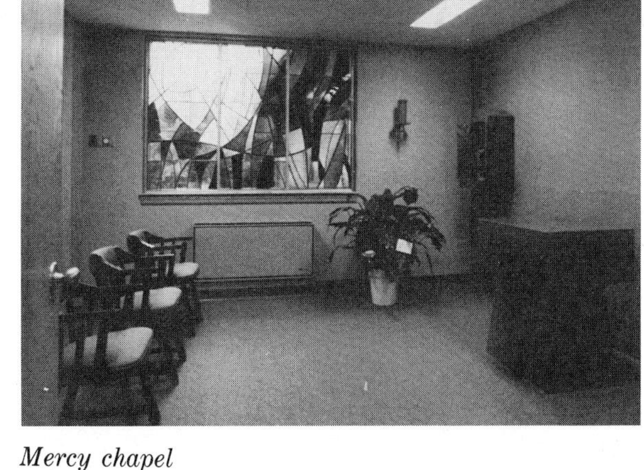

Mercy chapel

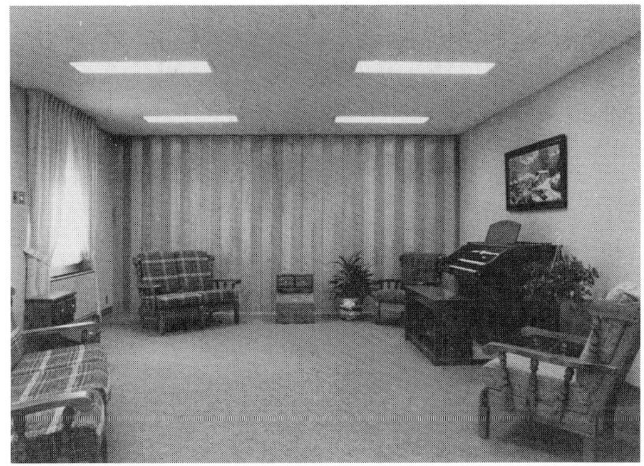

Multipurpose family lounge

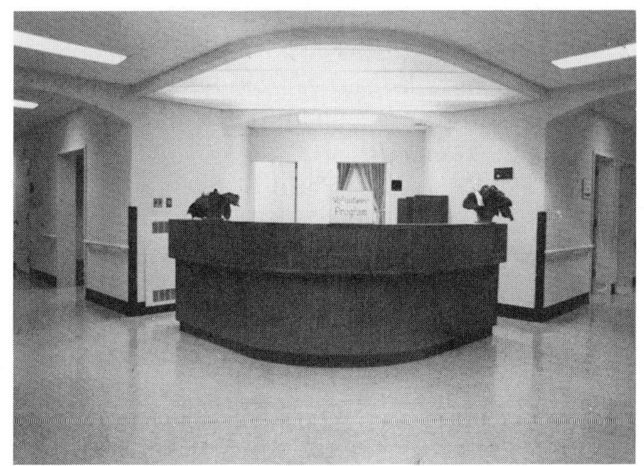

Nurses' station

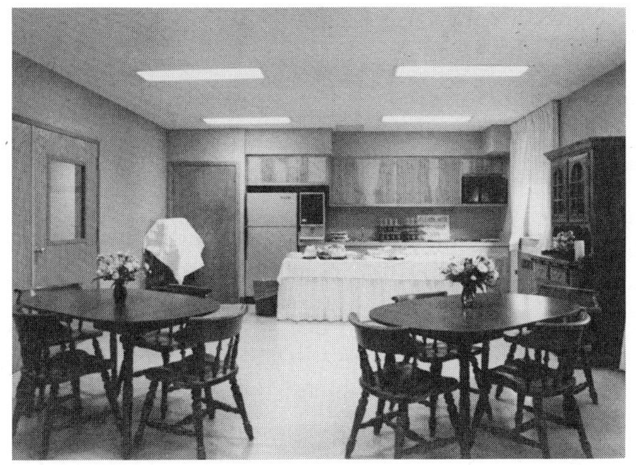

Kitchenette

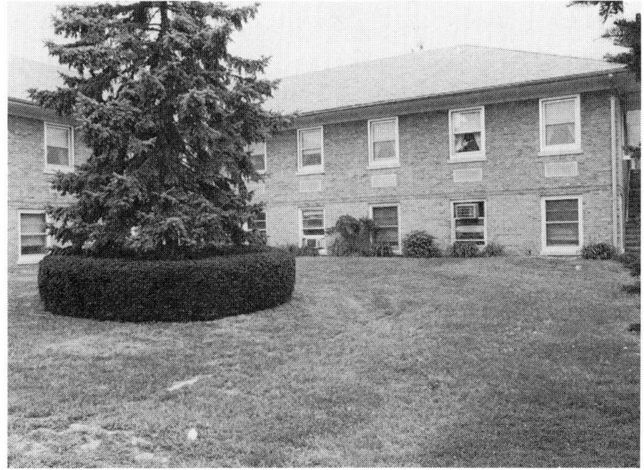

Front yard of hospice

• NATHAN ADELSON HOSPICE

3201 South Maryland Parkway
Las Vegas, Nevada 89107

Classification: Freestanding, nonprofit hospice
Sponsoring agencies: Nathan Adelson Hospice
Type: New construction
Area served: Las Vegas and environs
Inpatient population: 20
Established: July 1983; home-care program started
1979
Scope of work involved: New construction
    Architect: Nevada Archetronics
             801 S. Rancho Drive
             Las Vegas, NV 89106
Cost of work: over 2 million
    Interiors: Tamarind
           7961 West Third St.
           Los Angeles, CA 90048
*Comprehensive intention of building selection
and/or design:*
General intention: Homelike setting, light, secure,
handicap access, range of areas
Location: Campus of the University of Nevada,
Las Vegas
Description: Western organic style with tile, stucco,
berms, patios, clusters
    Community image: homelike institutional facility
    Interior image: light, warm, open, spacious, cozy,
    homelike
    Convenience: access by automobile, campus bus
    system
    Changes: nursing alcoves in country kitchens
Users:
    Outpatient staff: N/A
    Volunteers: 1 per patient, minimum
    Inpatient staff: (FTE) Approx. 6 RNs/shift, also
    6 LPNs or Aides
    Outpatients served: N/A
    Inpatient average population: not yet known
    Inpatient average length of stay: not yet known
    Family/visitors per week: not yet known
Services rendered: Home care, bereavement services, inpatient care, country kitchens, counseling,
family overnight stays in patient rooms.

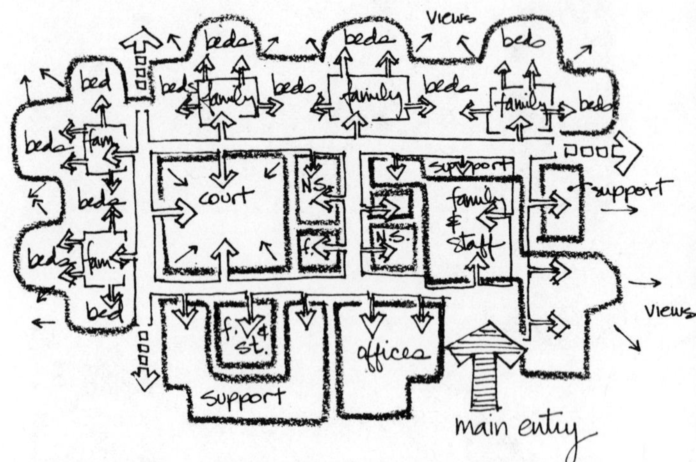

Parti drawing, Nathan Adelson Hospice

NATHAN ADELSON HOSPICE: ARCHITECTURAL COMPONENTS

Architectural Components	Notes	Wing/Total Number	Rough Dimensions or Size, Square Feet
1. Patient room			
	Single with bath	12	191 or 211
	Large single with bath	8	286
	Other (anterooms)	12	102/60
Bathrooms	Spa	1	165
2. Family lounge	Country kitchen	5	529 total
Child area	See country kitchen		
Eating area	Kitchenette	5	121
Other	Nurses's alcove	5	25
Family private room	Scream room	1	90
Family other			
Bathrooms	Public W.C.	2	75
Conference	Counseling rooms	2	100 (avg.)
Parlor		1	325
3. Garden	Courtyard	1	3,000 total
Gardening area	Greenhouse	1	800
Garden patios		10	250
Chapel	See meditation room		
Transition room	N/A		
Meditation room		1	300
Chaplain office		1	35
Meditation room	Multiuse garden area	1	420
4. Nurses' station		1	120
Medication room	Drug dispensary	1	100
Nurses' retreat	See greenhouse		
Staff room		1	210
Bathrooms	In staff room		
Central nurses' station		1	165
5. Daycare	Multipurpose room	1	345
Childcare	See family lounge		
Massage	See spa		
Physical therapy	N/A		
Occupational therapy	Play room	1	120
Library	See parlor		
Music/reading	See family areas		
Barbershop	Beauty shop	1	200
Tavern	N/A		
Store	N/A		
Game room	N/A		
6. Kitchen facilities	Part of institution	1	352
Storage			
Supplies			
Preparation			
Cleaning			
Office			
Dietary staff	See staff room		

Architectural Components	Notes	Wing/Total Number	Rough Dimensions or Size, Square Feet
Unit dining	Grill	1	480
Other dining	See family lounge		
Nutrition station	Near nurses' station		
7. Offices			
Director/administrator		1	130
Nurse coordinator		1	88
Social work coordinator		N/A	
Medical director		1	88
Conference room		1	180
Volunteer coordinator		1	80
Business office		1	72
Files		1	144
Volunteer work room		1	180
Home-care coordinator		1	80
8. Entry, front door			
Reception		1	225
Admitting	N/A		
Staff	Entry, front door		
Patient	Entry, front door		
Volunteer	Front door, hall doors		
Visitors	Front door		
Goods	Service entry, receiving	1	80
Other	See linen storage		
Hallways, main	Tiled		
Service	N/A		
Other	Court, pathways		
Exit goods	Service entry, kitchen	1	48
Laundry	Service entry		
Dead	Holding area	1	40
Service vestibule		1	48
Miscellaneous			
9. Parking	N/A		
Connections to other facilities	N/A		
Connection to neighborhood	N/A		
Street visibility	N/A		
Landscaping			
Front yard	N/A		
Back yard	N/A		
10. Services			
Laundry	Family and staff	1	80
Clean	Linen storage	1	120
Dirty	Utility room	1	64
Janitorial	Housekeeping	1	120
Closet	Janitor	1	64
General stores	Maintenance, air conditioning	1	208
Garbage pickup	Service entry		
Equipment storage	Bed storage room	1	120
Mail	Reception		
Miscellaneous	Sterile storage	1	64

NATHAN ADELSON HOSPICE: PROXIMITY MATRIX

| | | Variable Numbers | | | | | | | | | | | | |
Variables	1.	2.	3.	4.	5.	6.	7.	8.	9.	10.	11.	12.	13.	14.
1. Patient (bedrooms)	E													
2. Family (see 8 below)	A	E												
3. Meditation room	D	D												
4. Nature (gardens)	A	A	A	E										
5. Nurses' station	D	C	B	A										
6. Barbershop	C	C	B	A	A									
7. Kitchen (grill)	D	D	D	D	D	C								
8. Country kitchens	A	A	D	C	C	C	D							
9. Offices (admin.)	D	D	C	D	B	C	B	D						
10. Main entry/facility	D	D	B	C	D	B	C	D	A					
11. Bed entry/unit	D	D	D	D	D	D	C	D	D	D				
12. All parking	D	D	C	C	D	C	C	D	C	C	D			
13. Linen/laundry	C	C	D	D	C	C	C	C	C	C	A	D		
14. Janitorial	C	C	B	A	C	B	C	C	D	D	D	D	D	

Key: A = within 16-foot radius (based on 8-foot corridors)
B = within 32-foot radius
C = related areas (see plan)
D = distant
E = scattered, disparate association
blank = no relation

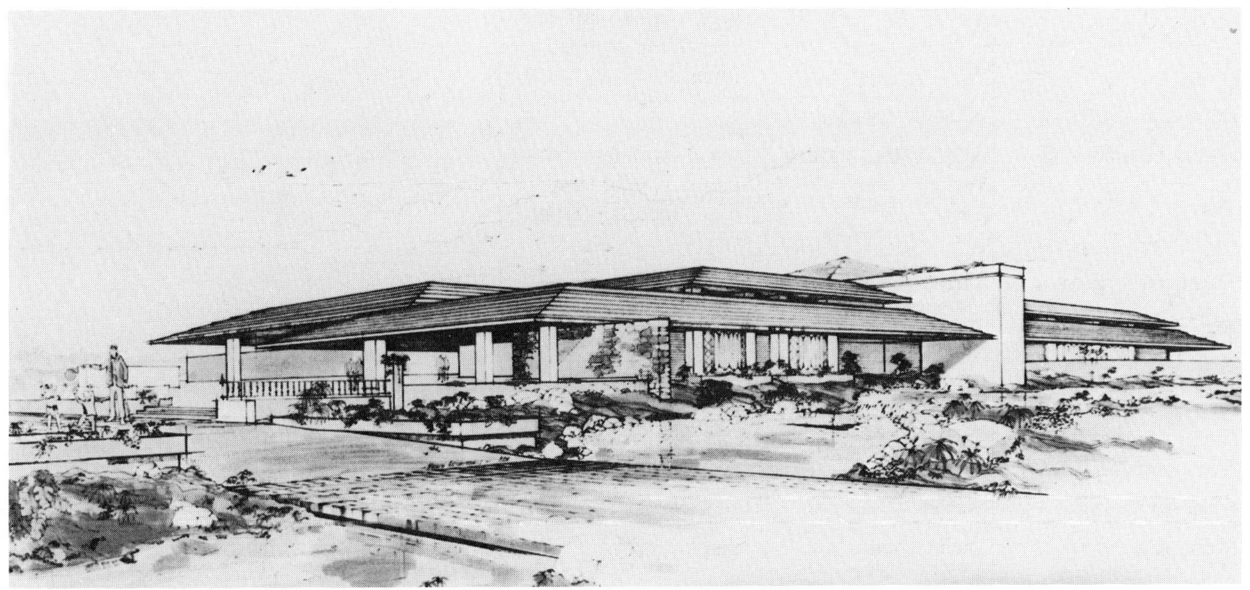

Rendering, Nathan Adelson Hospice

NATHAN ADELSON HOSPICE: DESCRIPTIVE MATRIX (Environmental Factors)

	Intent	*Existing*	
	General		
View			
Window	nonabandonment, view of nature	gardens, courts, through building view	
Doors	nonabandonment, privacy	action, passive views, relights	
Each bed	zoned for privacy	display, windows, country kitchen	
Other: artwork	nature, serene, variety	each cluster has different decoration	
Window			
Treatment	light, control	N/A	
Trim	N/A	N/A	
Operation	N/A	operable, patio doors	
Covering	N/A	blinds, curtains, overhang	
Lighting			
Type	homelike, natural	incandescent, skylights	
Fixtures	homelike, decorative, varied	residential lamps	
Handicap access			
Bed and wheelchair	bed, chair, walker	wall bars, big doorways, open plan, tile corridors, grouped furniture	
Dominant colors	homelike, varied		
Dominant materials	coordinated, natural, varied	wood, wallpaper, paint, plastic laminate, metals, carpet, tile	
Furniture type	varied styles	lamps, tables, beds, etc., in many styles: Victorian, colonial, traditional, contemporary	
Ceiling height/treatment	varied	flat, skylights, acoustical tile, paint	
Floor surfacing	varied	tile, carpet	
Personalization	encouraged	display areas, plants, crafts	
Organization	courtyard	single-loaded cluster on courtyard	

| | General | | |
	Intent	*Existing*	
Equipment	practical, homelike, safe	kitchen, laundry, equipment, noninstitutional	
Signs	homelike, varied	eclectic styles	

General Notes

Nathan Adelson's courtyard scheme and single-loaded patient rooms suggest the monastery plans of the Middle Ages. The cluster design attempts to resolve the dispute over the merits of single rooms versus multibed rooms by providing a privacy gradient: the public corridors, the semipublic country kitchens, the semiprivate alcoves, and the private patient rooms. The patient rooms are all physically similar; diversity is to be provided through the use of five schemes of decoration: contemporary, traditional, colonial, Victorian, and provincial.

Nathan Adelson Hospice has a wide variety of family and staff areas, including the parlor, family room, greenhouse, and courtyard. Involvement and nonabandonment are encouraged through the series of windows that view the courtyards and greenhouse, rather than by proximity of the nurses' station to patient areas. This visibility extends to the country kitchens, not as much to the patient rooms. In addition, small nurses' desks are located at each country kitchen cluster, to prevent isolation if the country kitchens are empty.

Hallways seem too extensive and room provision too similar, even with the variety of decorative schemes that are used. The outdoor court is large and should be pleasant when filled with trees and fountains, but may also obscure the view through the building. Overall, however, the patient and family space per square foot at this facility is the greatest of all hospices in the compendium. This hospice, too, is the first new freestanding facility in the United States since the Connecticut Hospice and was scheduled to be completed in the summer of 1983.

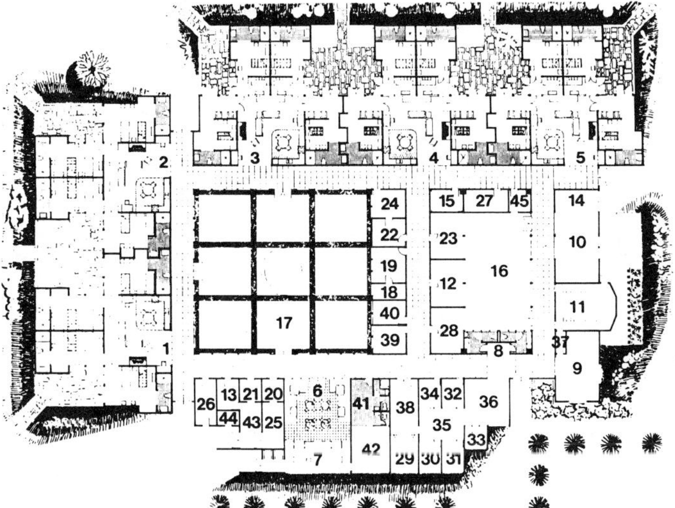

Early plan of the hospice

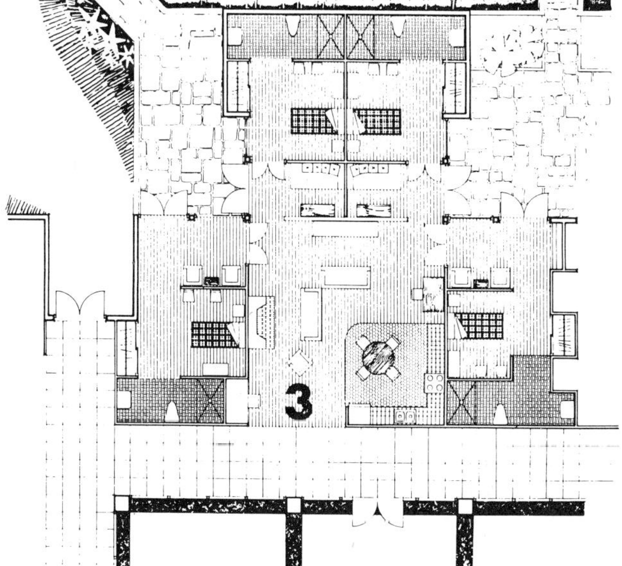

Cluster arrangement of family lounge and kitchen

• PINECREST HOSPITAL HOSPICE

2415 De La Vina Street
Santa Barbara, California 93105

Classification: Hospice in hospital
Sponsoring agency: Pinecrest Hospital
Type: Remodeled inhouse unit
Area served: Santa Barbara
Inpatient population: 26 maximum
Established: 1975
Scope of work involved: N/A
    Formerly: Skilled nursing facility
    Architect: Inhouse
Cost of work: N/A
    Build: N/A
    Furnishings: N/A
Comprehensive intention of building selection and/or design: N/A
General intention: Homelike, clean, economical
Location: One wing of hospital's skilled nursing facility
Description: Ground floor, double-loaded institutional patient wing with residential touches
    Community image: part of hospital complex
    Interior image: long double-loaded corridor, family areas and offices at entry
    Convenience: ground-floor location with nearby entry
Other: Hospital was sold in 1981
    Changes: More office space, larger private rooms located off main thoroughfare. Large family areas also needed.
Users:
    Outpatient staff: N/A
    Volunteers: N/A
    Inpatient staff: (FTE) N/A
    Outpatients served: N/A
    Inpatient average population: N/A
    Inpatient average length of stay: N/A
    Family/visitors per week: N/A
Services rendered: Inpatient, outpatient care, bereavement counseling, overnight sleeping for family in private rooms.

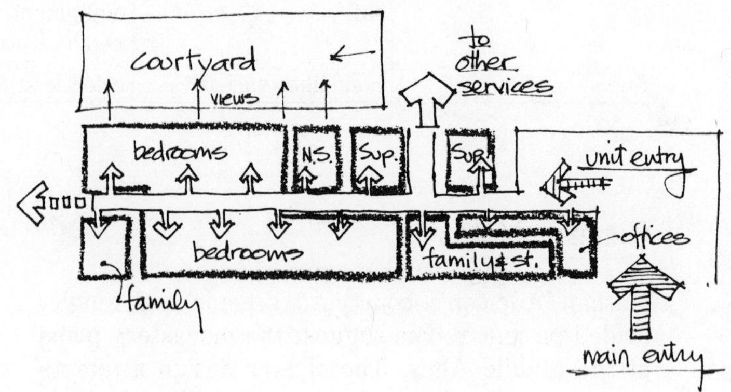

Parti drawing, Pinecrest Hospital Hospice

PINECREST HOSPITAL HOSPICE: ARCHITECTURAL COMPONENTS

Architectural Components	Notes	Wing/Total Number	Rough Dimensions or Size, Square Feet
1. Patient room			
	Single (east)	14	158
	Double (west)	6	300
Bathrooms	Showers	1	158
	W.C. singles	14	18
	W.C. doubles	6	32
2. Family lounge	Living rooms, kitchenette	1	190
Child area	N/A		
Eating area	See family lounge		
Family private room	None		
Family other	None		
Bathrooms	Unit	1	35
Conference	None		
3. Garden	Patio	1	35' × 100'
Gardening area	No specific area—many plants		
Chapel		1	158
Transition room	Patient room or chapel		
Meditation room	None		
Chaplain office	None		
4. Nurses' station		1	270
Medication room		1	154
Nurses' retreat	Staff lounge	1	45
Staff rooms	Off unit		
5. Daycare	See family lounge		
Childcare	N/A		
Massage	N/A		
Physical therapy	Off unit		
Occupational therapy	N/A		
Library	N/A		
Music/reading	See family lounge		
Barbershop	N/A		
Tavern	N/A		
Store	Off unit		
Game room	N/A		
6. Kitchen facilities	Off unit		
Unit dining	Patient rooms, living room/kitchen		
Other dining	Off unit, staff lounge		
7. Offices			
Director	N/A		
Nurse coordinator	N/A		
Social work coordinator		1	40
Boardroom		1	158
Conference room	See boardroom		
Volunteer coordinator		1	48
Business office	N/A		
Files	See nurses' station		

Architectural Components	Notes	Wing/Total Number	Rough Dimensions or Size, Square Feet
8. Entry, front door	Lobby	1	500
Reception	At entry		
Admitting	At entry		
Staff	Back door		
Patient	Lobby		
Volunteer	Lobby or back door		
Visitors	Lobby		
Goods	Service entrance		
Other			
Hallways, main	Lobby		
Service	Hospice wing		
Other	Unit entry		
Exit goods	SNF service entry		
Laundry	Off unit		
Dead	Entry or back door		
9. Parking	SNF parking		
Connections to other facilities	N/A		
Connection to neighborhood	N/A		
Street visibility	N/A		
Landscaping			
Front yard	N/A		
Back yard	N/A		
10. Services			
Laundry	Utility room	1	160
Clean linen		1	128
Dirty linen		1	96
Janitorial	N/A		
Closet	N/A		
Stores	Basement		
General stores	Closet	1	64
Offices	N/A		
Garbage	Off unit		
Garbage pickup	Service		
Equipment storage	N/A		
Mail	N/A		
Miscellaneous	N/A		

PINECREST HOSPITAL HOSPICE: PROXIMITY MATRIX

	Variable Numbers													
Variables	*1.*	*2.*	*3.*	*4.*	*5.*	*6.*	*7.*	*8.*	*9.*	*10.*	*11.*	*12.*	*13.*	*14.*
1. Patient	C													
2. Family (lounge)	C	A												
3. Chapel	C	D												
4. Nature (patio)	C	D	B											
5. Nurses' station	C	B	D	C										
6. Inpatient services	D	C	D	C	C									
7. Kitchen	D	D	D	D	D	D								
8. Kitchenette	C	A	D	D	B	C	D							
9. Offices	D	A	D	D	C	C	D	A						
10. Main entry/facility	C	C	D	D	D	D	D	D	C					
11. Bed entry/unit	C	A	D	C	C	B	D	B	A	C				
12. All parking	C	C	C	D	D	D	D	D	C	B	C			
13. Linen/laundry	D	B	D	D	B	C	C	B	B	D	A	D		
14. Janitorial	*	*	*	*	*	*	*	*	*	*	*	*		

Key:
    A = within 16-foot radius (based on 8-foot corridors)
    B = within 32-foot radius
    C = related areas (see plan)
    D = distant
blank = no relation
    * = no information available

PINECREST HOSPITAL HOSPICE: DESCRIPTIVE MATRIX
(Environmental Factors)

Patient (Bedrooms)		
	Intent	*Existing*
View		
Window	view of nature, activity	east entry, A.M. sun; west patio, P.M. sun
Doors	existing, nonabandonment	bed faces doors
Each bed	existing, privacy	hall, window behind each bed
Other: artwork	homelike	pictures, plants
Window		
Treatment	existing	small east window, larger west patio
Trim	existing	N/A
Operation	N/A	N/A
Covering	homelike	drapes
Lighting		
Type	homelike, flexible	incandescent, fluorescent
Fixtures	N/A	N/A
Handicap access		
Bed and wheelchair	bed, recliner, wheelchair, walker	large doors, little furniture, built-ins
Dominant colors	homelike	warm colors
Dominant materials	homelike, practical	paint, plastic laminate, fabrics, plants, afghans
Furniture type	homelike, institutional mix	hospital beds, tables, chairs, built-in closets, residential chairs, lamps
Ceiling height/ treatment	N/A	N/A
Floor surfacing	N/A	N/A
Personalization	some	closets in rooms
Organization	existing, active	located near entry of hospital, double-loaded hall with family, nurses' station at one end, chapel at other end
Equipment	homelike, flexible, use existing	lights, HVAC, telephones, television, oxygen/suction
Signs	N/A	N/A

• RIVERSIDE HOSPITAL HOSPICE

500 J. Clyde Morris Boulevard
Newport News, Virginia 23601

Classification: Hospice in hospital
Sponsoring Agency: Riverside Hospital
Type: Remodeled inhouse separate unit
Area served: Local community
Inpatient population: 7 beds, room for 8
Established: 1979
Scope of work involved: N/A
   Formerly: Mental rehabilitation unit
   Architect: Inhouse
Cost of work: N/A
   Build: N/A
   Furnishings: N/A
Comprehensive intention of building selection and/or design: N/A
General intention: Homelike, small, personal comfortable, flexible, secure
Location: Fifth floor, rehabilitation ward (connected to hospital by causeway)
Description:
   Community image: part of hospital
   Interior image: homelike, peaceful, small unit
   Convenience: far from entry
Other: Walls were not moved in this remodeling
   Changes: More living space needed
Users:
   Outpatient staff: N/A
   Volunteers: N/A
   Inpatient staff: N/A
   Outpatients served: N/A
   Inpatient average population: N/A
   Inpatient average length of stay: N/A
   Family/visitors per week: N/A
Services rendered: Home care, inpatient, bereavement counseling. Provider member, National Hospice Organization.

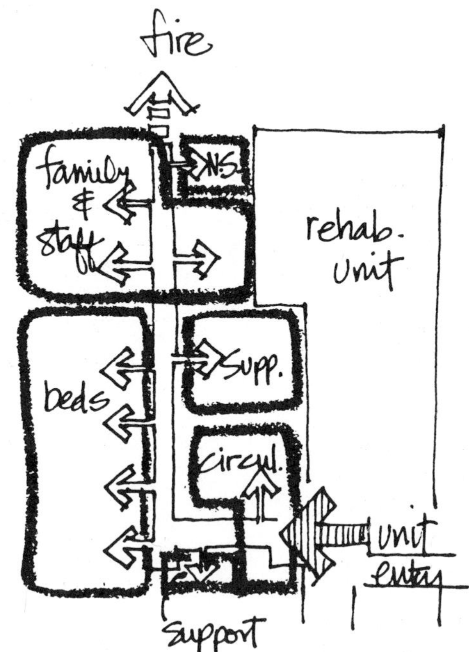

Parti drawing, Riverside Hospital Hospice

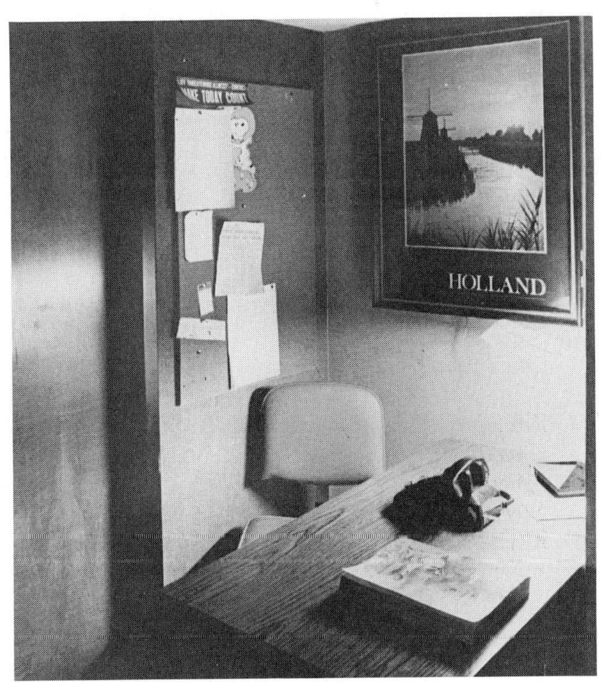

Volunteer's desk

RIVERSIDE HOSPITAL HOSPICE: ARCHITECTURAL COMPONENTS

Architectural Components	Notes	Wing/Total Number	Rough Dimensions or Size, Square Feet
1. Patient room			
	Convertible single	1	229
	Double	3	229
Bathrooms	W.C.	4	25
	Bath/shower room	1	72
2. Family lounge	Living room	1	229
Child area	N/A		
Family eating area	Dining room	1	229
Other	N/A		
Family private room	N/A		
Family other	N/A		
Bathrooms	W.C.	2	25
Conference	See dining room		
3. Garden	N/A		
Gardening area	N/A		
Chapel	N/A		
Transition room	N/A		
Meditation room	N/A		
Chaplain office	N/A		
4. Nurses' station		1	71
Medication room	N/A		
Nurses' retreat	Off unit		
Staff rooms	N/A		
Bathrooms	N/A		
5. Daycare	N/A		
Childcare	N/A		
Massage	N/A		
Physical therapy	Off unit		
Occupational therapy	N/A		
Library	N/A		
Music/reading	Living room		
Barbershop	Off unit		
Tavern	N/A		
Store	N/A		
Game room	N/A		
6. Kitchen facilities	Off unit		
Unit dining	N/A		
Other dining	See family dining		
Nutrition station	N/A		
Kitchenette	Pantry	1	63

Architectural Components	Notes	Wing/Total Number	Rough Dimensions or Size, Square Feet
7. Offices			
Director	N/A		
Nurse coordinator	N/A		
Social work coordinator	N/A		
Boardroom	N/A		
Conference room	N/A		
Volunteer coordinator	N/A		
Business office		1	135
Files	Nurses' station		
Other	Volunteer desk	1	75
8. Entry, front door	N/A		
Reception	N/A		
Admitting	N/A		
Staff	N/A		
Patient	Elevators	3	6′ × 8′
Volunteer	Elevators		
Visitors	Elevators		
Goods	From hospital		
Hallways, main	Causeway to rehabilitation wing		
Service			364
Other	N/A		
Exit goods			
Laundry	N/A		
Dead	Elevator to hospital basement morgue		
Miscellaneous	N/A		
9. Parking	N/A		
Connections to other facilities	N/A		
Connection to neighborhood	N/A		
Street visibility	N/A		
Landscaping			
Front yard	N/A		
Back yard	N/A		
10. Services			
Laundry	Off unit	1	21
Clean	Linen room		
Dirty	Off unit		
Janitorial			43
Closet	General storage	2	86
Stores	N/A		
General stores	Supplies	1	28
Offices	N/A		
Garbage	Off unit		
Garbage pickup	N/A		
Equipment storage	See storage		
Mail	N/A		

RIVERSIDE HOSPITAL HOSPICE: PROXIMITY MATRIX

Variables	*Variable Numbers*													
	1.	2.	3.	4.	5.	6.	7.	8.	9.	10.	11.	12.	13.	14.
1. Patient	A													
2. Family	C	A												
3. Chapel (see 2 above)														
4. Nature (artwork)	E	E		E										
5. Nurses' station				E										
6. Inpatient services	*	*		*										
7. Kitchen	*	*		*	*	*								
8. Kitchenette	C	A			A	*	*							
9. Offices (volunteer)	B	B		E	B	*	*	B						
10. Main entry/facility	D	D			D	*	*	D	D					
11. Bed entry/unit	B	C		E	D	*	*	C	A	D				
12. Parking/staff	D	D			D	*	*	D	D	C	D			
13. Linen/laundry	C	A			B	*	*	A	A		B			
14. Janitorial	B	D			C	*	*	C	C		A		C	

Key:
- A = within 16-foot radius (based on 8-foot corridors)
- B = within 32-foot radius
- C = related areas (see plan)
- D = distant
- E = scattered, disparate association
- blank = no relation
- * = off unit

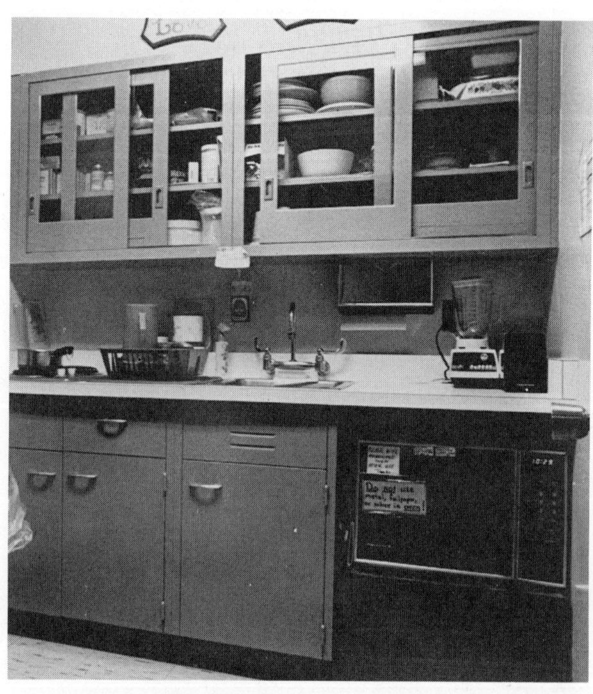

Kitchenette, Riverside Hospice

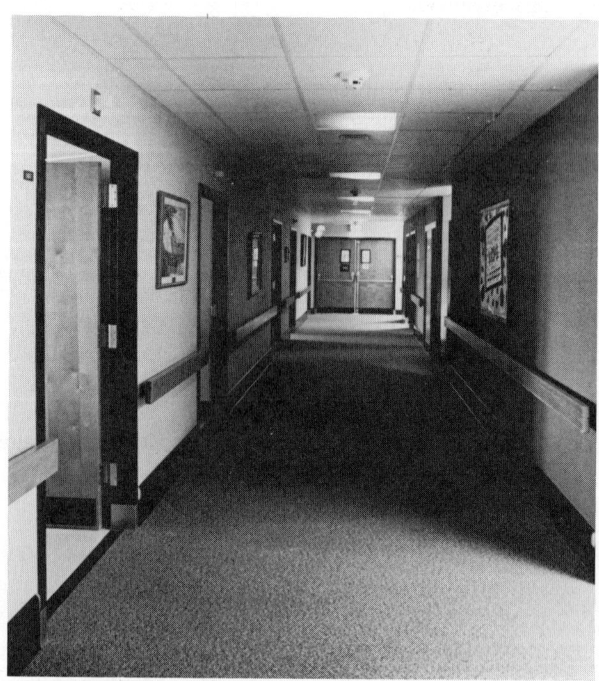

Hallway

RIVERSIDE HOSPITAL HOSPICE: DESCRIPTIVE MATRIX
(Environmental Factors)

	Patient (Bedrooms)		Family (Lounge)	
	Intent	*Existing*	*Intent*	*Existing*
View				
Window	light, nature	treetops, 5th floor	light, nature	treetops, 5th floor
Doors	nonabandonment, privacy	partial hall view	existing, privacy	grouped family activities
Each bed	privacy, light, adaptable	curtains, room for personalization	N/A	N/A
Other: artwork	visible, comforting	at foot, nature prints, etc.	homelike, comforting	framed nature prints, drawings
Window				
Treatment	N/A	N/A	N/A	N/A
Trim	homelike	wallboard, windowsill	homelike	wallboard, windowsill
Operation	existing	casements	existing	casements
Covering	homelike, adaptable, light	drapes	homelike, special, adaptable	floral print drapes, leaded glass in dining room
Lighting				
Type	flexible, homelike	fluorescent/ incandescent	homelike	incandescent
Fixtures	practical, background	head wall up/down fluorescent/ incandescent lamps	homelike, special	residential lamps, wall lamps
Handicap access				
Bed and wheelchair	bed, recliner, wheel-chair, walkers	large doors, linoleum floors, solid furniture	recliner	large doors, carpet
Dominant colors	background, clean, cheerful	no patterns; white, brown, pastels	homelike, peaceful, flexible	floral patterns, warm tones, green, blue, brown
Dominant materials	background, clean, practical	paint, plastic lami-nate, fabrics, lino-leum, metal	homelike, comforta-ble, elegant	paint, rich wood, car-pet, fabrics, brass, glass
Furniture type	background, clean, practical	hospital beds, over-bed tables, institu-tional desk, chairs, tables, built-in closet	homelike, dignified, comfortable, flexible	residential dining set, buffet, china cabinet, sofa, rocker, chairs, lamps, cabinets
Ceiling height/ treatment	existing	8′ 6″ approximately, with curtain track; painted	existing	8′ 6″ approximately; painted
Floor surfacing	clean, durable	linoleum	homelike	low-pile carpet
Personalization	encouraged in back-ground room design	pictures, afghans, plants, rocking chairs, furniture	limited, adaptable	contribution of art, plants, books, etc.

| | Patient (Bedrooms) | | Family (Lounge) | |
	Intent	Existing	Intent	Existing
Organization	existing, contiguous	4 rooms on double-loaded corridor (core)	existing, contiguous	2 rooms on dining room corridor (core type)
Equipment	nonabandonment, homelike, choice	telephone, lights, HVAC, wall television, privacy curtains, oxygen/suction	homelike, privacy, flexibility	telephone, television (living room), lights, HVAC, no intercom
Signs	practical, existing	room numbers, call lights	practical, existing	room numbers, call lights

| | Kitchenette | | Unit Hallway | |
	Intent	Existing	Intent	Existing
View				
Window	none		none, but some variety	has alcoves, elevator entry, volunteer desk
Doors	open to family area	open to hallway, through to dining room, living room	existing, privacy	open to main hall one end only
Each bed	N/A	N/A	N/A	N/A
Other: artwork	cheerful	homemade signs, a few cartoons	homelike, special	abstract, nature, artwork, pictures
Window				
Treatment	none	N/A	none	N/A
Trim	N/A	N/A	N/A	N/A
Operation	N/A	N/A	N/A	N/A
Covering	N/A	N/A	N/A	N/A
Lighting				
Type	practical, efficient	fluorescent	practical, homelike	fluorescent
Fixtures	area	overhead fluorescent	low-wattage light; economical	overhead fluorescent in center hallway
Handicap access				
Bed and wheelchair	walker	not equipped for handicap access	bed, wheelchair, walker	wide, with wall bars, low-pile carpet
Dominant colors	homelike, cheerful, economical	colored enamel, paint	homelike, light, varied	peach and white walls, dark carpet, blond trim, light wood doors
Dominant materials	homelike, clean, economical	metal, paint, glass, linoleum, plastic laminate, dishes, utensils	homelike, special, durable	paint, acoustical tile, carpet, wood, metal, artwork

(Environmental Factors)

	Kitchenette		Unit Hallway	
	Intent	*Existing*	*Intent*	*Existing*
Furniture type	homelike, clean, economical	built-in cabinets, countertop, also lockers	none	N/A
Ceiling height/ treatment	existing	8′ 6″ approximately; painted	existing	8′ 6″ approximately; acoustical tile
Floor surfacing	clean, durable	linoleum	homelike, practical	low-pile carpet
Personalization	limited	participation by family encouraged	limited	artwork, bulletin board (volunteer)
Organization	contiguous	small room across living room, dining room, near nurses' station	existing	double-loaded
Equipment	homelike, clean, flexible	sink, microwave, blender, refrigerator, stove, toaster, etc.	protection, fire safety, direction	wall bars, sprinklers, telephone
Signs	existing	homemade directions, room number	safety, homelike	N/A

Riverside has several unusual architectural aspects. The location of the volunteers' desk central to the patient rooms deemphasizes the supervisory role of the nurses' station, in stressing the function of the volunteers. The dining room is decorated in an elegant and formal manner, making it homelike but also dignified and special, as well as suitable for the conferences that also take place there.

The patient rooms, supplied with a minimum of beds and tables, are purposely not decorated. Patients are encouraged to bring their own furniture, decorations, and personal items. However, the bedrooms are rather sparse; carpeting, for example, would be a welcome addition. Moreover, each patient room is organized in exactly the same way. The arrangement of beds affords the patients privacy, but does not allow both patients a view of the windows and door.

An attempt has been made to enliven the corridor areas with various paints, alcoves, and artworks. The patient rooms are positioned at the unit entry, which brings them near to the comings and goings of the unit. The location of the family areas together and across from one another helps, too, to dispel corridor monotony, as does the small size of the unit and its shortened hallway.

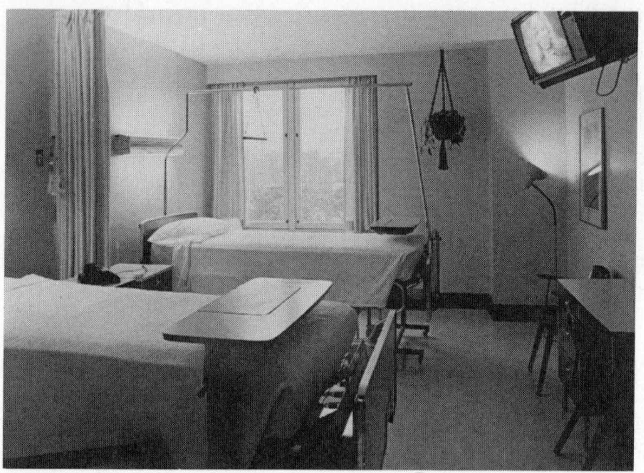

Double patient room

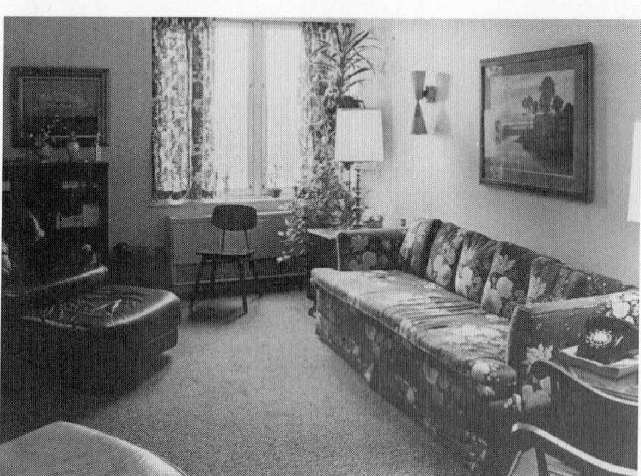

Family lounge

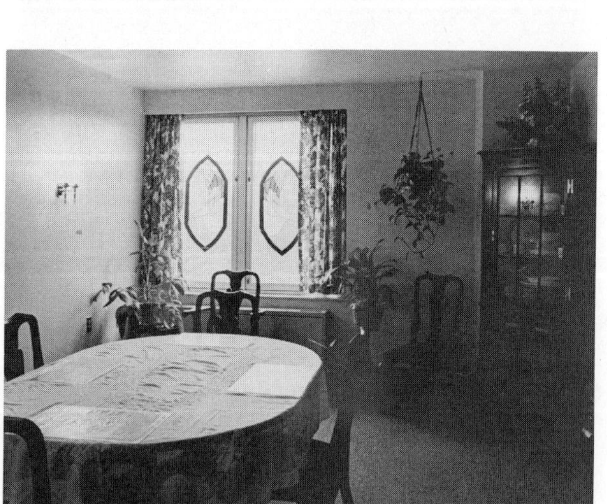

Dining room

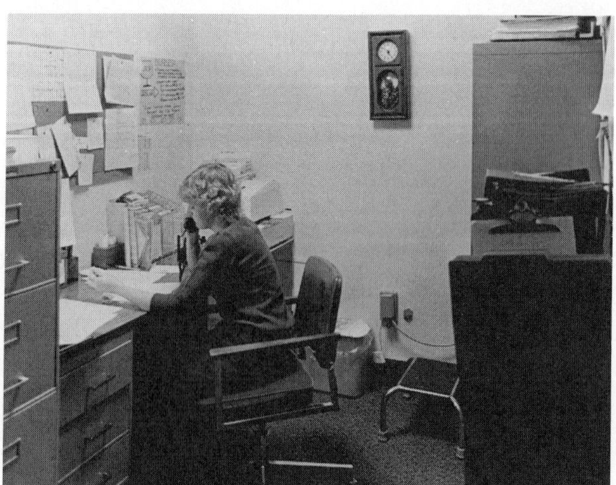

Nurses' station

• ROSARY HILL HOME

600 Linda Avenue
Hawthorne, New York 10532

Classification: Freestanding, pre-hospice skilled nursing facility for the terminally ill

Sponsoring agencies: Dominican Sisters of Hawthorne (Congregation of St. Rose of Lima or Servants for the Relief of Incurable Cancer)

Type: New construction, 1927; addition built 1983

Area served: Westchester County, New York City

Inpatient population: 72 maximum. Inpatients have no money or family to care for them at home, are incurably ill, and must be mentally sound and nondisruptive.

Established: 1901

Scope of work involved: 1983 construction included demolishing all but the chapel, and building nursing units and convent. Current size of facility is 100,000 square feet.

    Formerly: Same
    Architect: The Eggers Group, P.C.
             Two Park Avenue
             New York, New York 10016

Cost of work: $12,000,000
    Build: N/A
    Furnishings: N/A

Comprehensive intention of building selection and/or design: N/A

General intention: Homelike, noninstitutional, peaceful, reassuring

Location: Over 15 acres of mature wooded hillside overlooking valley and hill range

Description: Harmonized modern mission style, open, spacious, bright, serene
    Community image: mission hospital on the hill
    Interior image: light, comfortable, clean, cheerful, efficient, warm skilled nursing facility
    Convenience: access by car, ambulance

Other: Convent areas will not be included in take-offs (square footage derived from plans)

Users:
    Outpatients staff: None
    Volunteers: Yes; number not known
    Inpatient staff: 60 (approx.)
    Outpatients served: none

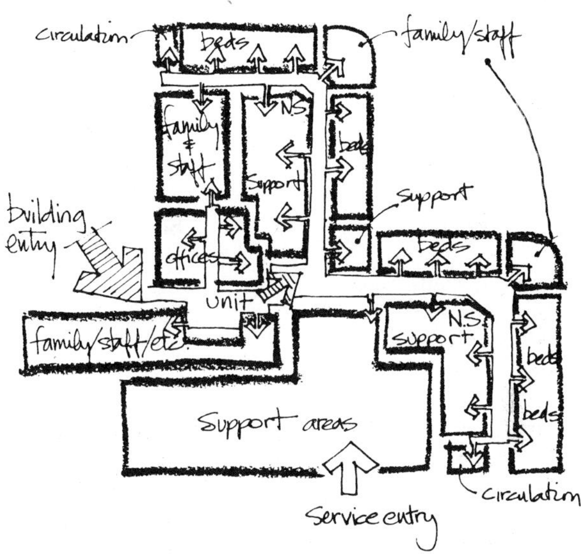

Parti drawing, Rosary Hill Home

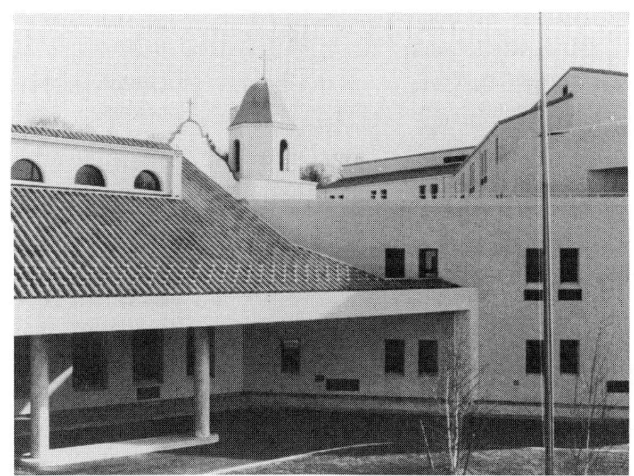

Hospice entrance and driveway

Inpatient average population: not known
Inpatient average length of stay: longer-term care
Family/visitors per week: Varies, but not as many as in short-term hospice care

Services rendered: Inpatient care, including crafts, physical therapy, family counseling

ROSARY HILL HOME: ARCHITECTURAL COMPONENTS

Architectural Components	Notes	Wing/Total Number	Rough Dimensions or Size, Square Feet
1. Patient room			
	Single with W.C.	11/22	160/30
	Isolation with bath	1/2	270/70
	Other: four with W.C.	6/12	465/50
Bathrooms	Bath with whirlpool, shower, W.C.	2/4	490
2. Family lounge	Dayroom	2/4	345
Child area	N/A		
Eating area	See guest dining, kitchenette		
Other	Heritage room	1	192
Family private room		1	150
Family other	See kitchenette		
Bathrooms	M/F W.C.s in lobby	2/4	130
Conference	See multipurpose room		
3. Garden	Roof terrace	1	1,712
Gardening area	Dayrooms, patient rooms		
Chapel	Off unit		
Transition room	N/A		
Meditation room	N/A		
Chaplain office	Rectory, 1st floor	1	825
Solarium	With 124 sf storage	1	1,155
4. Nurses' station		2/4	165
Medication room		1/2	143
Nurses' retreat	Lounge	2/4	115
Staff rooms	Lockers	2/4	30
Bathrooms	W.C.	2/4	38
5. Daycare	See dayroom		
Childcare	N/A		
Massage	N/A		
Physical therapy	Treatment room	1/2	140
Occupational therapy	Recreation room	1	440
Library	Medical	1	120
Music/reading	See dayroom		
Barbershop		1	192/98
Tavern	Waiting room		
Store	N/A		
Game room	N/A		
Other	Multipurpose room	1	1,120
6. Kitchen facilities			
Storage	Dry	1	320
Supplies	Refrigerator/freezer	1	305
Preparation		1	1,070
Cleaning		1	235
Office		1	128
Dietary staff	M/F W.C.s	2	212
Unit dining	Staff dining	1	380

Architectural Components	Notes	Wing/Total Number	Rough Dimensions or Size, Square Feet
Other dining	Guest dining room	1	242
Nutrition station	Nurses' station		
Kitchenettes		2/4	190
7. Offices			
Director		1	218
Nurse coordinator		1	218
Social work coordinator	N/A		
Boardroom	See multipurpose room		
Conference room	See multipurpose room		
Volunteer coordinator			
Business office	Administration	1	132
Files	Nurses' station		
Other	See reception		
Volunteer	Workroom with W.C.	1	110/39
Service	Receiving office	1	84
Office storage	Administration	1	155
8. Entry, front door	Level B vestibule	1	142
Reception	Off level B	1	153
Admitting	Lobby, level B	1	400
Staff	Service entry, convent		
Patient	Main entry		
Volunteers	Main entry/chapel hall		
Visitors	Main entry/chapel hall		
Goods	Service entry (corridor)	1	500
Other	Loading dock	1	264
Hallways, main	Patient hallways	1/2	2,720
Service	Kitchen, laundry		1,528
Other	Waiting/lounge/grand stair		2,880
Administration hall		1	376
Exit	Hallway to Level C	1	8' × 84'
Dead	Morgue, service entry, level B	1	270
Miscellaneous	Elevator lobby/elevators	1/2	475/153
	Fire stairs/lobby stairs	2/1	176/176
9. Parking			
Connections to other facilities	Yes; specific data N/A		
Connection to neighborhood	N/A		
Street visibility	N/A		
Landscaping	N/A		
Front yard	N/A		
Back yard	N/A		
10. Services			
Laundry		1	1,628
Clean linen	Storage	2/4	85
Dirty linen	Storage	2/4	99
Janitorial	Main closets	1/2	40
Closets			24
Work room		2/4	80

ROSARY HILL HOME: ARCHITECTURAL COMPONENTS (*cont'd.*)

Architectural Components	Notes	Wing/Total Number	Rough Dimensions or Size, Square Feet
General stores	Level C service storage		2,015 total
Offices	See offices		
Garbage incinerator		1	312
Water closet	Service level B	1	25
Equipment storage	Nurses' station	1/2	36
Boiler room	Chiller, switch gear		1,940
Misc. maintenance			648
Laundry room		1/2	126
Pharmacy		1	418
Cart storage	Stretcher alcove	2/4	26
Other storage	In patient corridors		275 min.

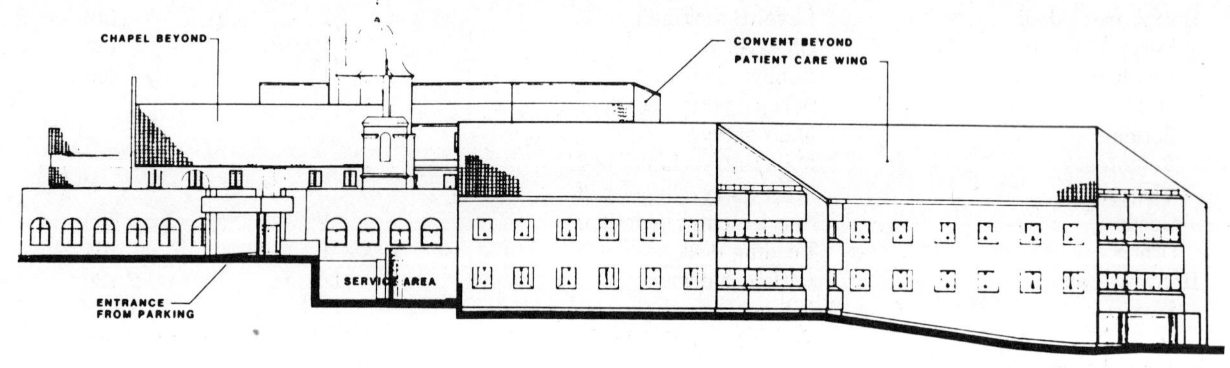

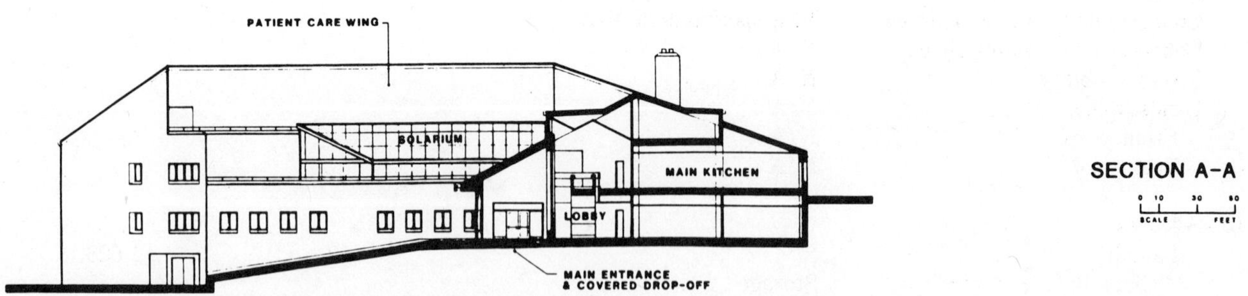

Elevation and section, Rosary Hill Home

ROSARY HILL HOME: PROXIMITY MATRIX

	Variable Numbers													
Variables	1.	2.	3.	4.	5.	6.	7.	8.	9.	10.	11.	12.	13.	14.
1. Patient	C													
2. Family (dayrooms)	C	C												
3. Chapel	D	D												
4. Solarium, terrace	C	D	C											
5. Nurses' station	B	A	D	E	C									
6. Treatment room	C	D	D	D	C	E								
7. Kitchen	D	D	C	D	D	D								
8. Kitchenette	C	C	D	C	B	C	D							
9. Offices (admin.)	C	D	D	D	D	E	D	D						
10. Main entry/facility	C	D	C	C	D	B	D	D	B					
11. Bed entry/unit	C	D	C	C	C	A	C	B	C	B				
12. All parking	D	D	C	D	D	D	C	D	C	C	D			
13. Linen/laundry	C	B		D	B	C	D	C	D	D	D	D		
14. Janitorial	C	C	C	C	C	C	C	C	C	C	C	D	C	

Key: A = within 16-foot radius (based on 8-foot corridors)
      B = within 32-foot radius
      C = related areas (see plan)
      D = distant
      E = scattered, disparate association
  blank = no relation

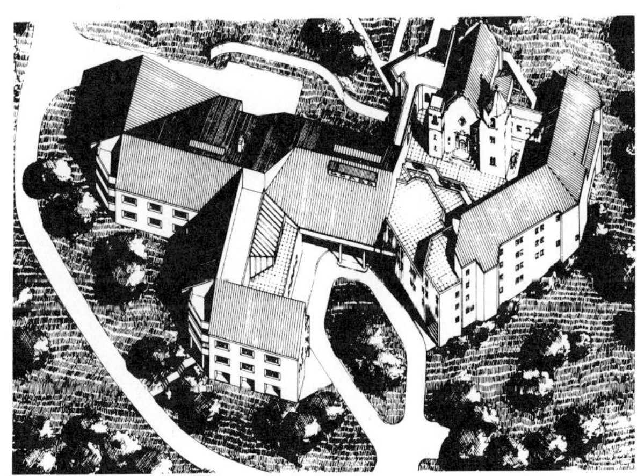

Rendering, Rosary Hill Home

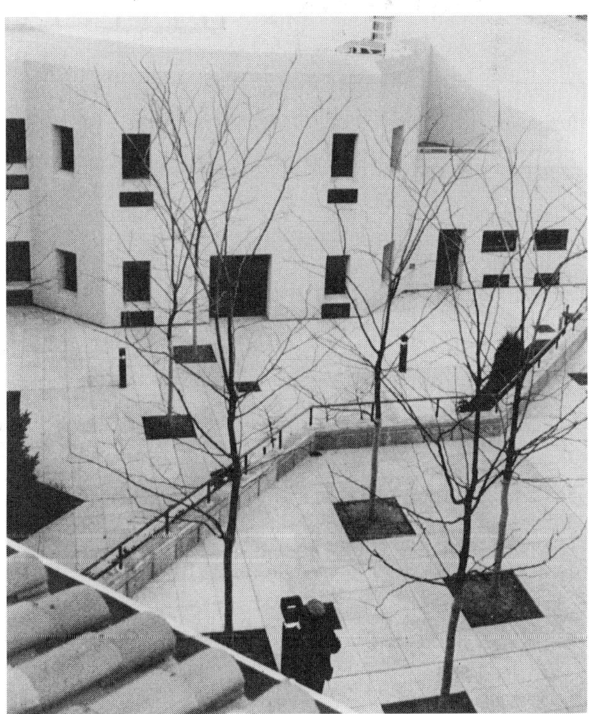

Courtyard

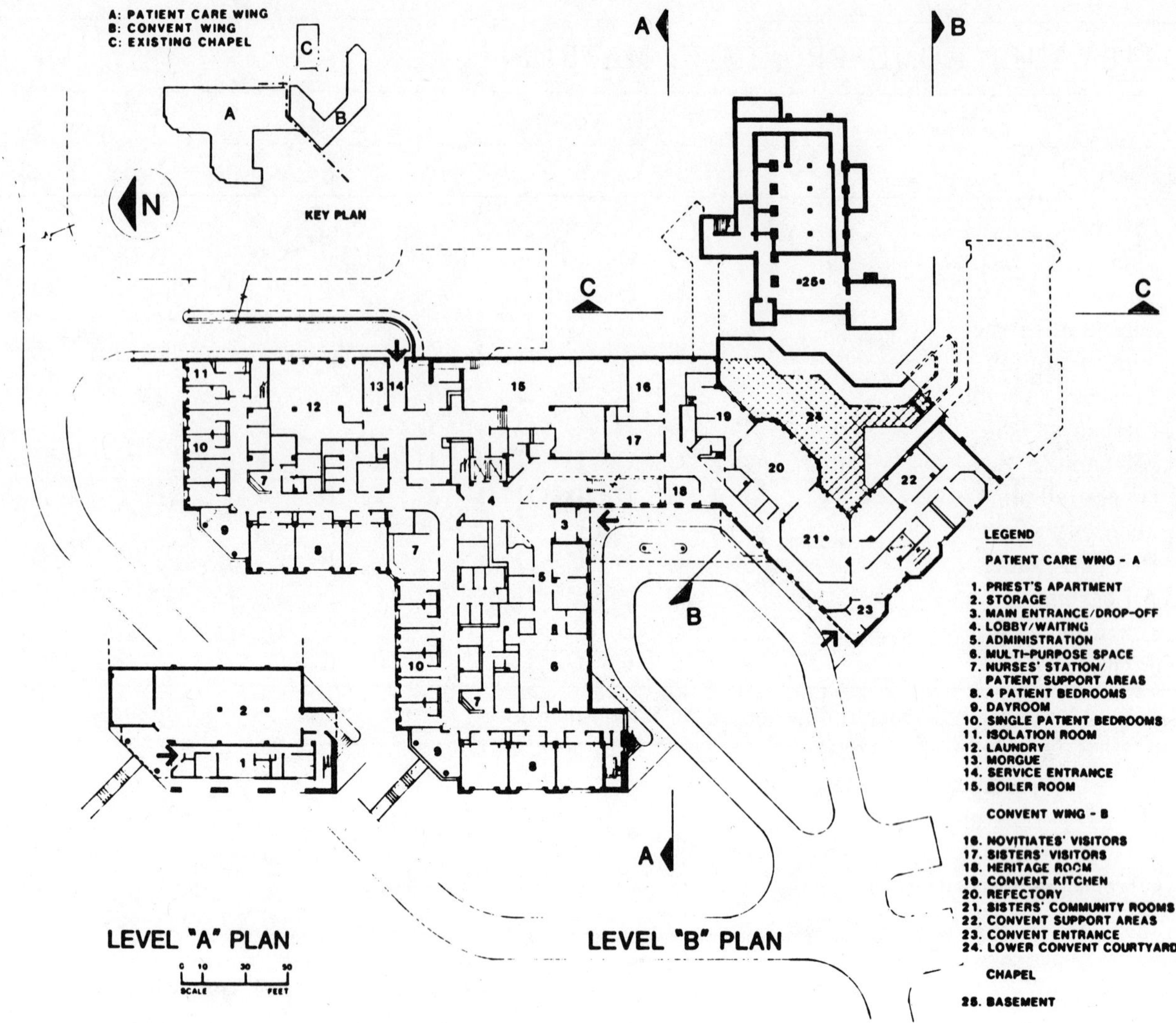

Plans, levels A and B of Rosary Hill Home

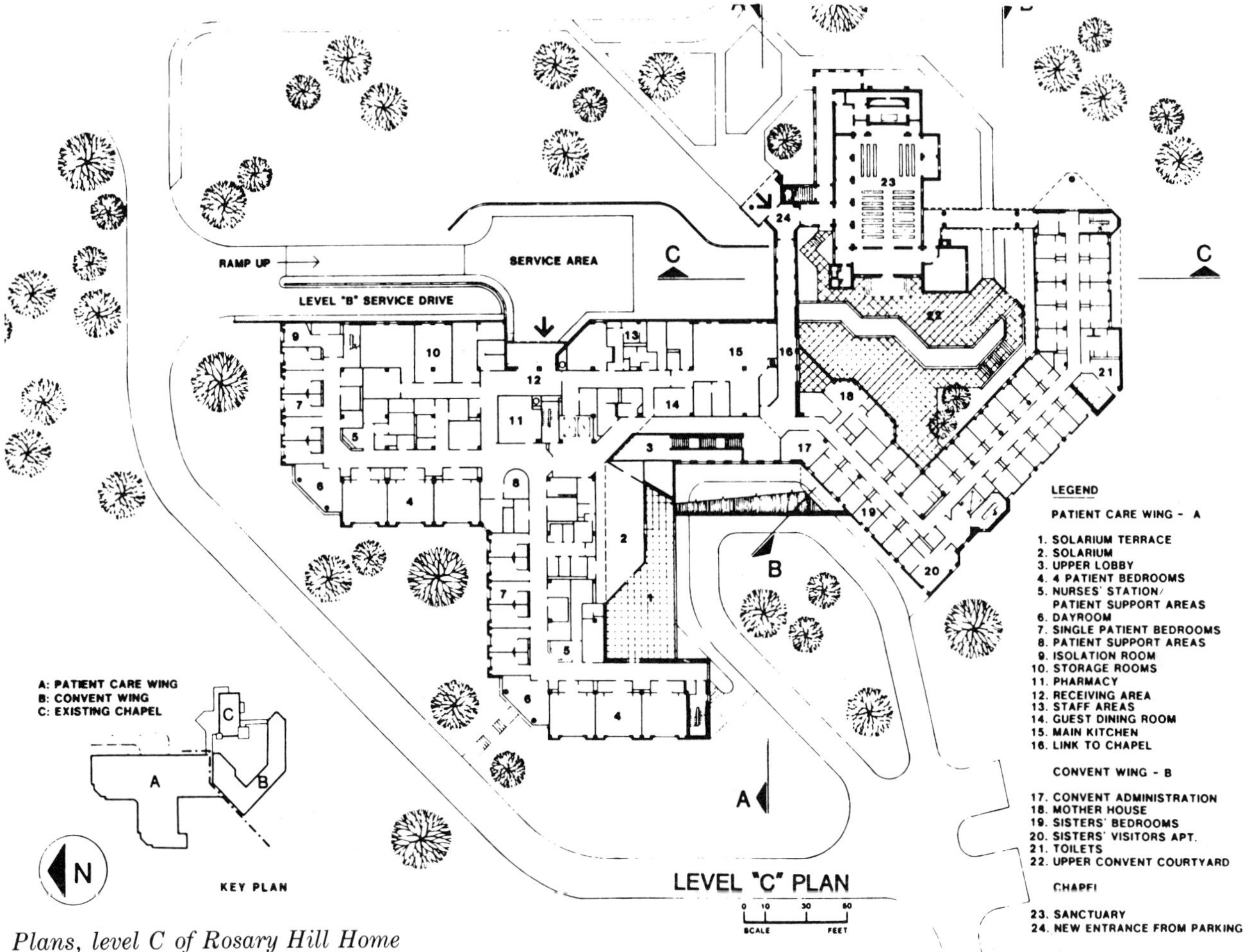

Plans, level C of Rosary Hill Home

• SACRED HEART HOSPITAL

900 East Clairmont Avenue
Eau Claire, Wisconsin 54701

Classification: Hospice in hospital
Sponsoring agencies: Sacred Heart Hospital and home health agencies
Type: Remodeled unit on general medical floor
Area served: Eleven counties
Inpatient population: 10 maximum; German and Norwegian ethnic background, Catholic and Protestant, middle-class
Established: 1980
Scope of work involved: N/A
    Formerly: General medical institution
    Architect: Inhouse
Cost of work: N/A
    Build: N/A
    Furnishings: N/A
Comprehensive intention of building selection and/or design: N/A
General intention: Homelike, clean, well-kept facility
Location: Fifth floor of hospital
Description: Small, private, special, clean, light
    Community image: part of hospital
    Interior image: remodeled unit
    Convenience: difficult to reach because of fifth-floor location
Other: Used Bellin Hospice as a model for remodel
    Changes: Relocation to ground floor with sun porch and garden next to hospital daycare play area
Users:
    Outpatient staff: N/A
    Volunteers: N/A
    Inpatient staff: N/A
    Outpatients served: N/A
    Inpatient average population: 4–6
    Inpatient average length of stay: N/A
    Family/visitors per week: Varies
Services rendered: Inpatient contract with home health agency for home care, bereavement counseling. Family can sleep in patient rooms on hide-a-beds.

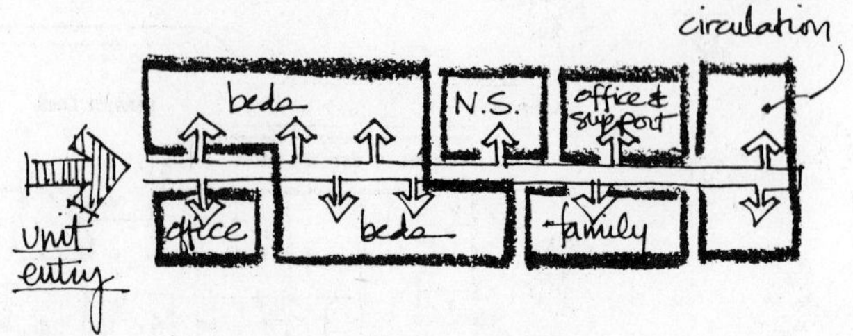

Parti drawing, Sacred Heart Hospice

SACRED HEART HOSPITAL: ARCHITECTURAL COMPONENTS

Architectural Components	Notes	Wing/Total Number	Rough Dimensions or Size, Square Feet
1. Patient room	Double	5	14′ × 20′
Bathrooms	W.C.		N/A
2. Family lounge		1	N/A
Child area	N/A		
Eating area	In lounge		
Other	See kitchenette		
Family private room	See conference room		
Conference	For staff, families	1	N/A
3. Garden			
Gardening area			
Chapel	Off unit; televised services		
Transition room	None		
Meditation room	None		
Chaplain office	Off unit		
4. Nurses' station		1	N/A
Medication room	N/A		
Nurses' retreat	Nurses' conference room	1	N/A
Staff rooms	N/A		
5. Daycare	N/A		
Childcare	N/A		
Massage	N/A		
Physical therapy	N/A		
Occupational therapy	N/A		
Library	N/A		
Music/reading	See family lounge		
6. Kitchen facilities	Off unit		
Unit dining	Staff eats with hospital staff		
Kitchenette		1	N/A
7. Offices			
Director	N/A		
Nurse coordinator		1	N/A
Social work coordinator	None		
Boardroom	None		
Conference room	None		
Volunteer coordinator	None		
Business office	None		
Other	Bereavement counseling	1	N/A

Architectural Components	*Notes*	*Wing/Total Number*	*Rough Dimensions or Size, Square Feet*
8. Entry, front door	N/A		
Reception	N/A		
Admitting	N/A		
Staff	Medical unit/service elevator		
Patient	Service elevator (bed)		
Volunteer	Through medical unit		
Visitors	Through medical unit		
Goods	Hospital entry		
Hallways, main	Medical unit		
Service	Hospice unit		
Exit goods	Hospital units		
Laundry	Hospital units		
Dead	Service elevator to basement		
9. Parking	Hospital parking		
Connections to other facilities	N/A		
Connection to neighborhood	N/A		
Street visibility	N/A		
10. Services			
Laundry			
Clean	Linen	1	N/A
Janitorial	N/A		
General stores	Off unit		
Garbage	N/A		
Equipment storage	See linen		

SACRED HEART HOSPITAL: DESCRIPTIVE MATRIX (Environmental Factors)

Overall Unit

	Intent	*Existing*
View		
Window	add light to room, view outdoors	east and west views of sunrise, sunset, university gardens
Doors	privacy, existing	N/A
Each bed	nonabandonment, privacy	window and door
Other: artwork	comforting, accessible	nature scenes
Window		
Treatment	existing; top half of each outside wall is window	plants
Trim	N/A	N/A
Operation	N/A	N/A
Covering	N/A	N/A
Lighting		
Type	natural	N/A
Fixtures	homelike	N/A
Handicap access		
Bed and wheelchair	bed access	service elevator
Dominant colors	homelike	N/A
Dominant materials	homelike, cleanable	N/A
Furniture type	homelike, institutional	hospital beds, with lounge, chair, love-seats, etc.
Ceiling height/ treatment	N/A	N/A
Floor surfacing	N/A	N/A
Personalization	encouraged	space at bedside stands, windowsills, closets
Organization	existing; mixed functions	double-loaded corridors, patient rooms at entry, nurses' station in middle of corridor
Equipment	N/A	N/A
Signs	N/A	N/A

• ST. MARY'S HOSPICE

1601 West St. Mary's Road
Tucson, Arizona 85705

Classification: Proposed new hospice, affiliated with hospital

Sponsoring agency: St. Mary's Hospital

Type: New facility adjoining existing hospital complex

Area served: Tucson and environs

Inpatient population: 20 beds

Established: Proposed facility. Existing hospital has 10 remodeled acute-care beds for hospice patients

Scope of work involved: New construction

    Architect: Anderson De Bartolo Pan, Inc.
              6339 East Speedway Blvd.
              Tucson, Arizona 85710

Cost of work: $2,252,350 (est. 1981)
    Build: $1,772,000
    Furnishings: $215,000

Comprehensive intention of building selection and/or design: N/A

General intention: Homelike ambience within institution, patient and family consided unit of care, patient's right of choice emphasized

Location: Between residential and hospital areas

Description: Contempory, long, low profile with courtyards, gardens to soften institutional environment

    Community image: part of new SNF, hospital health care center campus

    Interior image: light, contemporary, spacious, clean insitution

    Convenience: maximized for hospital, SNF patients, good visibility, entry

Other: No funding at this time

    Changes: Design somewhat predicated on the skilled nursing facility building; no kitchen facilities in hospice design, for example

Users:
    Outpatient staff: N/A
    Volunteers: N/A
    Inpatient staff: N/A
    Outpatients served: 50 (projected)
    Inpatient average population: N/A
    Inpatient average length of stay: 2 weeks (projected)
    Family/visitors per week: N/A

Services rendered: Home care, inpatient care, bereavement counseling

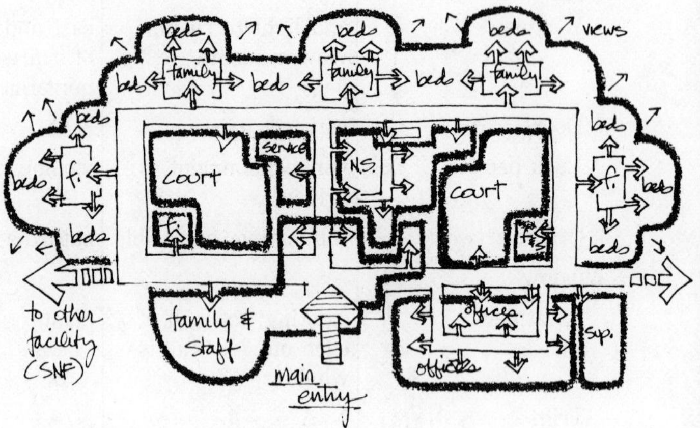

Parti drawing, St. Mary's Hospice

ST. MARY'S HOSPICE: ARCHITECTURAL COMPONENTS

Architectural Components	Notes	Wing/Total Number	Rough Dimensions or Size, Square Feet
1. Patient room	Single with W.C.	20	230 (min.)
Bathrooms	Tub and shower rooms	2	150 (each)
2. Family lounge	One for each 4-bed cluster	1/5	400 (each)
Child area	See nursery		
Eating area	See kitchen		
Other	None		
Family private room	Family room	1	250
Family other	Counseling rooms	2	100
Bathrooms	Public W.C.s	2	160
Conference	See clinical conference		
3. Garden	Interior courts	2	2,500
Gardening area	Patient room courts	15	100–180
Chapel		1	250
Transition room	Viewing room	1	200
Meditation room	See chapel		
Chaplain office		1	175
4. Nurses' station		1	150
Medication room		1	40
Nurses' retreat		1	125
Staff rooms	Clinical conference	1	250
Bathrooms	Public W.C.s	2	60
Nurses' workroom	Inpatient and home care	1	300
Medical storage		1	120
5. Daycare	Multipurpose room	1	1,000
Childcare	Nursery with W.C.s	1	360
Massage	See physical therapy		
Physical therapy	and personal care	1	350
Occupational therapy		1	200
Library	See family room		
Barbershop	None		
Tavern	None		
Store	Gift shop	1	150
Game room	See multipurpose room		
6. Kitchen facilities	Off unit		
Storage	N/A		
Supplies	N/A		
Preparation	N/A		
Cleaning	N/A		
Office	N/A		
Dietary staff	N/A		
Unit dining	Patient rooms/living rooms		
Other dining	Resident activity room		
Nutrition station		1	40
Kitchenette		1	180
7. Offices	Unassigned	1	175
Director	With W.C.	1	210

Architectural Components	Notes	Wing/Total Number	Rough Dimensions or Size, Square Feet
Nurse coordinator		1	175
Social work coordinators		2	175
Boardroom	See conference room		
Conference room		1	450
Volunteer coordinator		1	175
Business office	Secretary	1	160
Volunteer workroom		1	200
Other	Education coordinator	1	175
Bereavement coordinator		1	175
Medical director		1	175
Office supplies		1	80
Audio/visual room		1	150
8. Entry, front door	Outdoor court	1	2,000
Reception	Waiting area	1	450
Admitting	N/A		
Staff	Front door, SNF bridge		
Patient	Front door, entry court		
Volunteer	Front door, service		
Visitors	Front door		
Goods	Service, SNF bridge		
Other			
Hallways, main	Central axis, double loaded		8′ × 80′
Service	Rectilinear, single loaded		8′ × 500′
Other	Office area, double loaded		6′ × 110′
Exit goods	Service, SNF		
Laundry	Service, SNF		
Dead	N/A		
Miscellaneous	Service yard	1	2,500
9. Parking	Shared		10,500
Connections to other facilities	N/A		
Connection to neighborhood	N/A		
Street visibility	N/A		
Landscaping			
Front yard	N/A		
Back yard	N/A		
10. Services	Contracted		
Laundry	Contracted		
Clean		1	100
Dirty		1	100
Janitorial			
Closet		2	40
Stores			
General stores	Shared with SNF	1	150
Garbage	Incinerator		
Garbage pickup	Loading dock	1	550
Equipment storage		1	300
Mail	N/A		
Miscellaneous	Equipment alcoves	3	40
Equipment rooms		2	200

ST. MARY'S HOSPICE (PROPOSED): PROXIMITY MATRIX

Variables	*Variable Numbers*													
	1.	*2.*	*3.*	*4.*	*5.*	*6.*	*7.*	*8.*	*9.*	*10.*	*11.*	*12.*	*13.*	*14.*
1. Patient	E													
2. Family (living room)	A	E												
3. Chapel	D	D												
4. Nature (outdoors)	A	A	A	E										
5. Nurses' station	D	C	D	B										
6. Inpatient services	D	C	D	A	B									
7. Kitchen	D	D	D		D	D								
8. Kitchenette	D	D	D	B	D	D	D							
9. Offices	D	D	B	C	D	D	D	D						
10. Main entry/facility	D	D	C	A	C	C	D	C	B					
11. Bed entry/unit	D	D	C	A	C	C	D	C	B	A				
12. All parking	D	D	C	A	C	D	D	D	C	C	C			
13. Linen/laundry	D	D	D	A	A	C	D	D	D	C	C	D		
14. Janitorial	C	C	C		C	C		C	C	C	C		C	

Key:

- A = within 16-foot radius (based on 8-foot corridors)
- B = within 32-foot radius
- C = related areas (see plan)
- D = distant
- E = scattered, disparate association
- blank = no relation

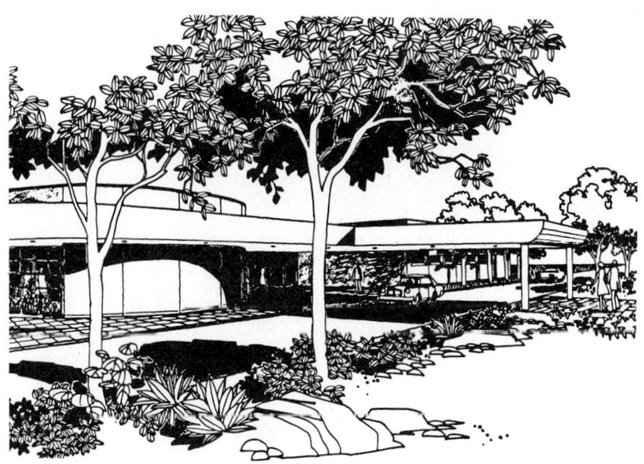

Rendering of the hospice entry

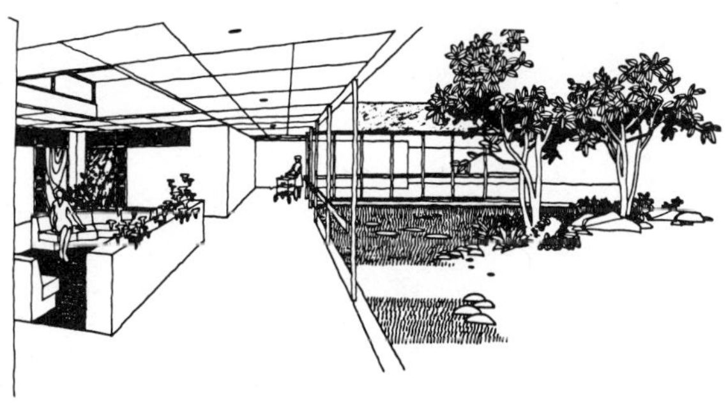

Rendering of the courtyard scheme

There are connections to the outdoors throughout the proposed design of St. Mary's Hospice, which is very appropriate to their Tucson climate. However, the extensive courtyard space is made available through single-loaded corridors that, in effect, extend the already long separation of patient rooms and nurses' station as well as other hospice functions. Overall, there is a great separation of function in this facility and little variety in room accommodation.

One note on the diagonal bed placement: although it is space-efficient, it does not allow much space around the patient's head, thereby making visiting, comforting, and simply being close to the patient difficult. This kind of bed arrangement cannot be recommended for hospice care.

The chapel and viewing room should be adjacent; other areas could be combined as well. If located together, the nursery, craft room, gift shop, cooking, and dining areas, for example, could provide an excellent central activity area. In addition, the nurses' station is too far from the patient rooms, in most cases, to promote nonabandonment of the patients, whose families cannot always be present. Patients often enter the hospice in beds or stretchers; the entry should be designed to accommodate the

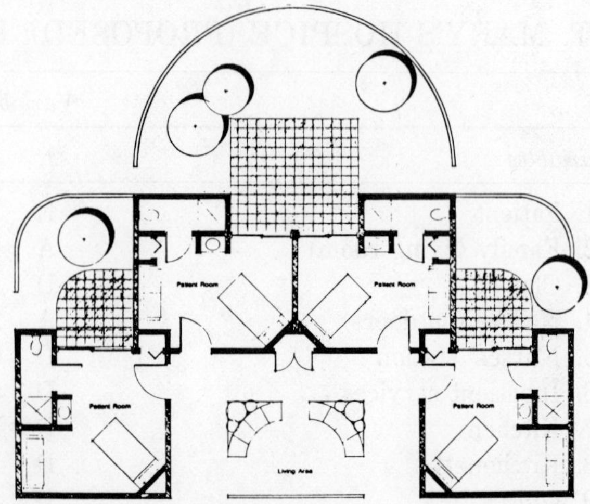

Typical patient room cluster

weak state of many of the patients. Bedrooms, too, should be located closer to the hospice entrance. Offices need not be located in a cluster, but could be spread throughout the hospice in appropriate areas, to integrate the functions of the unit with the patient and family areas.

On a positive note, the hospice design proposal's emphasis on space, light, and the outdoors is an admirable one; the idea itself is encouraging. This is a generous design.

• ST. PETER'S HOSPICE

315 South Manning Boulevard
Albany, New York 12208

Classification: Hospice

Sponsoring agencies: St. Peter's Hospital, Sisters of Mercy

Type: Remodeled hospital ward (intern's residence)

Area served: Albany and environs

Inpatient population: Maximum 10; all ages, Catholic, Jewish, Protestant

Established: 1981; home care, 1980

Scope of work involved:
  Formerly: Intern residence
  Architect: Quackenbush Wagoner & Reynolds
           22 Colvin Avenue
           Albany, New York 12208
  Interior designer: Fred Hershey
              Burlingame Interiors

Cost of work: $700,000
  Build: N/A
  Furnishings: N/A

Comprehensive intention of building selection and/or design: N/A

General intention: Remodel of two hospital floors, no longer up to code for acute care, to provide homelike "inn" atmosphere

Description: Fourth and fifth floors of hospital, double-loaded corridors
  Community image: part of hospital
  Interior image: resembles fine hotel, convivial, hospitable atmosphere
  Convenience: entry hard to find, circulation limited by location of stairs, elevators
  Changes: Connection to outdoors made difficult by fifth-floor location. Also needs staff lounge, probably on patient floor, and should remodel treatment room

Users:
  Outpatient staff: 4 nurses, 1 supervisor
  Volunteers: N/A
  Inpatient staff: (FTE) 14
  Outpatients served: N/A
  Inpatient average population: 6–8, approx.
  Inpatient average length of stay: 2–3 weeks
  Family/visitors per week: Varies

Services rendered: Consultation, home and inpatient care, day care, bereavement counseling, community education

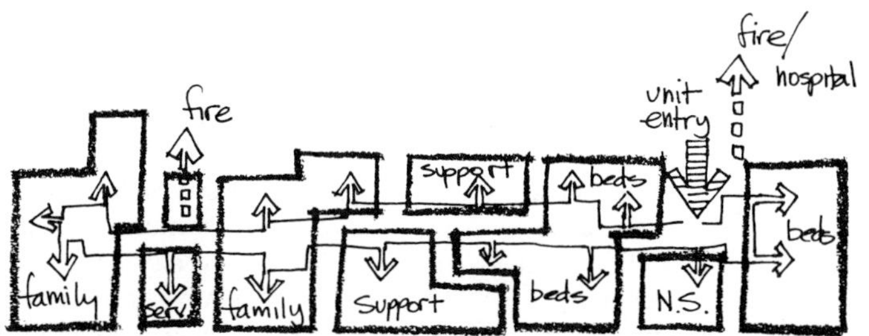

Parti drawing, St. Peter's Hospice

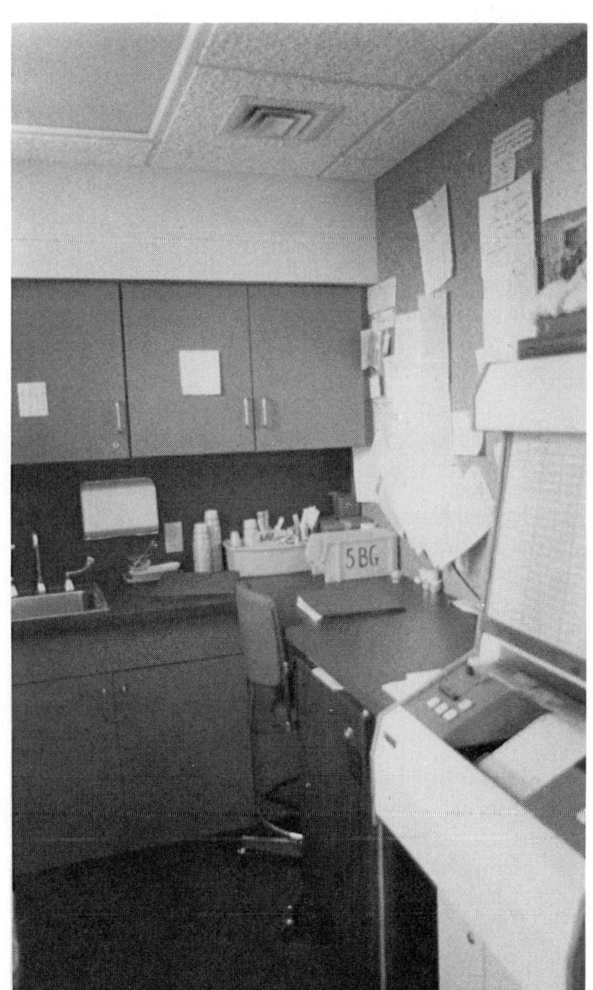

Nurses' station

ST. PETER'S HOSPICE: ARCHITECTURAL COMPONENTS

Architectural Components	Notes	Wing/Total Number	Rough Dimensions or Size, Square Feet
1. Patient room			
	Single	4	196
	Triple with sink	2	430
Bathrooms	Each single and triple	6	45
	Shower/bath	1	78
2. Family lounge	Dayroom	1	1,352
Child area	In multipurpose room		104
Eating area	In dayroom		
Other	Alcoves in dayroom		195
Family private room	Overnight room	1	156
Family other	Many areas off corridor		200
Bathrooms	In overnight room	1	25
	General	1	169
Multipurpose	With bar, child area, and television	1	1,086.5
Conference		1	322
3. Garden	N/A		
Gardening area	In dayroom		
Chapel	Off unit		
Transition room	No		
Meditation room	See multipurpose room		
Chaplain office		1	135
4. Nurses' station	Alcove	1	270
Medication room		1	60
Nurses' retreat	N/A		
Bathrooms		1	24
Supervisor's office		1	80
5. Daycare	See family lounge	1	
Childcare	See multipurpose room		
Massage	See overnight room		
Physical therapy		1	180
Occupational therapy	Dayroom		
Library	Dayroom alcove	1	154
Music/reading	Dayroom/multipurpose		
Barbershop	Beauty shop	1	195
Tavern	N/A		
Store	Off unit		
Game room	N/A		
6. Kitchen facilities	Off unit		
Storage	Off unit		
Supplies	Off unit		
Preparation	Off unit		
Cleaning	Off unit		
Office	Off unit		
Dietary staff	Off unit		
Unit dining	Staff kitchenette	1	136
Other dining	Dayroom		
Nutrition station	N/A		
Kitchenette	In dayroom	1	182
Bathroom		1	48

ST. PETER'S HOSPICE: ARCHITECTURAL COMPONENTS (*cont'd.*)

Architectural Components	Notes	Wing/Total Number	Rough Dimensions or Size, Square Feet
7. Offices	Fourth floor		
Directors		2	726 (total)
Nurse coordinator		1	374
Social work coordinator			
Boardroom			
Conference room		1	363
Volunteer coordinator		1	135
Business		1	135
Home care		1	135
Research		1	135
Hospice library	with W.C.	1	196
Office storage			40
8. Entry, front door			
Reception	Fourth floor	1	312
Admitting	Fourth floor (exam)	1	135
Staff	Fourth floor		
Patient	Fourth or fifth floor		
Volunteer	Fourth or fifth floor		
Visitors	Fourth or fifth floor		
Goods	Hospital route		
Other	N/A		
Hallways, main	In pavilion, fifth floor	1	1,296
Service	Fourth floor	1	736
Other	Hospital connections		
Exit Goods			
Laundry	Off unit		
Dead	Off unit		
Miscellaneous	N/A		
9. Parking		2 lots	
Connections to other facilities			
Connection to neighborhood	N/A		
Street visibility	N/A		
Landscaping	N/A		
Front yard	N/A		
Back yard	N/A		
10. Services			
Laundry	Off unit		
Clean	Fifth floor	1	136
Dirty			104
Janitorial			
Closet	Fifth floor	1	24
Stores	Equipment, fifth floor	1	96
General stores	See stores		
Office	Off unit		
Garbage	Fifth floor	1	48
Garbage pickup	Off unit		
Equipment storage	See stores		
Mail	At nurses' alcove		
Miscellaneous			

ST. PETER'S HOSPICE: PROXIMITY MATRIX

Variables	Variable Numbers													
	1.	2.	3.	4.	5.	6.	7.	8.	9.	10.	11.	12.	13.	14.
1. Patient (bedrooms)	C													
2. Family (multipurpose room)	C													
3. Chapel	*	*												
4. Nature (greenhouse)	D	C	*											
5. Nurses' station	C	D	*	D										
6. Beauty shop	D	A	*	C	D									
7. Kitchen	*	*	*	*	*	*								
8. Kitchenette (dayroom)	D	B	*	B	D	A	*							
9. Offices (admin.)	C	D	*	D	C	D	*	D						
10. Main entry/facility	D	D	*	D	D	D	*	D	C					
11. Bed entry/unit	B	D	*	D	A	D	*	D	C	D				
12. All parking	D	D	*	D	C	D	*	D	C	C	C			
13. Linen/laundry	B	C	*	D	C	D	*	D	D	D	C	D		
14. Janitorial	D	B	*	A	D	B	*	B	C	D	D	D	D	

Key:

- A = within 16-foot radius (based on 8-foot corridors)
- B = within 32-foot radius
- C = related areas (see plan)
- D = distant
- blank = no relation
- * = off unit

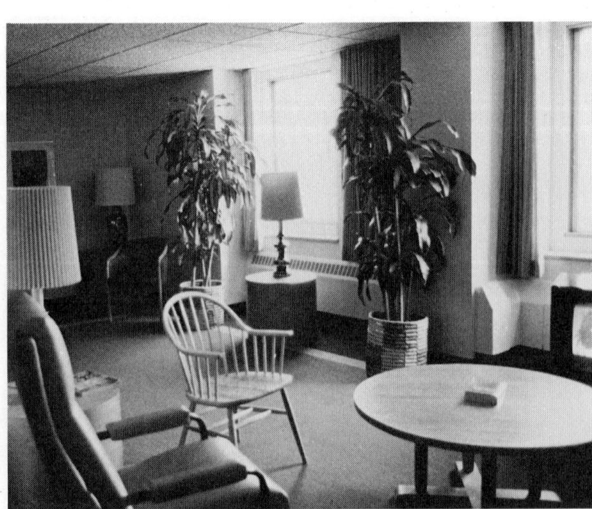

Multipurpose family room

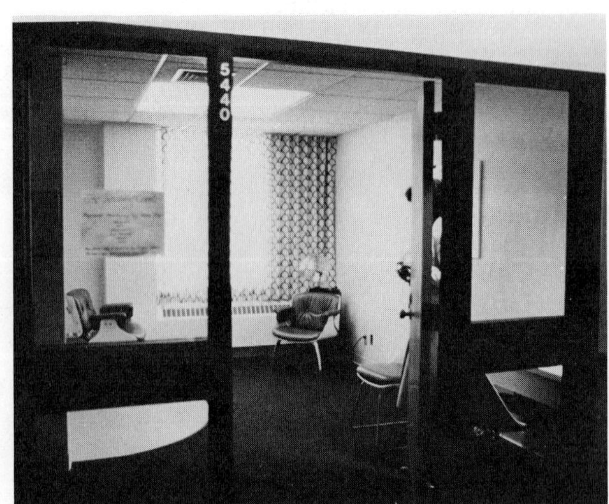

Barbershop

ST. PETER'S HOSPICE: DESCRIPTIVE MATRIX (Environmental Factors)

	Patient (Bedrooms)		Family (Dayroom)	
	Intent	*Existing*	*Intent*	*Existing*
View				
Window	light, nature	views of neighborhood	homelike	cross light
Doors	nonabandonment, privacy	staggered doors near nurses' station, entry	residential, open plan	changing vistas of outdoors
Each bed	private, territorial	zoned view of neighbor	convenient	minimized obstruction
Other: artwork	variety	donated nature scenes and abstracts	variety	donated nature scenes and abstract prints
Window				
Treatment	big lights	new windows for remodel	big lights	dayroom greenhouse, stained glass
Trim	homelike	wood, painted	homelike	wood, painted
Operation	control	operable in emergency	control	operable in emergency
Covering	choice, homelike	drapes with cord	choice, homelike	drapes with cord
Lighting				
Type	flexible, homelike	task lighting, incandescent	flexible, homelike	fluorescent/incandescent
Fixtures	homelike	patients operable lamps and switches	homelike, low level	overhead; some lamps
Handicap access				
Bed and wheelchair	yes; noninstitutional	roomy furniture separations and room sizes	yes; noninstitutional	roomy furniture groups, solid pieces
Dominant colors	residential, contemporary style	rich, deep patterned blues, reds, greens	contemporary style, residential	light colors: blue, beige, off-white
Dominant materials	residential	wallpaper, wood, paint, drapes	residential	paint, wallpaper, wood, drapes
Furniture type	residential (revised institutional)	modified wood, bedboards; overbeds and recliners; colonial style built-in dressers	residential, contemporary, wood and "leather look"	wood and woven materials, "natural" colors, some furniture built-in
Ceiling height/treatment	residential	2 × 2 grid tile with concealed grid	residential	2 × 2 grid tile with concealed grid
Floor surfacing	residential	carpet, ceramic tile in baths	residential	carpet, ceramic tile, vinyl in kitchen
Personalization	encouraged	each room different; shelves for personal items	homelike	plants, artwork, hall telephone
Organization	innlike	short, double-loaded corridor	innlike	nodes and nooks along linear corridor

ST. PETER'S HOSPICE: DESCRIPTIVE MATRIX (Environmental Factors)

	Patient (Bedrooms)		*Family (Dayroom)*	
	Intent	*Existing*	*Intent*	*Existing*
Equipment	individual control	oxygen/suction, sinks, individually controlled HVAC, hospital beds	minimal	oxygen/suction, lighting, television, clocks, telephones
Signs	homelike	small, discreet room signs only	homelike	none

	Nurses' Alcove		*Kitchenette*	
	Intent	*Existing*	*Intent*	*Existing*
View				
Window	light, airy	two large windows, sky/street view	homelike, light, airy	window "wall," sky/street view
Doors	openness	no door at alcove, cabinet door at office	openness	part of dayroom
Each bed	open	open	N/A	N/A
Other: artwork	innlike	clock, abstracts	N/A	little wallspace
Window				
Treatment	large	N/A	large	N/A
Trim	homelike	wood, painted	homelike	wood, painted
Operation	control	operable	control	operable
Covering	choice, homelike	drapes with cord	choice, homelike	drapes with cord
Lighting				
Type	flexible, homelike	task lighting, incandescent/fluorescent	flexible, homelike	incandescent/fluorescent
Fixture	homelike	lamps and wall wash overheads	homelike	overhead fixtures
Handicap access				
Bed and wheelchair	little access	small areas for temporary visitor seating only	openness	no obstructions, but not handicapped-equipped
Dominant colors	contemporary style, residential	beige, yellow, with oak trim	clean, modern, residential	beige, brown, off-white; yellow/red accents
Dominant materials	innlike	paint, wood, drapes, "leather" and woven seats	clean, modern, residential	paint, wood, plastics
Furniture type	residential	rolltop oak desk, couch and chairs, clock	residential	built-in cabinets, countertops, room for chairs
Ceiling height/ treatment	typical, residential	2′ × 2′ grid tile	typical, residential	2′ × 2′ grid tile
Floor surfacing	residential	carpet	residential	vinyl flooring (roll)

ST. PETER'S HOSPICE: DESCRIPTIVE MATRIX (Environmental Factors)

	Nurses' Alcove		Kitchenette	
	Intent	*Existing*	*Intent*	*Existing*
Personalization	some	plants	family use	for cooking individual dishes
Organization	added where needed	spread out; office adjacent to separate alcove	convenient, open	triangle with open countertop, sink
Equipment	minimal	locked medical cabinets, counter, telephone, clock, no intercom	fully equipped	plus microwave, coffee machine, etc.
Signs	residential	none	residential	none

	Fifth-Floor Hallways	
	Intent	*Existing*
View		
Window	light, open, homelike	windows in hall alcoves, family rooms
Doors	open, private, noninstitutional	wood patient-room doors, open family rooms
Other: artwork	variety, homelike	watercolors, oils, of nature scenes, etc.
Window		
Treatment	light, homelike	new windows
Trim	homelike	wood, painted
Operation	control	operable in emergency
Covering	choice, homelike, control	drapes with cord
Lighting		
Type	homelike, natural, low-level	incandescent/fluorescent
Fixtures	homelike, flexible	residential lamps, indirect wall wash
Handicap access		
Bed and wheelchair	bed, chair, walker	wide hall, grouped furniture, wood wall bars, light, soft
Dominant colors	contemporary, residential	light colors with dark accents, beige, blond wood
Dominant materials	homelike, clean, quiet, durable	carpet, wood, paint, acoustical tile, fabrics, metal

ST. PETER'S HOSPICE: DESCRIPTIVE MATRIX (Environmental Factors)

Fifth-Floor Hallways		
	Intent	*Existing*
Furniture type	lasting, homelike, contemporary, clean	Colonial and Danish, couches, many chairs, tables, lamps, etc.
Ceiling height/treatment	typical, fireproof	8′ acoustical tile
Floor surfacing	quiet, homelike	carpet
Personalization	encouraged	plants, gifts, etc.
Organization	homelike living space, variety	series of short halls with nodes, open turns
Equipment	fire, life-safety	concealed but clear
Signs	homelike	none

General Notes

Overall, the hospice has several positive features. The hallways were successfully designed to be used as living space. Various nodes draw activity along the corridor, establishing a more residential organization, permitting cross lighting through opposing windows and relieving the corridors of the oppressiveness common to double-loaded halls. The lighting systems were deliberately designed to provide indirect (wall wash) lighting throughout. Handcrafted bed boards and alcove desks were added, which provide homelike touches. Some areas, such as the multipurpose room, may seem to have been allocated an overly generous amount of space, yet this extra space will allow the hospice to be flexible with their use of space over time—a feature that many of the smaller hospices lack.

At the time of the survey, the fourth floor had not yet been remodeled, and contrasted unfavorably with the patient floor. The style shop (hairdresser) was placed farther away from the unit entry in order to draw people from all over the hospital, and has been a mixed success because of its distant location. The nurses' alcove is another mixed success. The alcove is small, to encourage nurses to remain in the patient room, but is awkwardly designed: guests and visitors, seated in the adjacent waiting area, face the back of the alcove desk. The nurses' station is also too small for nursing activities. In addition, the alcove is not accessible to the handicapped; neither is the kitchenette. More custodial-equipment storage is needed along the corridors and more hospice signs are needed, either in the hospital or on hospital grounds.

This ward was selected to be remodeled into a hospice unit because the previous acute-care space was available (despite the ward's above-ground location, which precludes the possibility of having a garden). Because the bed space was available, no patients had to be moved on the floor below during construction. The mechanical remodel involved converting a central radiator system to a local system with hot-water baseboards and a separate control room.

Throughout, the hospice needs the new elevator that they have planned to install, a better entry from outside the unit, and more staff space on the patient floor. The unit could also use bulletin boards, for personalization by staff, family, and other hospice users. These changes will probably occur over time, however.

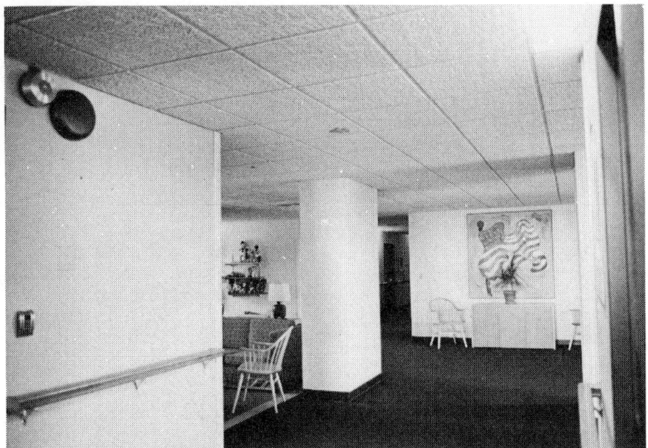

Fifth-floor hospice entrance

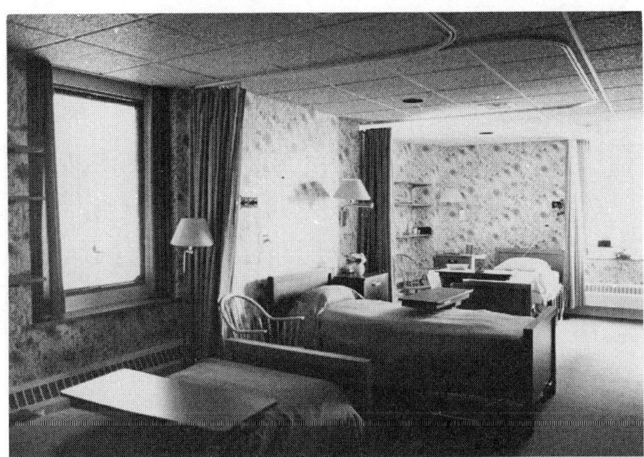

Triple patient room

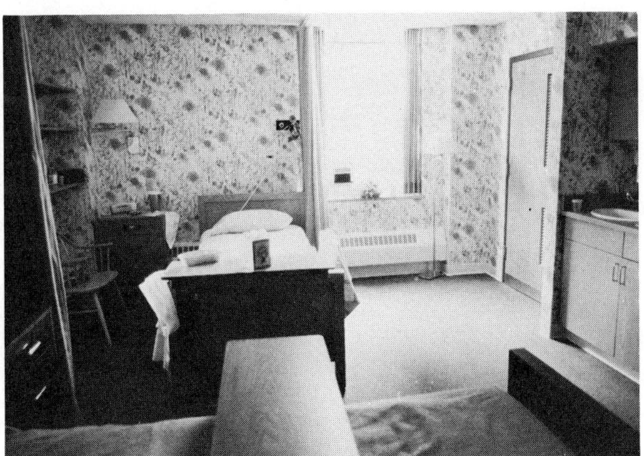

Detail of patient room

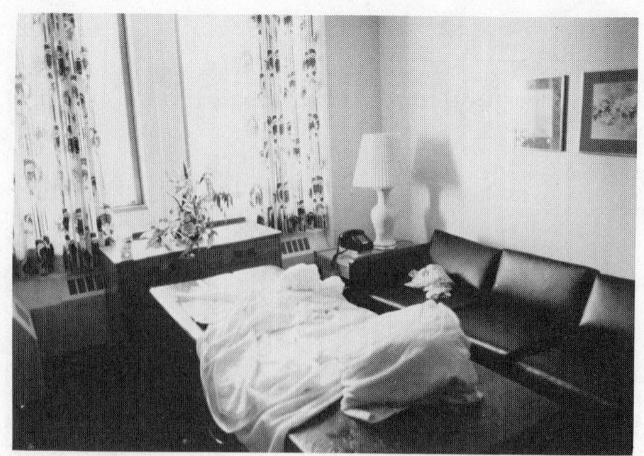

Private family room, with cot for overnight stays

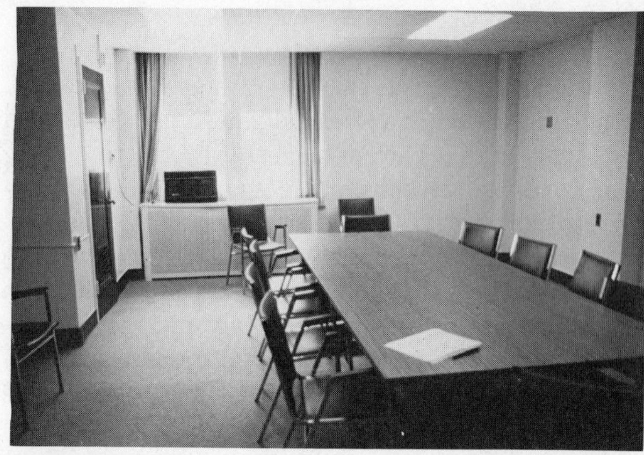

Conference room

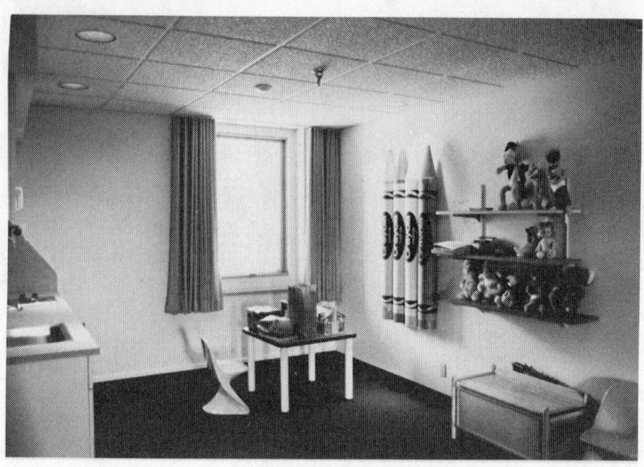

Childcare area of family lounge

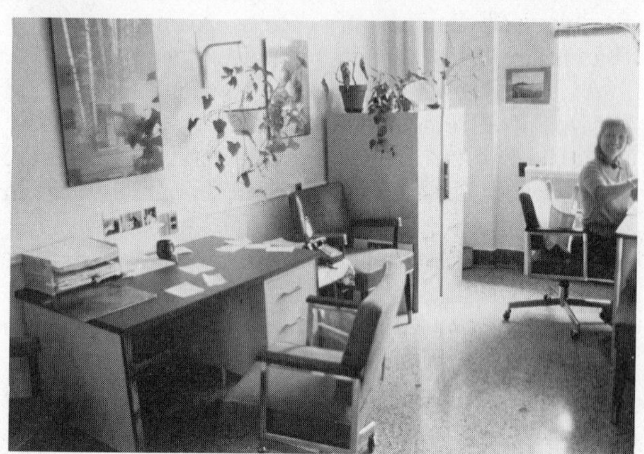

Sunny administration office

• ST. ROSE'S HOME

71 Jackson Street
New York, New York 10002

Classification: Freestanding, pre-hospice skilled nursing facility

Sponsoring agencies: Dominican Sisters of Hawthorne (Congregation of St. Rose of Lima)

Type: New construction

Area served: New York metropolitan area

Inpatient population: Designed for 100 (modified for 50)

Established: May 1957

Scope of work involved: N/A
   Architect: The Eggers Group, P.C.
            Two Park Avenue
            New York, New York 10016

Cost of work: N/A
   Build: N/A
   Furnishings: N/A

Comprehensive intention of building selection and/or design: N/A

General intention: Comfortable, modern, clean facility

Location: Urban area, facing Corlears Park, East River

Description: Modern six-story building
   Community image: skilled nursing facility
   Interior image: clean, bright, modern
   Convenience: freestanding facility: has its own entrance; bus and car transportation available

Other: There is reason to believe modifications have taken place, changing rooming to double, four- and six-bed rooms from original plans and reducing total number of patients to fifty

Users:
   Outpatient staff: N/A
   Volunteers: N/A
   Inpatient staff: (FTE) 17
   Outpatients served: N/A
   Inpatient average population: N/A
   Inpatient average length of stay: N/A
   Family/visitors per week: Varies

Services rendered: Inpatient care of indigent terminal cancer patients

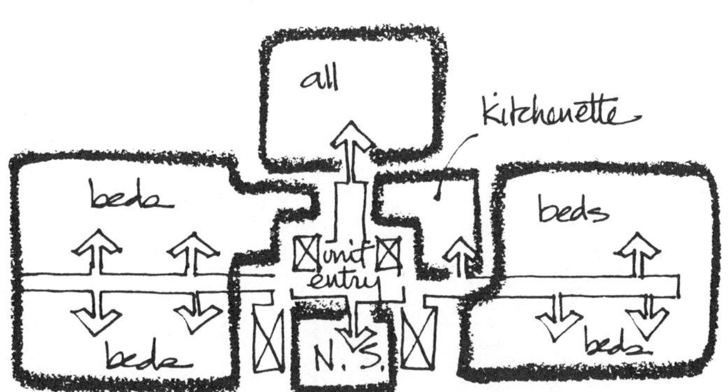

Parti drawing of patient floor, St. Roses' Home

ST. ROSE'S HOME: ARCHITECTURAL COMPONENTS

Architectural Components	Notes	Wing/Total Number	Rough Dimensions or Size, Square Feet
1. Patient room			
	Single (Isolation)	2/6	128
	Four-bed	2/12	382
	Other: eight-bed	1/6	700
Bathrooms	W.C.s for four-bed	2	180
	W.C. for eight-bed	2	112
	Patient bath/shower	2	50
2. Family lounge	N/A		
Eating area	N/A		
Other	N/A		
Family private room	N/A		
Family other	Parlor	2	150
Bathrooms	M/F W.C.	1 each	25
Conference	See parlor		
3. Garden			
Gardening area	See daycare		
Chapel	Sacristy	1	1,452
Transition room			
Meditation room	2nd-floor dayroom		
Chaplain office	See sacristy		
4. Nurses' station		1/3	136
Medication room	N/A		
Nurses' retreat		1	1,080
Staff rooms	N/A		
Bathrooms		1/3	26
5. Daycare	2nd floor	1	422
	3rd floor with outside deck	1	473/300
	4th floor with outside deck	1	270/200
Physical therapy			
Occupational therapy	See dayroom		
Library	N/A		
Music/reading	N/A		
Barbershop	N/A		
Tavern	N/A		
Store	N/A		
Game room	N/A		
Other	Treatment rooms	1/3	148
6. Kitchen facilities		1	960
Storage		1	190
Supplies		1	119
Preparation	N/A		
Cleaning	N/A		
W.C. and vestibule		1	55
Dietary staff	N/A		
Unit dining	N/A		
Other dining	N/A	1/3	304
Kitchenette			

Architectural Components	Notes	Wing/Total Number	Rough Dimensions or Size, Square Feet
7. Offices			
Director		1	270
Nurse coordinator	N/A		
Social work coordinator	N/A		
Boardroom	N/A		
Conference room	N/A		
Volunteer coordinator	N/A		
Business office	N/A		
Files		1	120
8. Entry, front door	Vestibule/lobby	1	528
Reception	N/A		
Admitting	1st floor with W.C.	1	210
Staff	Use front or service door		
Patient	Patient vestibule	1	98
Volunteer	N/A		
Visitors	Entry vestibule		
Goods	Service vestibule (kitchen)		
Other			
Hallways, main	1st floor		748
Service		3	1,230 each
Other	Elevators	2	6 × 8
Exit Goods	Service vestibule (see kitchen)		
Laundry	Basement		
Dead	Patient vestibule		
Miscellaneous	Stairs	2	8 × 20
9. Parking			
Connections to other facilities	N/A		
Connection to neighborhood	N/A		
Street visibility	N/A		
Landscaping			
Front yard	N/A		
Back yard	N/A		
10. Services			
Laundry			
Clean linen		1/3	8 × 11
Dirty linen		2/6	3 × 4
Janitorial			
Closet	1st floor	1	4 × 4
Stores		1/3	4 × 4
General stores	Medical	1	246
Garbage	Garbage chute	1	3 × 4
Garbage pickup	N/A		
Equipment storage	Wheelchair	1/3	5 × 14
	Stretcher	1/3	84
Miscellaneous	Pharmacy and narcotic storage	1	400
Laboratory		1	96
Sterilizing area		1	98

ST. ROSE'S HOME: PROXIMITY MATRIX

Variables	1.	2.	3.	4.	5.	6.	7.	8.	9.	10.	11.	12.	13.	14.
1. Patient	C													
2. Family (parlors)	D													
3. Chapel	C	C												
4. Nature (large windows)	A	C	C											
5. Nurses' station	B	D	D	A										
6. Inpatient services	C	D	C	A	B									
7. Kitchen	D	D	A	D	D	D								
8. Kitchenette	C	D	D	D	A	A	C							
9. Offices	D	A	B	D	D	D	C	D						
10. Main entry/facility	D	A	B	D	C	D	C	D	B					
11. Bed entry/unit	C	D	A	D	C	B	D	C	A	C				
12. All parking														
13. Linen/laundry	C	D	D	D	A	C	C	B	D	D	C			
14. Janitorial	C	A	D	D	B	C	D	A	B	C	D		C	

Variable Numbers

Key: A = within 16-foot radius (based on 8-foot corridors)
  B = within 32-foot radius
  C = related areas (see plan)
  D = distant
  blank = no relation

ST. ROSE'S HOME: DESCRIPTIVE MATRIX (Environmental Factors)

Patient Floors 2, 3, and 4

	Intent	*Existing*
View		
Window	light, nature	very large views, river and park
Doors	connection to nature	on floors 3 and 4, dayroom connects to outdoors
Each bed	privacy within community	private curtain, multibed rooms
Other: artwork	cheerful, homelike	religious art and sculpture
Window		
Treatment	N/A	N/A
Trim	N/A	N/A
Operation	N/A	N/A
Covering	privacy	curtains
Lighting		
Type	natural, practical	large windows, incandescent/fluorescent light
Fixtures	N/A	overbed incandescent/fluorescent lights
Handicap access		
Bed and wheelchair	beds, wheelchairs, walkers	wide doorways to chapel and dayrooms
Dominant colors	homelike, comforting, cheerful	pastel, floral, and pattern sheets
Dominant materials	clean, comfortable, long-lasting	paint, linoleum, wood, brick, plaster, stone
Furniture type	flexible, comfortable	hospital beds, tables, patient lockers
Ceiling height/ treatment	N/A	N/A
Floor surfacing	N/A	N/A
Personalization	encouraged	plants, flowers, crafts, in patient rooms and dayrooms
Organization	centralized, communal	cruciform plan; patients on one axis, entry and n.s. on the other axis
Equipment	homelike, clean, modern	radios, television, patient lights, HVAC
Signs	N/A	N/A

Chapter Five

Comparisons and Analysis

Chapter 4 provides the raw data for the analysis of hospice units. From the tables, we can determine the distinctive or unique hospice elements; the more specific information is used to contrast and compare similar-sized units. The hospice information thus identifies the overall priorities of hospice inpatient architecture and the more specific needs of special groups within the continuum of hospice inpatient facilities.

In this chapter, general results of the total sample of forty-eight hospices and palliative-care units are included. The bulk of the chapter is given over to comparisons of the twenty-one detailed units, organized by size and type. In addition, remodeled oncology units and nonautonomous hospice areas are examined and two examples of an innovative and as yet untried approach to hospice units are isolated. The conclusion of this chapter sums up the preceding information, reviewing the hospice-specific architecture deduced from the sample and the variability of provision in different types of hospice units. Specifically, size and scale are discussed as factors that influence hospice architecture priorities, by forcing trade-offs and competing with established institutional norms. Finally, the summary concludes with comments on the current state of hospice inpatient development and the limits of a study of this kind.

General Results

The combined data from the total sample of the twenty-one detailed facilities and the twenty-seven additional units reveal four architectural elements at the top of the list: family rooms, kitchenettes, indoor gardening, and artwork. These four items were present in most hospice settings. They were followed in frequency by the two items representing a separate or semiautonomous functioning of the hospice: a separate hospice nurses' station; and a separate wing, unit, or floor. Of lesser frequency, but still represented in over half of the facilities, were the following: outdoor garden; dining room; and multipurpose room.

Several elements or room types in the listing were not found in great numbers because their functions were performed in multipurpose rooms. Conference or counseling rooms, for example, or the family private room, were often combined in a multifunctioning small room and titled with only one function. Such a room could have other, less common uses, such as physical therapy or boardroom meetings, depending on its location or furniture. Moreover, although chapels or meditation rooms were not provided on many of the units, other rooms were commonly used for weekly or special services; often, the parent facility chapel was available. This adaptive functioning will be discussed in greater detail at the conclusion of this chapter and in Part Three.

The general sample of data reveals some surprises in the number of facilities that lack transition or viewing rooms, or a staff retreat on the unit. One explanation for the absence of viewing rooms is the greater representation of small remodeled units that have a large proportion of single bedrooms. These single rooms are most often used for viewing after death. The lack of staff retreats is not so simply explained, however. Perhaps staff feels that areas off the unit are sufficient for grieving and stress-relief purposes. More likely, staff negotiation with hospital administrators for patient and family areas includes capitulation of nurses' and volunteers' retreat areas.

The compendium sample also includes more dependent units, those without their own nurses' station or a complete separation from the oncology, medical/surgical, or rehabilitation units in which they are found. This may explain the general lack of inpatient services provided in the remodeled areas. There are few physical therapy or occupational therapy services, libraries, beauty shops, and so on, available in most hospice settings in the sample. Usually, these facilities may be found, like the formal chapels, in the parent establishment. However, the short-term nature of hospice inpatient stays together with the weakness and debilitation experienced by many of the dying patients suggests that should these activities occur at all, they may take place in the patient rooms, or as an alternate function within the existing areas provided. Certainly, duplication of these areas may be necessary if the hospice patient is to take part in this kind of activity.

One issue in hospice design, the final answer on bedroom population, is not completely resolved by this general data. There seems to be no unanimity with regard to patient bedroom populations. The majority of these forty-eight hospices and palliative-care facilities have, however, provided a variety of accommodation. Sixty percent, or twenty-nine out of the forty-eight, have everything from one-, two-, three-, and four-bed rooms to six- and eight-bed rooms available. Most of these units provide two types of accommodation; only four of the twenty-nine have three kinds of rooming arrangements. The remaining nineteen hospices have either single or double rooms; no facility supplies only large multibed rooms. The English group of facilities provides a variety of bedroom accommodations, as do the Canadian hospices. Calvary Hospital in the United States is unique among the large care providers in having only one kind of bedroom, the single room, for all 200 patients. Of the American freestanding units in the sample, only Nathan Adelson supplies all single rooms in patient cluster arrangements. All the other freestanding facilities have at least two kinds of bedrooms. Variety is provided for units as small as the six-patient Hospice of the Monterey Peninsula, and as large as the 72-patient Rosary Hill Home and St. Joseph's Hospice in the United Kingdom.

The total number of patients in the sample varies, from 2 beds at Westchester's United Hospital to 200 at Calvary Hospital. The total number of beds documented in the sample is over 1,259 for forty-three of the hospices, making an average inpatient population for the palliative units of just under 30 beds per facility or unit. The units are almost evenly divided on location, with twenty-five having ground-floor access and twenty-three located above ground. Almost all of the hospices and palliative-care units have places for the family to sleep, with bedside chairs being the most common accommodation, and private rooms for the family the least common.

Specific Data Analysis

More specific discussion of the data is best organized by a separation of the inpatient palliative-care facilities into five groups, representing their population, status, and type (new or remodeled). These groups are as follows:

1. Large longer-term facilities (new construction), examples of which are Calvary Hospital in the Bronx, Rosary Hill Home in Hawthorne, New York, and St. Rose's Home in New York City.
2. Medium freestanding hospice facilities (new construction), including the Connecticut Hospice and Nathan Adelson in Las Vegas, Nevada.
3. Medium freestanding hospice facilities (remodeled), of which there are four in this sample— Hospice of Cincinnati, Hospice of the Good Shepherd (proposed) in Waban, Massachusetts, Hospice of Northern Virginia in Arlington, and Hillhaven (now closed).
4. Medium parent-based hospice units (remodeled), such as Cabrini Hospice in New York City, Kaiser Permanente in Norwalk, California; Mercy Hospice in Rockville Centre, New York; and Pinecrest Hospital Hospice in Santa Barbara, California.
5. Small parent-based hospice units (remodeled), represented by Bellin Hospice, Green Bay, Wisconsin; Clover Hospice, Auburn, Maine; Lutheran Hospital Hospice, Moline, Illinois; Riverside Hospital Hospice, Newport News, Virginia; Sacred Heart Hospice, Eau Claire, Wisconsin; and St. Peter's Hospice, Albany, New York.

These five categories represent the architecturally distinct and autonomous or semiautonomous hospice inpatient unit. This discussion would not be complete without including the very common solutions that have less architectural significance: the remodeled oncology unit and the hospice-designed beds on a medical/surgical ward, skilled nursing facility, or rehabilitation setting. These solutions are represented in the sample by two Washington State units—the Highline Community Hospital hospice/oncology unit in Seattle and Tacoma General Hospital Hospice—and by the Deer's Head Center Hospice in Salisbury, Maryland.

Finally, two innovative solutions suggesting a rare combination of inpatient resources—the newly constructed, parent-based, palliative-care unit—will be discussed. Examples include two proposed but not yet constructed schemes; the new floor addition to St. Mary's Hospital for Children in Queens and St. Mary's Hospice, proposed for Tucson, Arizona. These units attempt to combine the advantages of a parent association with the possibilities inherent in new construction, creating a campus-like environment. Although new to the United States, this palliative-care unit type already existed in Great Britain; a 1978 article discussed the continuing-care unit at the Royal South Hants Hospital in Southampton (Sartain 1978, 291–95).

Larger Longer-term Facilities.

The oldest established special facilities for the terminally ill are represented by Calvary Hospital and the Rosary Hill and St. Rose's Homes. All three were begun (in different original buildings) at the turn of the century as places for the incurably ill, in the tradition of the early religious Irish and English hospices. These newly reconstructed facilities are the most recent examples of their type. Calvary Hospital was constructed anew in 1978 at a cost of 12 million dollars. Rosary Hill's newest construction was completed in 1983, also for 12 million, and comprises 72 patient beds and a large convent. St. Rose's Home is of older vintage, having been completed in 1957 and now remodeled to house fewer than the original hundred patients.

As longer-term facilities that often become the institutional homes of their patients, these units have need of more support services—laundry and physical and occupational therapy, to name a few. The goal of longer-term facilities is significantly different from that of the shorter and intermittent stays provided by hospice inpatient units. Moreover, family participation has historically played a less significant role in the longer-term palliative-care facilities. For example, at St. Rose's Home, there are few spaces for family members to be alone with patients in privacy.

Rosary Hill, the newest of the three buildings, offers more family spaces and more variety than do either of the other two. However, Calvary has also responded to the need for more family and volunteer participation and is planning a 12-million-dollar addition to increase support services as well as the kind and number of family areas to be provided. An important difference in their facility, stressed by the Calvary administration, is the physical condition of Calvary patients, as opposed to St. Rose or Rosary Hill patients. Calvary claims their patients are often more severely debilitated than those at St. Rose's or Rosary Hill. This means, for Calvary, a different priority of support areas, increasing the need for specialists in ostomy and radiation therapy, and a different configuration for patient bedrooms. Calvary believes that their use of single-bed rooms in an intensive-care arrangement with the central nurses' station is necessary for these more severely debilitated patients. They feel that private rooms are necessary to provide the privacy and special treatments that their culturally heterogeneous, urban, and severely ill population needs.

Rosary Hill, St. Rose's and Calvary differ in one other very important way. Rosary Hill and St. Rose's are for indigent patients, for those who have exhausted their financial means. They receive no state or federal reimbursements and are not bound by insurance or Health Care Financing Administration regulations. Both are state licensed as skilled nursing facilities. Calvary, as an acute-care hospital for the terminally ill, receives sizable reimbursements from Medicare and others; the original facility was a Hill-Burton Hospital. (Under the Hill-Burton legislation, hospitals that received federal funds for construction had to dedicate a percentage of beds to patients who could not afford to pay for medical care.) This very different reimbursement situation is modified by the fact that all three facilities are Catholic organizations with substantial endowments. Calvary is sponsored by the Department of Health and Hospitals of the Catholic Charities of the Archdiocese of New York and has been favored with donated land, for example. The reimbursement situation has not affected the capital expenditures as much as the operating funds. It seems that the priorities of the caregivers have given form to the major architectural decisions and differences.

For purposes of architectural analysis, the two newest facilities, Rosary Hill and Calvary, are best compared. Calvary Hospital has a total bed component of 200, making it the largest terminal care facility in the United States. In contrast, Rosary Hill has a total population of seventy-two, less than half as large. Calvary and Rosary Hill are more similar in the number of patient beds under supervision by one nursing station, with twenty-five for Calvary and eighteen for Rosary Hill. Calvary has single rooms for all its patients, while Rosary Hill, more in keeping with the tradition of hospice care, has both 4-bed rooms and singles. In addition, both hospitals have isolation bedrooms, representing 2 percent to 4 percent of the total rooms. In patient rooms sizes, Calvary provides approximately 180 square feet per patient, including toilet, whereas Rosary Hill provides about 155 square feet, divided into their three types of bedding situations. Single rooms at Rosary Hill have about 190 square feet, and the four-bed rooms average an approximate 130 square feet per bed.

In terms of dayrooms on the patient floors, Calvary has 940 square feet per fifty patients for a total of 18.8 square feet per patient. Rosary Hill's dayrooms have 347 square feet for each group of eighteen patients, for a total of 19.17 square feet per patient. However, the dayrooms at Calvary represent the only family areas on the patient floors, in contrast to Rosary Hill, which also has kitchenettes, a family private room, and nearby multipurpose rooms. Moreover, Rosary Hill has provided other daycare areas for the patients in the bedroom areas, including a 440-square-foot recreation room, beauty parlor, treatment rooms, and a medical library. Calvary Hospital has patient and family areas on other floors, including the coffee shop and their multipurpose auditorium.

For large gatherings, Calvary's multipurpose room has been judged by its staff to be too small, at roughly 9.5 square feet per patient. Rosary Hill provides 16 square feet per patient and may better serve for large group assemblies. Rosary Hill also has a very large solarium and roof terrace for group assembly and connection to nature, the solarium having 16 square feet per patient, and both together providing about 40 square feet per patient. Calvary has little indoor/outdoor space, except for the coffee shop and its connection to the large outdoor terrace, much used for celebrations in warm weather. It is the largest gathering area available at Calvary, the terrace itself providing over 50 square feet (gross) per patient, although much is occupied by planters and steps. The coffee shop is an additional 8 square feet per patient, for less formal gathering by the more ambulatory patients and their family and staff.

Another measure of the two facilities can be seen in the comparison of their food-preparation and delivery areas. Calvary has pantry kitchens on each floor, helping to decentralize food preparation and provide hot, custom-prepared meals for each patient. Taken together with the kitchen areas, the total square footage is 1,900 for the pantries and 4,100 for the central kitchen, including staff cafeteria preparation, equaling 6,000 square feet. This has been found to be inadequate for the meals of over 500 persons; additional kitchen space will be added in the proposed remodeling. The space averages out to approximately 30 square feet per patient. Compare this figure with the kitchen area in Rosary Hill Home at 2,270 square feet and the four kitchenettes at 760 square feet, equaling approximately 42 square feet per patient. As the convent at Rosary Hill has its own kitchen, Rosary Hill's main kitchen need accommodate only patients, families, and a small percentage of staff. In contrast, Calvary's kitchen (30 square feet per patient) serves many more meals than does Rosary Hill's kitchen (42 square feet per patient). The patient areas at Rosary Hill are similar in form to one another, but provide a variety of accommodations, shortened and turned corridors, and vistas. Calvary's patient floors are all nearly identical except for decoration and colors; the corridor areas are dominated by the nurses' station with institutional linoleum and shiny surfaces.

Main entry areas at both facilities are welcoming and comfortable. The coffee shop at Calvary provides a comfortable, cheerful room for waiting and conversation. Rosary Hill's entry is celebrated with a formal open stair and seating areas, as well as their Heritage Room (where an exhibit of the history of the order is displayed). The main entry itself is at the opening of a Y-shaped intersection and is marked by the open stairwell and the large solarium and outdoor patio above. Calvary's entry is a chopped-off corner at the back of the V-shaped building, marked with an overhung drive-in area and the location of contiguous pedestrian and ambulance entries.

Calvary and Rosary Hill differ considerably in the style and appearance of their facilities. The Rosary Hill inpatient unit is detailed in mission style and is part of a campus that includes the convent and the older mission-style church. The whole facility is sited on parklike grounds in a rural community above the river. Calvary is a monolithic red brick building with no surface ornamentation, located in a hospital and near a train yard area of the Bronx. The decision to have the courtyard face south, thereby turning its back onto the street, was intentional; the courtyard is the private amenity of the hospital and the center of its outdoor views and activities.

Medium Freestanding Hospice Facilities (New Construction).

In this group fall two hospices, the prototypical and experimental Connecticut Hospice, constructed in 1980 for over 3 million dollars, and the newly constructed (completed June 1983) Nathan Adelson Hospice in Las Vegas, Nevada, built for more than 2.5 million dollars. These two facilities are the only examples of freestanding hospices in the United States that were constructed and planned from scratch at the time of survey; they also provide interesting contrast in organization and considerable material for postoccupancy evaluations. Both hospice groups initially provided home care only and had significant experience with hospice patients before their facilities were designed. Both draw from a well-educated and sophisticated population and have attempted to create a new kind of health-care facility.

Nathan Adelson is located on the University of Nevada campus, whereas the Connecticut Hospice chose to locate in the suburban neighborhood of Branford. Both facilities were designed with quality of environment foremost in mind, a connection to nature that was immediate and convenient, and with the family and patient as the focus of concern and care. Significant differences in the plans of the two facilities are the result of such factors as bedroom population and organization, size, climate, and office space.

Specifically, the Connecticut Hospice, firmly espousing traditional hospice values, has accommodated most patients in four-patient rooms, whereas Nathan Adelson provides single-bed rooms arranged in clusters. Connecticut offers some single rooms, for variety; Nathan Adelson seeks to provide contrast and variety by decorating the single cluster groups in several different decorative schemes. Nathan Adelson has a smaller inpatient population than does the Connecticut Hospice, with a total of twenty beds versus the Connecticut Hospice's forty-four. Moreover, although both facilities have outdoor areas that are convenient to patient bedrooms and family areas, Nathan Adelson has incorporated a large central courtyard, suitable for its hotter and dryer Nevada climate, and has provided a greater number and variety of outdoor areas.

Nathan Adelson has a total of approximately 20,000 square feet or a gross of 1,000 square feet per patient. Connecticut, with its larger patient population and infrastructure, still has approximately the same figure, with about 995 square feet per patient. The addition of outdoor terraces at both units again suggests parity, at 1,088 square feet per patient for Connecticut and 1,075 square feet per patient at Nathan Adelson. The units differ, however, in space allocation. Each bedroom at Nathan Adelson Hospice has its own bathroom, with handicap shower, toilet, and sink, for a total of 280 square feet per patient. Connecticut's four-bed patient rooms brings their total to 203 square feet per patient, but the addition of the central bath and tub rooms at Connecticut brings the figure up to 225 square feet per patient.

At Nathan Adelson, patient and family areas combined total an approximate figure of 550 square feet per patient. Connecticut has a lower figure of about 400 square feet per patient. These figures represent the difference in bedroom space allocation and the provision of large group space at Nathan Adelson. Kitchen facilities at the two hospices also show contrast. Nathan Adelson provides one area of 350 square feet, or 17.5 square feet per patient. Connecticut supplies a much greater proportion of kitchen space, about 32.5 square feet per patient, which is much closer to the larger hospitals. Nathan Adelson is not yet complete, so this discrepancy cannot yet be evaluated in operation. The dining and serving area at Nathan Adelson, the Grill, is approximately 480 square feet, whereas that at Connecticut is 1,364 square feet, with 918 square feet of seating. The kitchen space proportions are 24 square feet per patient at Nathan Adelson and 52 square feet per patient for Connecticut. However, Nathan Adelson is expecting more dining at their country kitchen areas.

Connecticut designated a greater proportion of its interior to offices than did Nathan Adelson, especially in home-care office space. Total office space at Connecticut is approximately 149 square feet per patient, while Nathan Adelson has a much smaller 63 square feet per patient, for administrative offices and volunteer and conference areas.

Gardens at Nathan Adelson are extensive and greatly varied. These include their courtyard, the smaller enclosed greenhouse, the meditation garden, and bedroom patios, for an approximate total of 6,420 square feet. The Connecticut Hospice has two terraces, the greenhouse corridors, and the dining terrace, for a total of 6,774 square feet; close in total overall space but widely different at 321 square feet per patient and 154 square feet per patient, respectively. However, both figures allow for considerable outdoor gathering space. Nathan Adelson's courtyard has 150 square feet per patient and Connecticut's has 50 square feet per patient. Both facilities display outdoor fountains in their plans.

Indoors, all patients can gather in several areas at both facilities. Nathan Adelson has a small meditation room with 300 total square feet, or 15 square feet per patient. At the Connecticut Hospice, religious services can be attended by patients in the adjoining commons room, with 21 square feet per patient. The greenhouse at Nathan Adelson is another large gathering room, with a total of 800 square feet, or 40 square feet per patient. Also provided at Nathan Adelson is a large multipurpose room of 465 square feet, or 23 square feet per patient. Connecticut has two large living rooms for gathering. Each is approximately 1,048 square feet, or 24 square feet per patient. Together, they provide 48 square feet per patient for smaller gatherings at two locations off the main spine.

From this data, it might be suggested that Nathan Adelson may have problems with too small a kitchen and tight allocation of office space. The comparative data does little to suggest a right and wrong approach in this type of facility, however. The most significant difference between Nathan Adelson and Connecticut is not in space allocation, but in the ordering of the spaces and the style and appearance of the buildings. The generous family areas at Nathan Adelson, like the courtyard and greenhouse, may be overlarge for a facility of this kind and remain mostly empty, but they may instead foster more activity and new uses as the hospice changes over time. Nathan Adelson has some adaptability by virtue of its generous provision of family space, more so than the Connecticut Hospice was able to provide. It remains to be seen whether the country kitchens will work to encourage communication and comfort and promote nonabandonment of the patient or whether they will simply function as another threshold to cross to the private rooms beyond. This arrangement certainly adds to the corridor length and distance from the central nurses' areas to the patient rooms.

Reference should be made to the different typological ordering of the two hospices. Connecticut can be read as a variant on the traditional hospital cross-ward pavilion plan; each of the two wings meet at a central seating and observation area. The multibed and single rooms are placed along a double-loaded corridor, but are arranged in a linear fashion rather than across from one another. The provision of two corridors per wing, one for service functions and the other (the greenhouse hall) for family, patient, and staff traffic, attempts to separate the institutional and homelike functions of the facility. The nurses' station at the living room is small and does not overwhelm the living or patient bed areas, thereby minimizing its controlling image and function. This was done intentionally to deinstitutionalize the nursing station and to emphasize the need for nurses to work the floors rather than remain in the nursing areas. In use, however, these areas have been judged too small for the necessary activities of the staff, although their location has not been considered a drawback.

In appearance, the Connecticut Hospice has drawn from the local suburban school, using brick and wallboard for wall surfaces, and an elevation and a plan reminiscent of the same cross-ward, single-story pavilion commonly used for hospitals, schools, nursing homes, and so on. The use of such durable but natural materials as brick and wood, the provision of outdoor areas, the large expanses of glass and skylights, and the considerable attention to finishing details and ornament suggest a first-class institutional building rather than a typical long-term-care facility. This use of an institutional motif, albeit a suburban school one, was intentional; it is plain that this is a building housing forty-four hospice beds. As Paul Goldberger commented, in his *New York Times* review of the building:

> . . . had the budget been unlimited, one wonders if this building should have been permitted to take on a more residential feeling anyway. Perhaps not; this is, in the end, an institution, not a house. It is a place of comfort for the dying, but not a place of illusion; to have pretended that this building was a house and not a hospital might well have been patronizing to its occupants (Goldberger 1980).

The suburban school appearance of the hospice continues to the interior, where the architecture becomes a backdrop for the personalization encouraged by the caregivers and their hospice philosophy. The building is decorated with blond woods, woven fabrics, and carpet, and is designed as a stage for activities. A sort of neutral Scandinavian style predominates. Over time, personalization may increase the homelike feeling of the hospice, as at St. Christopher's, where hand-crocheted afghans have contributed to a homelike atmosphere.

In contrast to the wing pavilions of Connecticut Hospice, Nathan Adelson has, perhaps unconsciously, adopted a variation on another great hospital scheme from the past—the courtyard plan. A similar organization can be found in the early Carthusian monasteries; it is part of the urban solution to the Ospedale Giustinian Di Venezia and the ordering of the modern Crittendon Nursing Home in Arkansas, among others (Weiss, 1969). The courtyard was, appropriately, part of the earliest hospital hospices, such as the second Hospital of the Knights of Rhodes, built 1440–89, and is a delightful solution to modern hospice design. Another new hospice facility, St. Anne's in Little Hulton, Manchester, is also organized around a court; there, however, the hallways are double-loaded with bedrooms away from the court, and the interior courtyard has a different relation to the patient rooms from that at Nathan Adelson (*Arch. Journal*, 1979, 169: 309). Like the early monastery plan, the Nathan Adelson Hospice has a single-loaded courtyard, defining the communal outdoor space and allowing for private patios on the other side of the bedrooms.

Nathan Adelson has modified the classic courtyard design with clustered living centers, similar to those used in university housing during the 1960s. These clusters provide a private living/dining room for the families and visitors of each group of four patients, as well as another gradient of privacy for the patient rooms themselves. Connection of these "country kitchens" to the hallway and courtyard beyond, as well as visual connections through the courtyard to the nurses' areas and active spaces, is designed to integrate the patient bedrooms with the rest of the facility. In order to minimize any abandonment of the patient made possible by a strung-out privacy gradient of this type, a small nurses' alcove has been added to the country-kitchen area. In this way, if family and friends are not present or the patient is too debilitated to leave the bed, a nurse is nearby. Inpatient services at Nathan Adelson are located on two sides of the courtyard in order to stimulate activity, to be viewed from the country kitchens, and to encourage circulation about the court.

As Gerald Moffit, the architect, describes the hospice:

> Since the basic psychological thrust of the hospice is to create a homelike atmosphere, it follows that the architectural response be consistent with the progressive domestic design practices of the region: What may be termed the western organic style, employing a long, low, horizontal building profile; familiar residential materials and roof pitches; dispersed conditions, patios, solar orientation with passive energy techniques,

landscape berms, individual scale are used (Gerald Moffit, Nevada Archetronics, in letter to the author).

Inside, the diversity missing from bedroom accommodations will be supplied by a complementary but unique decor in each cluster, designed in contemporary, colonial, Victorian, provincial, and traditional settings. It is hoped that this decoration will add a residential atmosphere and personalization to the cluster areas, in contrast to Connecticut's background interior design.

As Nathan Adelson was not yet complete at the time of this writing, an evaluation comparing the actual functioning of these two freestanding and prototypical hospices could not be undertaken. Such a study might help to resolve the divergence of opinion on bedroom populations and the relative efficacy of the cluster design for patient, staff, family, and visitors alike. Differences of view notwithstanding, the emphasis on light, choice, and community in both hospice designs embodies the hospice philosophy in bricks and mortar.

Medium Freestanding Hospice Facilities (Remodeled)

In this group fall two existing hospice inpatient units, the Hospice of Cincinnati and the Hospice of Northern Virginia; a planned facility, the Hospice of the Good Shepherd; and the now closed Hillhaven in Arizona. Because the hospices of Northern Virginia and the Good Shepherd have more in common with each other than with Cincinnati or Hillhaven, they will be discussed together; both are examples of remodeled school buildings in suburban locations. The Hospice of Cincinnati, in contrast, was remodeled from an unused nurses' residence that was part of a hospital complex in the urban center of Cincinnati. Hillhaven was a partially complete skilled nursing facility when it entered the National Cancer Institute pilot program and was remodeled for hospice inpatient care and, thus, shares some of the problems of the Cincinnati remodel design.

All four facilities have a medium inpatient population. Northern Virginia and Good Shepherd each have fifteen inpatient beds, there are eighteen beds at Cincinnati, and Hillhaven had thirty-nine. All have family areas; three of the four have ground-floor locations for patient beds. The four facilities have emphasized the use of natural lighting whenever possible, and all have attempted, with varying degrees of success, a homelike atmosphere. Each hospice provides a variety of bedroom accommodations, including single and double-bed rooms at Hillhaven and Cincinnati, single and four-bed rooms at Good Shepherd and Northern Virginia.

A comparison of the two remodeled health-related facilities, Hillhaven and Cincinnati, points out the difficulty in modifying institutional space. In most cases, the bedrooms are located across from one another on a double-loaded corridor, which is the arrangement most commonly associated with institutional design. Modification of this design, while possible, is difficult and costly and has the disadvantage of immediately cutting down on the number of existing bedrooms and thereby decreasing incentive for extensive remodeling. Cincinnati's remodeling was originally proposed by the landlord as an economical design, because it retained most of the existing walls. This proved to be less economical than had been thought, because of the extensive life-safety equipment and heating, ventilation, and air conditioning that needed to be added. As a result, the family areas and nurses' station on the patient floor, located on double-loaded corridors, are cramped and not at all homelike. The main office areas and family rooms on the lower floor do not provide a mix of function and make duplication of space necessary, as in the kitchenettes, for example, and the family rooms on both floors. Unfortunately, although the lower floor has many amply proportioned areas for family and meeting space, families are usually on the patient floor and so underuse these areas.

At Hillhaven, the patient areas remained grouped around a double-loaded corridor design, and one patient room was eliminated to provide space for the East Lounge. However, their double-loaded corridor is modified by the ground-floor location as well as the mix of all functions on one floor. Kitchen, chapel, office areas, and the outdoors are not far from the patient rooms. The variety of family and group gathering areas, such as the library, East Lounge, chapel, transition room, and activity room, are not substitutes for one another but allow a range of alternative areas for socialization and privacy. The outdoor patios and ground-floor location allow light and nature to reach the patients and promote a residential atmosphere. Unfortunately, Cincinnati is located on two above-ground floors in an urban area and has a firewall on one side of the hospice. Adding this firewall necessitated placing metal louvers over the windows that restrict light and view on one whole side of the hospice. The family areas on the other side share some view; one has been designated the garden room, with large windows, plants, and patio furniture. However, contact with the ground is restricted and absent from most of this scheme.

Perhaps the greatest difference between these two facilities is the entry. At Hillhaven, one enters through a garden, past patient windows and into a common activity area with kitchen, activity room, lobby, and physical therapy areas, then down a corridor, past the offices, chapel, and nurses' station to patient rooms. At Cincinnati, the entry is a newly constructed tower with stairs and elevator that lead to the office floor or directly up to the patient areas. This entrance is institutional and must be monitored by a tower security system.

In terms of space, Hillhaven and Cincinnati provide 108 square feet per patient and 126 square feet per patient respectively, for bedrooms, without including W.C. areas. Hillhaven provides more W.C. space so that if the baths are included, Hillhaven has 141 square feet per patient and Cincinnati 140 square feet per patient.

At Hillhaven, the family areas include the activity room, East Lounge, library lounge, kitchen, chapel and transition/viewing room, allowing a total of 1,962 square feet, or 50 square feet per patient. At Cincinnati, the family areas include the family lounge, the reading or garden room, the third-floor family room, and the two kitchenettes, for a total of 890 square feet, or 49 square feet per patient. Hillhaven adds the rose-garden patio at 670 square feet or 17 square feet per patient and the entry area, for approximately 1,200 square feet of additional garden area. Cincinnati does have an outdoor area at the base of the entry tower, surrounded by a cyclone fence and decorated by volunteers, but it is not at all convenient to the patient beds and is not part of the calculations. At the Hospice of Cincinnati, the kitchen is off the unit, but kitchenettes are available on the unit for nutrition breaks and gathering. At Hillhaven, the kitchen apparently functioned for patient meals as well as for the family cooking that is the hallmark of hospice care. A great difference in space allocation is conspicuous in the office areas. Hillhaven has a total of 1,694 square feet of administrative and office space, or 43 square feet per patient. The Hospice of Cincinnati has a total of 2,056 square feet of administrative and other offices, for a total of 114 square feet per patient. Should the patient load at Cincinnati be increased by the addition of another floor, another eighteen patients could be serviced by the same office areas, thereby decreasing the office proportion to a more moderate 57 square feet per patient. The Hospice of Cincinnati has a sizable homecare department of over 770 square feet, which Hillhaven apparently did not share. The homecare team at Cincinnati and provision of offices for fund raising and other volunteer activities seem to make up the main difference in the allocation of office space in these two hospices.

Hillhaven is no longer in use as a hospice, but Dale Lupu and Deborah Monahan provided us with some rare data in their postoccupancy evaluation of the facility. They concluded (Lupu and Monahan, 1980) that the patient room is a focus of much activity and must serve three purposes: it must be a personalized bedroom; it must be a medical support room; and it must be a visiting room for family and friends. Hospices should also provide symbolic areas, such as the chapel and viewing room, and a connection to nature. The overnight accommodations for family and friends at the patient's bedside or in separate lounges were very much needed and appreciated. Perhaps the most interesting data in Lupu and Monahan's study concerned the single/double room controversy. Patients reported that they preferred private rooms, but those who had roommates did not object to that situation. As Dale Lupu and Deborah Monahan report,

> The critical factor seems to be not whether there are one, two, or four beds per room, but whether the design of the room allows the patient privacy as desired and offers comfortable accommodations to visitors (Lupu and Monahan, 1980).

At Hillhaven, most patients spent the majority of their time in their rooms and appreciated dining with small groups on special occasions. The kitchen, family room, chapel, and gardens contributed much to the well-being of the families and staff. On the other hand, the floor plan, with its separation of social spaces and patient rooms, was not appreciated. It was reported that "most staff and volunteers preferred a circular floor plan giving patient rooms direct access to an activity or social area" and it was found that overall, the inpatient environment was important to the users of the building:

> . . . [patients, family, and staff] noticed comfortable and homelike aspects of the decor, they complained about the unsatisfactory aspects, such as the cramped staff lounge and hard-to-find entrances, and they used

general principles such as maximizing patient choice and providing opportunities for privacy when evaluating the environment (Lupu and Monahan, 1980).

Hospice of Northern Virginia and the soon-to-be-remodeled Hospice of the Good Shepherd provide very different solutions to the remodeled freestanding facility from that of Cincinnati and Hillhaven, as they are located in previously used school buildings. The most obvious advantages of converting a school into a hospice involve the inherent flexibility of a nonmedical building. Although schools are often designed in a double-loaded organization, they are not full of single-patient rooms, nor do they already have nurses' stations. Moreover, school buildings are accepted residential-scale institutions that offer a nonmedical image and a positive association for the neighborhood.

The Hospices of Northern Virginia and the Good Shepherd are designed with a smaller inpatient population of fifteen beds each. They have taken advantage of the flexibility of changing uses by providing both multibed and single rooms. Northern Virginia provides 189 square feet per patient for single bed rooms (including w.c.) and 160 square feet per patient for multibed rooms, for an average total of 166 square feet per patient bed. Good Shepherd is planning to provide 226 square feet per patient for single-bed rooms (including w.c.) and 163 square feet per patient for their total of 175 square feet per patient bed average. These rooms are interspersed among family and gathering areas, but have nearby nurses' stations. Northern Virginia has a family room, kitchenette, and meditation and conference rooms interwoven with the patient bedrooms, for an approximate total of 1,530 square feet of social spaces, or 102 square feet per patient. The Hospice of the Good Shepherd has a large living room with a large sun room, in addition to a family private room, family room/parlor combination, a social-work conference room, childcare rooms, and a large combined dining area, providing a total of over 2,739 square feet of social space, making an average of almost 183 square feet per patient total. If the sun porch is added to this figure, the total amount of gathering area space is over 225 square feet per patient, the largest amount for any hospice facility. Much of this space is multipurpose and can be set aside for various education and staff functions, family gatherings and celebrations, daily dining, private meetings, as well as religious services and private meditation.

The largest gathering area at Northern Virginia is the family living room, with 725 square feet in total, or 48 square feet per patient. Hospice of the Good Shepherd is planning their living room and sun room combination to have a total of 1,598 square feet, or 106 square feet per patient. Northern Virginia has one multipurpose room of 225 square feet, used for exam and lab activities and as a staff retreat room, located near the bedroom area. Good Shepherd provides a small physical therapy room with 80 square feet, for similar functions. The nurses' station at Northern Virginia, which includes a medication room and counter space, has a total of 155 square feet. Good Shepherd plans a nurses' station with a dictation area of 200 square feet and an additional medication room and utility storage area (100 square feet).

Office space for the two facilities is generous, as both have large home-care staff and volunteer programs. Northern Virginia gives over almost half of its total area to offices and kitchen, and the Good Shepherd is planning even more office and support space. Northern Virgina has a total office area of 2,390 square feet, including reception, administration, coordinating activities, facilities operation, and staff dining, equivalent to 160 square feet per patient. Good Shepherd has office areas for reception, home care, administration, coordinating activities, as well as the staff lounge located on the second and ground floors, for a total of 5,330 square feet, or 355 square feet per patient. Much of this space is devoted to the home-care component, without which the figure is approximately 3,237 square feet, or 215 square feet per patient.

Kitchen facilities at the two remodeled school hospices can also be contrasted. Northern Virginia has a kitchen of 600 square feet, designed to serve about 100 meals per day, and a dining area of 510 square feet. The kitchen space breaks down into 40 square feet per patient, which is similar to the kitchen facilities at the larger Rosary Hill and Connecticut hospices. The Hospice of the Good Shepherd has a total kitchen area of approximately 1,368 square feet with a dining room for the unit of 350 square feet and staff lounge of 220 square feet. The kitchen area is, therefore, more than twice that of Northern Virginia, with a space allocation of over 91 square feet per patient.

These large space allocations at the Hospice of the Good Shepherd are a function of at least five factors. First, it was determined that the patient beds would be best located together on the main floor for community and supervision reasons, and this limited the number of patient beds for the facility as a whole. Second, the size of the initial school building made possible generous allocation of spaces; the Hospice of the Good Shepherd simply had much more space to work with than Northern Virginia did. Third, the hospice had operated a large and successful home-care program and wanted room for growth, education, and organization. The fourth factor for the generous allotment of family and support space is a response to the increased need for meeting space and food provision anticipated by the inclusion of apartments. These apartments can contract for such services as meals, transportation, and laundry service from the adjacent hospice so that these other functions can be integrated with the hospice's other care activities. Inhouse physician suites will be convenient and accessible to the apartment dwellers, who will most likely be elderly and somewhat frail. Last, and perhaps most important, the HGS staff made a considerable survey of existing inpatient hospices in order to determine their own architectural space needs and priorities and has made an impressive effort to ward off the problems they observed at other locations. Therefore, space allocations at HGS are more generous and more adaptable than at any other hospice inpatient facility surveyed in this study. This flexibility together with the other services provided in conjunction with the hospice will make the Hospice of the Good Shepherd important to watch as a significant contributor to the hospice inpatient environment.

The Hospice of Northern Virginia, on the other hand, had a much smaller building to convert, with the same estimated need for beds. They also have a milder climate and can expect to use their outdoor spaces for assembly over a much greater proportion of the year. Hospice of Northern Virginia has added its own innovations to hospice inpatient design, especially in the areas of mulitpurpose space and entryways. Northern Virginia has attempted to resolve the difficult entry problems of hospice care by providing two main entries with different greeting areas. The family and staff entrance has a reception room and is near the parking lots, but it is not the formal front door of the building. The patient entrance, the building's formal entrance, is at grade for ambulance and bed entry and is served by reception from the nurses' station and family room. In this way, the hospice has provided a dignified entrance for the patient and separated the institutional functions (staff and family entrance) from the residential functions (patient entrance). Northern Virginia has also added to hospice design by incorporating a variety of spaces for multiple functions, thus allowing for change and growth and increasing the adaptability of a small building.

Comparison of the four freestanding remodel facilities shows clearly that Cincinnati and Hillhaven have less than half the family and social gathering space of Northern Virginia and the Hospice of the Good Shepherd. The patient bedroom space, too, is more generous at the remodeled school hospices, which provide beds in four-bed and single rooms. At both Northern Virginia and the proposed Good Shepherd, the bedrooms have a table and chairs for conversations, gathering, eating, and reading. At Cincinnati and Hillhaven, there was little room for these activities in the patient rooms.

Cincinnati had no large gathering space for celebrations. All the other facilities had some accommodation: Hillhaven had the activity room, with 23 square feet per patient; Northern Virginia had the living room, with 48 square feet per patient; Good Shepherd had the phenomenal living and sun room, with 106 square feet per patient. In addition, three of the four freestanding facilities had some accommodation for meditation; only Cincinnati seems to have no provision for that use. However, both the Hospice of the Good Shepherd and Northern Virginia have multiuse meditation areas and no formal transition or viewing room, whereas Hillhaven did have both a chapel and viewing room and found them both to be important.

Remodeling to provide a homelike environment was much more successful among the retrofit schools. Nonmedical but institutional buildings seem to provide more flexible design and decor than the adapted medical building types, though the overall organization may not be terribly different. To a large extent, the presence of numerous repetitively sized and populated single- and double-bed rooms adds to the difficulty of a homelike hospice remodeling. When these rooms are found together with a predominant nurses' station and the institutional separation of function, entries, and finishes, the retrofit is not a convincing modification of the original health-care facility.

Medium Parent-Based Hospice Units (Remodeled).

The four inpatient hospices represented in this section are all parts of larger hospitals. The parent hospitals have other specialized units, such as skilled nursing facilities, psychiatric units, or rehabilitation units. All are located in heavily populated regions; this sample includes facilities representing New York and California. Cabrini and Mercy Hospice are both part of a New York State demonstration project, and Cabrini is also part of the twenty-six-member Health Care Financing Administration demonstration. Kaiser Permanente Norwalk is one of the hospice inpatient units in the Kaiser (Health Maintenance Organization) system; they also have hospice beds at Hayward and in scatterbed locations. Pinecrest Hospice is not listed in the latest update of the National Hospice Organization's directory and may have ceased functioning since the compendium data was gathered in 1982.

Cabrini is the only hospice in this group not located on the ground floor. It is situated on a remodeled ward in the older section of the hospital, on the fifth floor. Mercy Hospital is not in the larger facility, but is instead located in a building with psychiatric and rehabilitation units on the campus of the parent hospital. Kaiser Permanente and Pinecrest are both loacted in wings on the ground floor of existing facilities; Kaiser is associated with an acute-care unit, whereas Pinecrest is a wing of a skilled nursing facility and on the campus with the larger acute-care facility.

All have a moderate number of inpatient beds, from fifteen at Cabrini, to seventeen at Kaiser Norwalk, eighteen at Mercy, and twenty-six beds at Pinecrest. All provide both single- and double-bed rooms and none has any larger groupings, although doubles at Kaiser share a doorway and some visibility. Although these four facilities represent the most autonomous of the parent-based units, none has its own kitchen facilities and most share other functions also, such as laundry and mechanical facilities. Most of these hospices also contract with visiting nurses for home-care visits; only Kaiser Norwalk has home-care offices. However, all of the other functions of hospice inpatient care are provided on the unit and most of these have a special, separate hospice entrance.

All four hospices have outdoor garden space and three out of four—Mercy, Pinecrest, and Kaiser Permanente—have chapel space on the unit itself. This occurs despite the radically different climates of Manhattan and Los Angeles, and the private and Catholic sponsorships of the hospices. All provide family space with a kitchenette, all allow the family to stay overnight if necessary, all have separate nurses' stations for the hospice patients, and all have a special decor.

Patient bedroom areas vary, from 88 square feet per patient at Cabrini, 93 square feet per patient at Kaiser, to 160 square feet per patient at Mercy, and 171 square feet per patient at Pinecrest. To some extent, these figures are greater for Pinecrest because that facility has proportionally more w.c. area included in the bedroom space figures.

Family space varies considerably in these four remodelings. Cabrini has a sun room and active lounge for a total of approximately 385 square feet, or 26 square feet per patient. Kaiser, in contrast, has a dayroom and family/guest private room, as well as chapel and viewing room, for a total of 1,200 square feet, or 71 square feet per patient. Mercy Hospital Hospice provides a family room and chapel and a family private room for a total of 1,118 square feet, or 62 square feet per patient. Pinecrest has a small family room, dining area, and chapel for a total of 730 square feet, or 28 square feet per patient. The three hospices with designed chapel space have similar-size units. Kaiser has a chapel of 220 square feet, whereas Pinecrest's is 158 square feet and Mercy's is the largest, at 238 square feet. However, Kaiser also has a transition/viewing room to double the total space, while Mercy's chapel has a wall separating it from the family room, which is removable for larger services and provides a total area of 969 square feet. Cabrini does not have a chapel on the unit, but the hospital has a chapel and services are also provided in the pavilion in the sixteenth-floor cafeteria.

Comparison of the office areas is as follows: Cabrini has a total of eight offices with 679 square feet, 45 square feet per patient; Mercy provides 510 square feet, 28 square feet per patient; Pinecrest has 246 square feet, 9 square feet per patient; and Kaiser has 1,115, or 66 square feet per patient, including staff conference space. Nurses' stations differ in size and functions in these units also. Cabrini's nurses' station (72 square feet) is located in the middle of the bedrooms and provides nonabandonment, medication, and location of charting. Mercy's nurses' station, at 193 square feet, is also the focus of the unit entry and provides a central check-in point as well as nursing support. Kaiser's nurses' station is located at the crossing of the unit and official entry into hospice functions and it is large at 410 square feet, though it shares the function of greeting with the waiting and reception area. Pinecrest has a large nurses' station for greeting

and supervision, although it shares this function with the family rooms across the hall and, at 424 square feet, still is proportionately only 16 square feet per patient.

The difficulties of remodeling medical space for hospice use are evident in these four units. Family areas have been carved out of groupings of patient rooms or existing dayroom areas. Only Mercy hired an architectural firm to remodel its hospice and was constrained by the existing structural system from combining bedrooms. Mercy's family and chapel areas were actually the nursery areas of a maternity ward. Kaiser Permanente kept one wing of patient bedrooms and a nurses' station intact and placed the new uses, such as the chapel, in another wing. Cabrini used the existing dayroom, adding adjoining areas for family rooms, and kept the existing bedrooms intact, except for the conversion of two bedrooms into an office area. Pinecrest was able only to carve out some area at the entry of the unit and set aside a patient room at the end of a long double-loaded corridor for the chapel. However, all the units tried their best to modify the environment. New furnishings and finishes were added, family rooms and kitchenettes were set aside, as were sacred spaces and connections to nature. Kaiser has extensive patio and outdoor space and Cabrini has decorated and planted a roof garden visible from the unit. Pinecrest has a large central patio area. However, Mercy Hospice was unable to add a convenient outdoor area because of the expense this would have necessitated; an outdoor room was to be provided and had been designed in the original plans.

Small Parent-Based Hospice Units (Remodeled).

In this group are six hospice inpatient units, representing the northeast, north central, and southern states; private, Catholic and Lutheran hospitals; and an intermediate-care-facility apartment complex. Also represented in this group is one Health Care Financing Administration demonstration hospice, Bellin in Wisconsin, and one New York State demonstration hospice, St. Peter's Hospital Hospice in Albany. The intermediate care facility (ICF) unit is Clover Hospice in Maine, and the remaining hospices are Lutheran Hospital Hospice in Illinois, Riverside Hospice in Virgina, and Sacred Heart in Wisconsin. They range in inpatient beds from five patient beds at Clover and seven at Riverside to ten at Bellin, Lutheran Hospital Hospice, Sacred Heart, and St. Peter's Hospice. Three of the remodelings were conducted by in-house teams of caregivers and hospital staff. The other three had either architectural, engineering, or interior design consultants.

Only one of these hospice conversions, Clover Hospice, was a ground-floor remodeling. The rest were remodelings of above-ground floors: Bellin on the second floor; Riverside and Sacred Heart on the fifth floors; Lutheran Pathway on the seventh; and St. Peter's on the fourth and fifth floors of a pavilion. These floors were chosen because they were adaptable for other uses at the time, not because they were above ground. Indeed, several of the proposed conversion plans listed a ground-floor location as far more desirable. Two, Clover and Lutheran, had convenient gardens; the others emphasized indoor gardening.

Only two of the hospices provide multibed (larger than double) rooms. Bellin has both single and four-bed rooms and St. Peter's has three-bed as well as single rooms. Clover and Lutheran Pathway provide only single rooms, Sacred Heart has only doubles, and Riverside has both singles and doubles. A list of their respective bedroom areas follows:

Hospice	Bedroom Area	Bedroom and W.C., Shower	Total Square Footage per Patient
Bellin	1,394 sf	1,624 sf	162.4
Clover	650 sf	802 sf	160.4
Lutheran Pathway	3,000 sf	3,177 sf	317.7
Riverside	916 sf	1,088 sf	155.4
Sacred Heart	1,400 sf	N/A	140.0
St. Peter's	1,644 sf	1,792 sf	179.2

Bedrooms at Lutheran Pathway are much larger than those at any of the other facilities—in fact, they are twice the size. They were originally double-bed rooms; increasing the square footage per patient was possible only by changing the occupancy of these existing rooms. Remodeling at St. Peter's allowed for a moderate increase in bedroom area space per patient, but walls and such were moved in this more extensive remodeling effort.

Each of these small hospice units has its own nurses' station and family areas. Family areas vary in use and disposition as well as in size, but all six have a general family lounge and kitchenette. Family space on the unit itself is sometimes augmented by additional multipurpose areas shared with other units or other uses. Total available family space is listed for each unit as follows:

Hospice	Family Room	Unit Family Areas	Total Square Footage per Patient
Bellin	448 sf	705 sf	70.5
Clover	360 sf	360 sf (1,450 total)	290.0
Lutheran Pathway	600 sf	1,164 sf	116.4
Riverside	229 sf	521 sf	74.4
Sacred Heart	yes	N/A	N/A
St. Peter's	1,352 sf	2,795 sf	279.5

The family rooms at Bellin, Clover, Lutheran Pathway, and Riverside range from 33 square feet per patient to 72 square feet per patient. St. Peter's has considerably more family space, and a large dayroom that is used by home-care patients on a daycare basis. St. Peter's also has a reading alcove, large kitchenette (182 sf), a dining area, and greenhouse/gardening space.

These six units also vary in amount of office space provided. As tabulated below, these spaces include only the offices near or on the units:

Hospice	Administrative Offices/Conference	Total Square Footage per Patient
Bellin	436 sf	43.6
Clover	196 sf	39.2
Lutheran Pathway	710 sf	71.0
Riverside	75 sf	10.7
Sacred Heart	N/A	N/A
St. Peter's	2,199 sf	219.9

St. Peter's has the most extensive home-care division of all of these hospices, in contrast with Clover, which manages the hospice for the intermediate care facility and apartment patients it has already. Riverside Hospital Hospice had only a volunteer desk and nurses's station on its unit, which renders doubtful the relative autonomy of its administration and organization. Sacred Heart has a large nurse-coordinator's office, conference room, and a bereavement counseling office on the unit, but the sizes were not given in the survey. Lutheran Pathway has a conference room, hospice office, director's and head nurse's office on the unit. Only St. Peter's Hospice had sizable nursing and staff retreat space, although most of the hospice plans suggested that off-unit staff retreats might be available. All had linen supply and dirty linen rooms, medication areas, and closet space.

Many of these units have multipurpose rooms, as they were often limited by available space and other constraints when remodeling. Riverside has a multipurpose room with a large table that is used for conferences, dining, bereavement, and viewing. Clover's living room is a dayroom for patients, a conference or meeting room, and a waiting and reception room. Their multipurpose room is shared with the rest of the facility, although it is located convenient to the hospice area. Clover's private family room is also used for retreats and overnight stays. St. Peter's has several large and small areas that function in different ways: the aforementioned dayroom; a private family room that is also used for patient massages and family overnight stays; and hallway alcoves, used for telephoning, resting, comforting, and so on. St. Peter's multipurpose room has a bar, television, and child area; it is used by family and staff and can be used for services, as can the dayroom. Bellin Hospice's patient rooms have lounge areas with tables and chairs. They also have a multipurpose room used for conferences, viewing, and private family space. Lutheran Pathway has set aside space for family and staff laundry, and has a conference area for both staff and family conferences. This living room/family lounge functions as a waiting and reception room as well as space for formal and informal gatherings, conversation, and dining off the kitchenette (which has a dining table as well). The family private room can be used as a meditation area, quiet reading room, and family gathering place or retreat. These small hospice units have to do a lot with the space available and they also recognize that mulitpurpose rooms make the hospice more homelike.

Several of these facilities have made a considerable effort to remodel the existing finishes, furnishings, and lighting. Lutheran Pathway has made not only generous space allocations for patient sleeping and family areas, but has eliminated all fluorescent fixtures from the unit, including the hallway and entry areas. Most of these units have added carpeting, new paint, plants, and homelike residential furniture. The Clover Hospice family room has a large brick fireplace. All have added artwork and Lutheran Pathway has a large photographic mural.

Special note should be taken of St. Peter's, the one small inpatient remodeled hospice to make ex-tensive renovations. St. Peter's has provided a large amount of family space and patient bedroom area, and has attempted to deal with the double-loaded corridor system by turning it into a series of short corridors with changing viewpoints and nooks for conversation. The remodeled corridor space has effectively transformed the hospice area. Other attempts to deal with the double-loaded corridors so typical in these facilities have been less extensive. Lutheran Pathway has distributed the patient rooms around family areas, and created a transverse axis and open area at the central living room area and entry. Bellin has made a similar attempt to counteract the double-loaded corridor with a family room at the unit entry and dispersed bedrooms. Riverside grouped patient bedrooms at the unit entry. The family areas, kitchenette, and nurses' stations are located in a quieter cul-de-sac away from the unit entry, in a plan organization most similar to St. Peter's scheme. Clover Hospice did not need to counteract the double-loaded scheme and was able to centralize most functions because of the small bedroom population and flexibility of building type.

St. Peter's also sets a standard for the design and decoration of patient bedrooms. The three patient rooms were designed for privacy and community and feature territorial bed arrangements, wallpaper, built-in furniture, as well as residential lamps and handmade, modified headboards on the hospital beds. St. Peter's nurses' alcove, placed at the entry of the patient floor, has a rolltop desk, carpeting, and indirect lighting. Bedrooms are dispersed around the entry, family areas, and the nurses' alcove. The remodeling of St. Peter's was ambitious and is very successful.

Small Parent-Based Hospice Areas (remodeled). In this group fall hospice units that are functionally not even semiautonomous. Such units include remodeled rooms on medical/surgical wards, sections of oncology units, and, in this case, an area of a skilled nursing facility. The small, parent-based hospice area is typically different from the scatterbed hospice in that the hospice area is specially decorated, and may have larger bedrooms, hospice offices, and family space. They differ from the small, parent-based units in that they have no separate nursing staff or stations and must share general nursing care, other services, and a common entry.

In general, these kinds of hospice facility are not recommended. As they have little or no autonomy, they are often the battleground for disagreements among care providers and contribute to the stigma of dying by architecturally segregating those who are no longer in active medical treatment. The dying realize that they are being "moved around the corner," from active treatment to palliative care, and may feel stigmatized and abandoned. Wholly remodeled oncology and medical/surgical units with the additional family rooms, conference, and staff support are a more appropriate solution. These are discussed below. Nevertheless, these nonautonomous hospice areas are a significant proportion of the architectural modifications of hospice inpatient settings, perhaps numbering as many as one quarter of the total inpatient facilities. One of the most thoughtful of these remodeled areas is found at the Deer's Head Center Hospice.

Deer's Head Center has addressed many issues of the larger and more autonomous units. Homelike modifications have been made to a six-bed area of a skilled nursing facility to revise it for hospice care with five basic design elements. First, a family room of 200 square feet (33.3 square feet per patient) has been set aside near the bedrooms. This family room includes donated residential furniture and a small kitchenette closet, and is located in an irregular-shaped room for variety and zoning purposes. A variety of bedroom populations sizes, and decor has also been provided, with each four-bed and single room decorated differently. Residential furniture and finishes have been added to the hospice bedrooms, family and office areas, and hallway. The rooms have been painted soft colors and the bedrooms wallpapered; donated residential chairs, art, mirrors, dressers, and lamps, as well as plants and personal items, decorate the rooms. The hospice bedrooms total 877 square feet, or 146 square feet per patient, as opposed to the rest of the facility, which has an average of 88 square feet per patient, almost doubling the square feet per patient for hospice care. Last, the area selected for the hospice is near the staff dining and wing entry areas and overlooks the garden and sunny balconies. All of these elements combine to maximize the available resources at Deer's Head Center, and typify the best of hospice area remodelings.

Remodeled Oncology Units. Although not the focus of this study, remodeled oncology units are a very prevalent type of inpatient hospice facility. Two examples of this approach point out differences in philosophy of care and architectural results. They are Highline Community Hospice and Oncology,

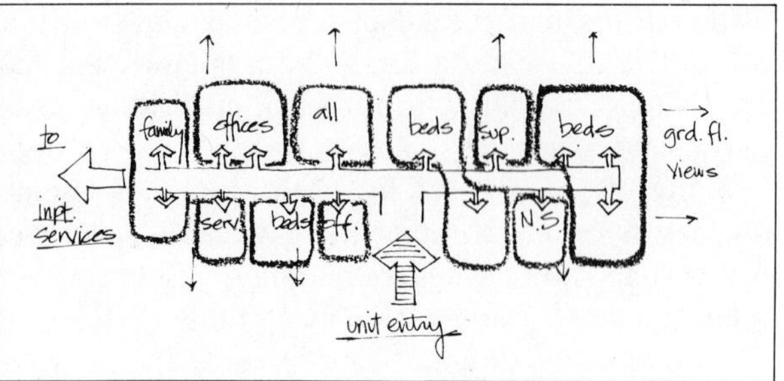

Parti drawing, Highline Community Hospital

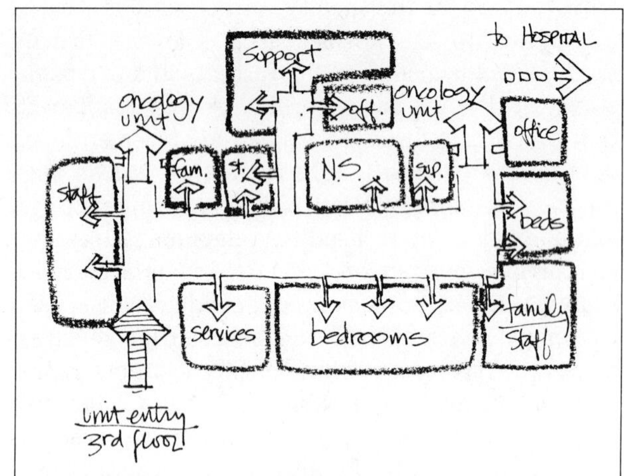

Parti drawing, Tacoma General Hospice

Seattle, Washington, and the hospice section at Tacoma General Hospital's oncology unit, Tacoma, Washington.

Highline Community Hospital is a small, community-based facility in an outlying suburban area of Seattle. It has recently undergone an extensive remodel, including additional medical/surgical units, and a redistribution of rehabilitation, physical therapy, and occupational therapy units, making these convenient to the oncology area. The oncology ward has been placed in its own older, ground-floor wing with an outside entrance. The twelve-bed combined oncology and hospice wing will have a conference room, a family area, a reception and waiting area for hospice and active care patients and family, offices, including hospice home-care and social worker offices, and an examination room. The unit itself will not separate hospice beds, but mix them among the active care patients in double-bed rooms. A standard nurses' station is at one end of the unit. The unit will provide areas for family overnight stays and it will encourage connections to the out-of-doors. Highline's oncology and hospice unit is located near the physical therapy/occupational therapy section for the use of both hospice and active therapy patients. It will be decorated with residential finishes and furnishings, warm, rich colors, incandescent lighting, artwork, and plants. In this way, a very small remodeling will improve the environment for all the patients without encouraging any stigma of the dying hospice inpatients. The nursing staff of this unit is trained in hospice philosophy and care, and will provide care for those who are dying as well as those who are recovering.

At Tacoma General, an area of the third-floor oncology unit is being remodeled as a separate, but nearby, hospice unit. It includes seven single-bed rooms with south and east views, a family lounge, waiting room and reception area, a staff lounge, a large nurse conference and education area, and an exam and chemotherapy room. The area has its own nurses' station, office, and utility rooms. The hospice area will function as an outpatient facility also, making use of chemotherapy and treatment for palliative purposes.

The unit will total 3,086 square feet or 441 square feet per inpatient (gross). The family lounge will be decorated with residential furnishings and include a kitchenette, children's furniture, and a place for family overnight stays. Family overnight facilities will also be provided off the unit. The total cost of the remodel has been estimated at $44,967 (1981 dollars) for equipment including nurses' station, patient rooms, the utility room (with an area for family and patient personal laundry), and the family lounge and kitchen (Consolidated Hospitals, 1981, 12). Patient rooms are similar in size to the existing oncology bedrooms, and will have reading lights, pictures, cork display boards, drapes, shelves, magazine racks, clocks, television, and institutional over-bed tables, beds, and bed-lounge chairs. Each room is also being provided with a straight-back chair and contributed furniture.

The hospice area will be next to the twenty-eight-bed oncology area, with its own nurses' station and family lounge. No remodeling is expected to be done on the oncology side of the floor. The large bath and shower facilities for the hospice are located on the oncology side, as will be the lobby connection to the rest of the hospital and the stairs. Although there is a bridge connection to the hospice, it is too bad that Tacoma General was unable to provide the family and other support areas on the oncology side. One wonders if the close proximity of the hospice area to the oncology unit will promote or negate the stigma associated with dying in a hospital.

Medium Parent-Based Palliative-Care Units (New Construction). The last group of facilities covered by this survey is composed of a rare and, as yet, unbuilt hospice type in the United States. England has at least one good example, the Royal South Hants Hospital Continuing Care Unit. These facilities are new additions or separate new palliative-care buildings added to the campus of large umbrella organizations. At Royal South Hants Hospital, for example, the twenty-six-bed continuing care unit has been added to a hospital complex that already has facilities for acute care, community primary care, and a children's health division. This new building has four five-bed rooms, four single rooms and one double suite for overnight visitor stays— the patient is moved next door to the suite when visitors stay overnight. An attempt has been made to create a homelike or domestic environment rather than a clinical one. There are family rooms, day room, quiet rooms, courtyards, and a kitchenette, called the *tea bar* and *ward pantry.*

In the United States, the building of new facilities for hospice care is rare. There are only two free-standing new-construction facilities at this time, the Connecticut Hospice and the Nathan Adelson Hospice. There are plans for two new parent-based palliative-care units, a separate building at St. Mary's Hospital in Tucson, Arizona, and a new floor addition at St. Mary's Hospital for Children in Queens. Both are in the planning stages, but some details can be discussed now.

The hospice planned for St. Mary's in Tucson is a twenty-bed unit affiliated with a skilled nurses' facility, located across the street from the main hospital grounds. This facility, designed by Anderson, De Bartolo and Pan of Tucson in 1981, is remarkably similar to Nathan Adelson Hospice, designed by Nevada Archetronics, although the architects were not aware of one another's designs at the time, according to Gerald Moffit of Nevada Archetronics. Both are based on a four single-room cluster around a family area, housing a total of twenty patients. The St. Mary's scheme would replace a current ten-bed hospice unit in the acute-care hospital, but plans are not now being pursued.

Under the plans for St. Mary's, the twenty patient rooms would each be approximately 230 square feet including a private water closet, smaller than the approximate 280 square feet at Nathan Adelson.

The cluster family lounges at St. Mary's average 400 square feet, versus the larger 529 square feet of Nathan Adelson's country kitchens. St. Mary's was planned around two smaller outdoor courtyards, whereas Nathan Adelson has one large courtyard and a sizable covered greenhouse. St. Mary's proposal includes a chapel and viewing room, a gift shop, craft room, and nursery for childcare. Also included are a personal care room (for physical therapy) and various size family areas, including the above-mentioned cluster family lounges, as well as a separate family room, counseling rooms, a large thousand-square-foot multipurpose activity room, and a kitchenette. Nathan Adelson has similar family and support spaces, without a viewing room or gift shop, but including a large dining area and beauty/barber shop. The St. Mary's plans do not detail any nurse desk in the cluster area as Nathan Adelson has done. St. Mary's plans also call for the use of an angled patient bed that is inappropriate for hospice comforting and visiting, as discussed later. The largest programming difference of these two very similar designs is the amount of space set aside for the offices. St. Mary's proposal allots a sizable office area, approximately 2,475 square feet, or 123.75 square feet per patient. At Nathan Adelson, the office area totals about 1,040 square feet, or 52 square feet per patient, less than half of the other facility. Nathan Adelson's office area has been found to be small when compared to that at Connecticut Hospice, too, and may well become a problem for staff.

A comparison of the general organizing schemes represented in the partis of St. Mary's and Nathan Adelson suggests that they are surprisingly similar. As St. Mary's was to function with a parent facility and Nathan Adelson is freestanding, this similarity may indicate that the hospice unit itself, whether autonomous or parent based, may be amenable to a uniform architectural solution.

It is notable that these two units were designed in the arid West, where the courtyard design is indigenous to the climate and Spanish-Indian culture. Locale and culture are important to consider in the adaptation of hospice architecture to the United States; using a regional style can help the facility blend in with the neighborhood and promote a residential atmosphere. Nathan Adelson and St. Mary's hospices have also supported a compromise to the single and multibed room controversy with their single-room clusters. However, both facilities have provided this sole type of room throughout their building, without adding other kinds of rooming, and so are uniform in their solution. The cluster serves to promote socialization outside the patient room, but not within it; the four one-bed rooms are single rooms still, and the corridor has been modified. St. Mary's proposal does suggest, however, that the walls of adjoining bedrooms could be movable, to allow some double-room accommodation.

Since the designs of St. Mary's proposed facility and Nathan Adelson's existing hospice are so similar, it would be interesting and valuable for St. Mary's to conduct a post-occupancy evaluation of the Nathan Adelson Hospice.

At St. Mary's Hospital for Children, a small, modest skilled nursing facility in Queens, the addition of a new palliative-care floor on the existing building will allow the flexibility of new construction with the advantages of a parent facility. The parent organization is particularly significant because this will be the first United States palliative-care unit for children. Children have different trajectories of illness and dying from adults, and often respond to treatment in idiosyncratic and erratic ways, partly as a function of their rapid growth. Providers of palliative care for children must be alert to subtle and rapid changes in the child's illness, and thus need access to alternative therapies. Moreover, children are our dearest resource; the terminal illness of a child is fraught with our deepest anguish and helplessness in the face of death. A palliative-care facility for children must be especially sensitive to the rights of the dying and their loved ones. Two other aspects particular to children will affect the design and its function of this palliative-care unit. First, children do not have full legal rights in this society. They are subject to the wishes of their parents and guardians, which makes the family an even greater element in the palliative care of dying children. Second, children have a range of interests and abilities that depends upon their stage of development; the whole spectrum of interests must be accommodated at any children's facility. The palliative-care unit will be a microcosm of the parent facility, but in a very small area. It must be flexible.

St. Mary's Hospital for Children is attempting to deal with these consideration in their plans for an additional palliative-care floor on top of their existing facility. In addition to palliative care, home care, day care, bereavement care, and education and research will be provided. As stated by Dottie C. Wilson, director of the palliative-care center at St. Mary's, the intent of the facility is "to provide a wide variety of choices of lifestyle and activities to accommodate children of various ages (birth to 16) who are terminally ill . . . and their families (who are permitted unlimited visiting and overnight stays) in an environment also supportive of staff and volunteers."

The hospital will provide one single room, one triple room, and three double rooms. There will be a raised tub room, a shower room accessible to wheelchairs, and several staff and public toilets, including a children's washroom area, all on the same floor. Family space will include a lounge with public toilets on the floor below the patients' rooms, a chapel on the ground floor, and a quiet room and daycare area for crafts and general activities on the patients' floor. The unit will have a combined viewing/exam room, with a different entrance for each function. There will be a pantry for snacks and hospital food, with a refrigerator, microwave, and other electrical appliances. The staff lounge will be located on the patient floor, staff retreat areas located on lower floors. The facility will be decorated with homelike furnishings and will include a greenhouse and gardening area. There will also be a game room, perhaps with video games. Offices, conference rooms, and the volunteer area will be set up on the floor below the patient rooms. (Note: the facility became operational as of 1984; the proposed modifications listed above were current at the time of the survey.)

Conclusion

This survey of forty-eight existing, planned, or programmed palliative-care units found the following minimum elements to exist in the majority of facilities:

- A variety of bedroom accommodations and decor
- More square feet per patient in bedroom areas than is provided in traditional medical facilities
- Family rooms that include at least one large gathering area and may include private areas in patient rooms, private family rooms, and access to multipurpose rooms for conferences and dining, and a chapel or meditation room
- Kitchenette facilities, usually in conjunction with family rooms, for family, patient, and staff use
- Indoor gardening areas with operable windows and skylights
- A considerable amount of artwork, especially nature and representational scenes
- A separate and specially designed nurses' station for hospice use
- A separate and distinctive entry for the unit, building, or both
- Outdoor areas for hospice use
- A dining room that may be used for various purposes
- A multipurpose room suitable for large-scale gatherings
- An average, overall, of just under thirty beds per unit
- Family overnight accommodations

In addition, most hospices and palliative-care units intended to provide a homelike atmosphere, lots of natural light, and both privacy and activity for the patients. The patients, staff, and family were encouraged to participate in care, decoration, and activities. Sacred space or meditation areas were also included.

Contrary to their literature, however, many hospices did not have a significant number of retreat areas available to staff. Often, patients entered the facilities through emergency entrances or back doors. Many remodeled units were unable to transform double-loaded corridor areas into homelike space. There was no unanimity as to the "right" colors for the units, although carpeting was a frequent addition, as were lighting changes and the addition of residential furniture and window curtains. Many units also added flowered and print sheets. Most units had several multipurpose areas and some duplication of services, such as kitchenettes located close to the bedrooms. The larger-scale remodeled units had oxygen and/or suction in the walls and had modified hall lighting and signs. Virtually all the units used hospital beds, overbed tables, and lounge chairs. Few hospices had childcare and most had no space allocation for occupational therapy, physical therapy, or beauty shops on the unit.

Office space in these palliative-care units varied widely, as did the sizes of patient rooms and nursing areas. The kitchen areas, when provided on the unit, were larger than most institutional design formulas would allot. These were used to serve additional meals and foods tailored to the needs of the patient, such as breakfast. Meals were recognized as a time for patients to socialize—the hospices made an effort to serve meals that were visually interesting and manageable for the patient.

In general, most facilities allocated too little space for group meetings, for hall storage, and for changes in function that will occur in any new kind of care.

Locale and Design. Hospices tried to respond to the specific needs or characteristics of their populations and locales. Furniture was selected to match the prevailing residential style of the neighborhood, or a modified contemporary design was adopted. The need for larger or more noisy families to have privacy was a consideration in some hospice's choice to use certain room configurations, such as a large percentage of single rooms; the age and condition of the majority of their patients were also taken into account. Hospices in milder climates often relied more upon outdoor meeting space and had greater amounts of outdoor space for recreation. Some hospice designs reflected the climate, such as Nathan Adelson; others were less successful in dealing with wind and sun, such as Calvary Hospital. Urban hospices, with a greater number of poor and dependent elderly patients, had a larger social work contingent, and also had more security problems and difficulty in finding space for outdoor gardening.

Overall, the hospices and palliative-care units were very attentive to changes in their population bases and to the needs of the local community. The attempt by hospices to provide local services was matched, as much as possible, by an architectural adaptation to their local conditions.

Size and Scale Considerations. Size and scale of the facility affected each of the hospice designs.

Large units—those with ten beds or more—often separated functionally different areas by substantial distances. This made replication of services necessary: more family rooms, kitchenettes, and nurses' stations, for example, were needed. In general, the larger the unit, the more standardized the design, and the greater the reliance upon economies of scale and formulas of institutional design. This trend was broken, however, by examples from each type of hospice discussed earlier: by Rosary Hill, by Nathan Adelson and the Connecticut Hospice, and by Northern Virginia and the Hospice of the Good Shepherd. The smaller facilities, by virtue of their size, had different-purpose rooms closer together. Some smaller units were more innovative in design than others, such as St. Peter's and Clover Hospice.

Smaller units provided multibed rooms, but they were more likely than the larger units to have single rooms or doubles, and were more likely to have only one kind of rooming accommodation.

In the group of units having more than twenty-five beds, only the Hospice of Grenada Hills, Nathan Adelson, St. Mary's Tucson, and Calvary Hospital had single rooms for all patients. The rest of the large facilities had a variety of rooming accommodations. In general, the larger the unit, the more support services were included. Laundry rooms were seldom part of any facility with fewer than fifteen patient beds, and no unit with a population under fifteen had its own kitchen facilities. Larger units, such as that at Cincinnati, often contracted for laundry services.

Chapter Six

Alternatives and Constraints

The preceding information about existing, planned, and programmed hospice and palliative-care units in the United States and elsewhere has revealed a unanimity of purpose in their design, if not always in the implementation of that design. Hospices and palliative-care units have, without a uniform federal standard, developed a consensus of priorities in design and decor, though their circumstances vary widely. As a result of the efforts of the caregivers, an identifiable hospice unit is emerging. Some of the basic elements of hospice design can be found in the remarks of Dr. William E. Gibson, in his 1978 address to the Institutes on Hospices of the Catholic Hospital Association:

> The requirements in any health facility or unit dedicated to the care of the terminally ill include both design and function. Institutional appearance should be avoided, and a residence-like environment should be adopted. Whether it be a freestanding building or incorporated within an existing structure, it should provide for ease of mobility, adequate security, and any amount of desired privacy. At the same time, it should be easily accessible to the family from the outside and, if possible, homelike gardens should be readily available (Gibson 1978, 8).

The intentions of hospice caregivers and proponents, however, have not been uniformly met at each hospice location. Discrepancy is evident in the matching of intention to execution at the most expensive as well as the most humble of inpatient units. To some extent, this discrepancy is the result of honest differences of opinion; in other cases, it results from a limit of ability. There are, however, major constraints in the design of hospice units, and little information is available as to the effects of those constraints or other possible options that could be considered.

Constraints

In hospice inpatient architecture, the three main constraints on the translation of intention into physical form are simple: existing resources and remodeling limitations; building codes, payment regulations, and licensing procedures; and the existing medical establishment as well as the institutional forms that translate its intentions. These three main constraints are the environment in which inpatient hospice care must develop.

Hospice Architecture and Remodeling

In the United States, most of the hospices that provide architecturally distinct and functionally semiautonomous units for inpatient care do so in remodeled facilities. Remodeled units have distinctly different problems from hospices able to construct totally new facilities. The goal of creating a homelike environment, for instance, is much more difficult to achieve when the original medical facility was equipped with double-loaded corridors, smaller patient bedrooms, fluorescent lighting systems, harder finishes and furnishings, large, domineering nurses' stations, above-ground locations, sealed windows, and antiseptic conditions. Little has been written about these converted units; previously, hospice literature has, for philosophical reasons, dwelt mostly upon the possibilities of freestanding design for hospice care. However, the financial considerations and practicality of remodeled parent-based units have increased their number greatly over the free-standing hospices.

Remodeled units are found in many places. Although some hospices have seen fit to remodel nonmedical buildings, they are a distinct minority. Most remodeled or converted facilities are found in acute-care oncology or medical/surgical areas, in older acute-care wards of various types, in acute-care support spaces, such as nursing residential rooms or intern areas, or in skilled nursing or intermediate care facilities. The nursing facility space may be converted from rehabilitation areas or from relatively new or older code-restricted wings or wards. In several cases, nursing facility space has been put back to its original use after some experimentation with hospice use, such as at Hillhaven in Arizona.

Conversion of acute-care space for hospice purposes has been prevalent in the last decade, for several reasons. As pointed out by Antoinette Newman, Kenneth Schwartz, and James Diaz, "There is currently an excess of acute beds nationally, and . . . acute care facilities in older buildings have the best chance of being converted to skilled nursing facilities as the 'next step down' in health facility sophistication, as generally now defined by licensure" (Newman et al. 1980, 1). Although the authors are discussing the conversion of acute care space to skilled nursing facilities, not hospices, their point applies to hospices as well. Updated fire and safety regulations have rendered some of this acute-care space below standard, making these units available for conversion.

Older hospital wards, which usually have a lower debt, are also likely candidates for conversion, especially if they are part of a multiservice system, such as a public health hospital. Remodeled units can provide additional services to a larger facility and reduce excess capacity. Although terminal-care facilities do not bring in as much money as acute-care units do, they do not require as intensively the services that acute care demands, such as large diagnostic and treatment areas.

However, although there are positive aspects to making use of existing space and resources in developing hospice facilities, there are drawbacks as well. As Newman, Schwartz, and Diaz point out,

> . . . it may well be impossible in many conversions to provide for the most essential needs of the residents, to appropriate spaces for socializing and for developing social competence. Unless the proposed SNF can offer

these design features, the psychological needs of the resident are not likely to be met (Newman et al., 1980).

This point is perhaps even more applicable to hospices than to SNFs. Hospices require even more space per person than do most SNFs, for retreat, family, and meeting areas. In addition, most of the surplus space in acute-care conversions is above the ground floor, adding to its unsuitability for hospice use.

Overall, however, a case can be made to support conversions as the best use of existing and limited resources in some circumstances. Certainly, the practical nature of the remodeled units has resulted in a great number of inpatient settings located here in the United States. The compendium provides examples of the efforts of existing hospices to deal with the constrictions of their buildings. More specific strategies for implementing hospice design intentions in these restrictive remodel units are discussed later.

Current Economic and Regulation Effects

Hospice-specific architecture has been developed since the early 1970s without uniform regulation, licensure, or payment procedures. The Tax Equity Act, passed in the summer of 1982, contained hospice reimbursement legislation that went into effect January 1, 1983. It provides Medicare funds for hospice home and inpatient care, for hospices that choose to receive the benefit. At the present time, the Medicare benefit has a ceiling of $6,500 for the duration of care, not to exceed six months. A further provision of the law is that 80 percent of this money, or $5,200, must be used for home care; only $1,300 can be applied to inpatient care for respite or pain control. As of November 1985, only 220 hospices have applied for Medicare certification; however, eleven hospices applied in October 1985 alone. The National Hospice Organization is looking into legislation that will increase the money from Medicare and remove the "sunset provision," so that Medicare funding can continue after it is scheduled to run out. In addition, hospice care is proposed to become an optional Medicaid benefit, which would allow states to offer a comprehensive hospice benefit. At present, although many parts of hospice care are covered by Medicaid, there is no comprehensive coverage.

How does this reimbursement situation affect home-care and inpatient hospice units? Currently, the money made available by the federal government is inadequate for most hospices. Most home-care hospices are not applying for inpatient status until they see whether the National Hospice Organization's proposals will pass. The existing legislation also limits reimbursement of inpatient stays to five consecutive days of one inpatient stay, although the current average length of inpatient visits is two weeks. This restriction will have an extreme effect on architecturally distinct remodeled units when all inpatient beds are not occupied. Traditionally, hospice care has been made available to everyone, including those who have little ability to pay; reimbursement has been supported by acute-care provisions under a larger umbrella of health-insurance payment. The advent of the diagnostic-related groups (DRGs), in which all federal payments will now be prospective, rather than retrospective, means that this kind of supported payment will no longer be possible. Hospice regulations for Medicare certification, as established by the Health Care Financing Administration, include a range of services not seen at the pre-law hospices surveyed in the compendium, such as extensive pharmacist and physician participation. However, the regulations do have a protective effect; regulations will maintain the integrity of hospice care as an alternative to the current modes of caregiving for the dying.

The reimbursement law has set up different rates of payment for the inpatient component, based on whether inpatient care is required for pain and symptom control, or for respite for the patient and family. The law has implied that respite care is not as valuable as pain-control care, by giving less money for respite. This, too, has prompted hospice care providers to wait and see whether a change in this aspect of the law will be forthcoming.

Hospitals are getting into the act of providing hospice inpatient and home care, however, as the payment system for them also has switched into a prospective one. Existing hospices have found that they are entering a world of competition in the medical field. However, most hospices are confident that they will continue to provide quality care for the dying in the future.

Converting Institutional Space for Hospice Use

As discussed in chapter 1, "The Hospice Alternative," and in light of the difficulties that current reimbursement legislation presents, it seems likely that parent-based facilities and hospices that provide only home care will predominate in the future growth of the hospice movement. Because it is usually more cost-efficient and expedient to remodel than to begin new construction, it also seems likely that a large percentage of future parent-based hospices will be located in converted institutional space.

The layout and materials of existing hospitals and skilled nursing facilities have a great influence on the design of converted hospice units. The hard, shiny finishes, institutional double-loaded corridors, and the existing arrangement of rooms and services make remodeling the facility to accord with hospice standards very difficult.

Acute-care facilities are organized for short-term, medically intensive care. Nursing facilities are organized for long-term custodial care. Neither has developed an appropriate atmosphere for the terminally ill and their families. One report, mentioned earlier (Newman 1980), explored the typical configurations of hospital buildings. Few of these had surplus space on the ground floor for direct access to the outdoors, as would be suitable for a hospice. The typical acute-care unit has a cluster of thirty to forty beds, far too large for a hospice unit. Moreover, Newman's report stated that the typical skilled nursing facility ward is even larger, making conversion to hospice space even more difficult. The report notes that hospital buildings constructed after 1950 are probably the most economical to remodel, yet these units have the larger bed component, and have to be upgraded to meet life-safety requirements. If the skilled nursing facility requires more area per bed (33 to 56 percent more space than in new acute-care facilities), then the even larger areas per bed needed by hospices make the acute-care units the least desirable for conversion.

There are subtle aspects of design, typical of acute-care and skilled nursing facility space, that could unconsciously undermine the intentions of the hospice operators in the conversion of institutional space for hospice use. One example can be taken from the current assumption that single rooms provide the best solution to the bedding problems of many hospitals. These private rooms, which are shallow, must be strung along a corridor system. In an attempt to minimize the length of the halls and maximize the patient's view through the doorway and window, a diagonal-bed placement has been adopted. (Angling the patient's bed diagonally permits the use of a narrower room, which shortens the necessary length of the hallway.) This bed placement can be seen in plans for the proposed

St. Mary's Hospice in Tucson. The diagonal placement of acute-care beds, however, does not translate into hospice use. A primary intent of hospice care is to provide comfort for the patient, a comfort of communication, touching, and choice, none of which is facilitated by placing the patient in a bed angled in a corner. In this bed configuration, the patient's head is given the least amount of space around it, so that it is very difficult to sit near the head of the bed and visit, write letters, eat with, feed, brush the hair of the patient, or otherwise give comfort. In addition, this diagonal-bed arrangement makes it difficult to move the bed nearer or farther from the window, nor is it a typical homelike configuration. In this case, the intention of hospice care has been confounded by a "progressive" acute-care bed arrangement; one that was instituted to solve previously existing problems with the institutional design of the hospital.

Another example can be taken from a larger organizational element of acute-care or skilled nursing facilities. The homelike qualities that hospices seek to provide in their inpatient units require more than changing a few articles of furniture, flooring, and light fixtures of an existing institutional unit. One of the basic needs of hospice units is multipurpose areas at all levels of organization, from family areas in the patient room, multiple uses for the nurses' station, to retreat and conference space, and outdoor gardens. Providing multipurpose areas in a hospice makes it possible for people to gather and activities to take place naturally and spontaneously, as they would in a residence. The institution, especially the medical institution, insists on economy of scale and specialization of function—activities occur in delegated areas at appointed times. Taking the concept of separation of function to an extreme, certain large institutions providing care for the terminally ill automatically opt for consistent treatment of each "section" of the facility. The offices are put together and separated from the patient rooms, which are identically organized and separated from the entry, which is separated from the nurses' stations, which are located far from the staff support areas, and so on. This methodology is simply not acceptable for hospice care, which seeks to deinstitutionalize the treatment of the dying. Obviously some order is necessary, but a functional understanding of architectural organization and elements must be achieved before form and detail solutions are applied to hospice inpatient care.

Alternatives

Experimental and Diverse Modes of Palliative Terminal Care

A few inpatient programs for the care of the dying should be added to the preceding material on hospices and palliative-care units. These are experimental and diverse programs with unusual requirements and architectural expression. In a kind of care so new and personal, a spectrum of hospice care philosophies, from the medically active care that includes radiation and chemotherapy treatment to the more traditional nonmedical palliation, can stimulate innovation; a continuum of care for all dying patients reminds the care provider and architect that flexibility is a keystone of hospice care.

Children's Hospice. One example of a new and experimental program of terminal care is St. Mary's Hospital for Children. The special problems faced by children's palliative-care units have been discussed earlier, but they bear repeating. Briefly, the palliative-care unit must manage the unique and erratic trajectories of children's illnesses, which often respond to treatment when an adult's would not; the societal anguish involved in the death of children; the rights of children, subsumed in the active role of the parents; and the developmental differences in the interests and abilities of children.

Another experimental unit is the neonatal hospice at the Children's Hospital in Denver. With terminally ill newborns, the emphasis in care is on the family members who need counseling and bereavement follow-up after the death.

Psychiatric Hospice. Another hospice program with special needs is the one established at St. Elizabeth's, a psychiatric hospital in Washington, D.C. The program was started in 1979 by the National Institute of Mental Health, which funded the hospital to set aside a six-bed area and family lodgings on hospital grounds for overnight stays. In this kind of care, terminally ill mental patients may be disruptive, nonverbal, and need confined spaces. Their families may need even more counseling and bereavement follow-up, because of their possible guilt associated with mental illness and confinement of the patient.

Nonmedical Palliative Care. The Hanuman Foundation, a nontraditional spiritual group, has run workshops on dying and its personal and religious implications, called the Dying Project. They now have a

> . . . suitable house, an appropriate location, and a full-time staff of three people . . . Located on six acres of secluded land in the hills ten minutes from Sante Fe, New Mexico, the Center is ready to receive participants . . . The Center itself provides no medical care but we have a close working relationship with some of the most open members of the Sante Fe medical community. We make no commitments in time, concerning how long participants may stay. The contract is moment to moment, trusting our hearts (Hanuman Foundation, 1981, 14–15).

The Foundation goes on to say that they will try not to have a rigid notion of the "correct" way to die: "for some people a quiet, meditative atmosphere would be optimum; for others, a more festive setting." Like the hospice inpatient units, the Center maximizes the patient's right of choice, but the organization's special need to be completely free of any sort of medical or institutional affiliation makes the Hanuman Center very different from most of the hospice inpatient units.

Long-term and Palliative Care. Other new approaches to the palliative care of the dying include the Lifecare Industry Nursing Center in Florida, where the elderly can relocate, as their needs and conditions warrant, from an independent apartment to an apartment with contracted services (housekeeping, meals, and so on) to an intermediate-care or skilled nursing facility. This model of community, from retirement apartments to terminal-care facility, is not as common in the United States as in countries with other forms of health-care financing. The Pilgrim Place Health Service Center, a California retirement community for former Christian workers, provides hospice care in apartment units located at the end of the three wings of their skilled nursing facility. However, the association of retirement community with hospice area is just beginning to be formed in the United States; no doubt existing resistance to this concept is supported by a deathhouse connotation, already associated with some intermediate care units.

Great Britain and the Netherlands have a socialized health-care system that provides various alternatives for the elderly and dying. At De Drie Hoven, Amsterdam, for example, architect Herman Hertzberger designed a residential complex for elderly and handicapped. The complex contains a variety of units, including fifty-five flats for married couples with disabilities; 171 apartment units and a 190-bed home for the aged; a sick bay with fifteen patient beds and five beds for guests; and an institution for the permanent care of 250 invalids and mentally ill people. There is also a daycare center for nonresidents, staff quarters with twenty-one two-room flats, and rooms for nurses and others. The complete complex includes kitchen, laundry, store, workshop, mortuary, meeting rooms, space for mechanical equipment, and communal areas. This facility was designed to make greatest use of views and connections to the outdoors and has decks, patios, loggias, and a proliferation of greenery. The complex is also equipped with a plant nursery, shed and compost areas, and cold frames. As one reviewer of the site noted, the architectural treatment of the hallways maximizes the units' connection to the outdoors:

> The living units in the different parts of the complex are situated along the passageways which may be regarded as streets. They also have their own front doors, porches, and, where possible, windows with a view over the street (*Architectural Review*, 1976, 159:68–82).

The nursing home has one, two- and four-bed rooms in each group of twenty-five. The whole complex was purposely left in an unfinished state, so that the contributions of the residents would be obvious, necessary, and provide the finishing. De Drie Hoven was designed so that relocation would not be necessary as the residents grew older and weaker. The attempt was to create a place where a sense of community could be fostered over time.

The British, notably Cicely Saunders, have added immensely to our understanding of the treatment of the dying. Facilities for hospice care in Britain have responded in creative ways to serve their clientele and communities. One noteworthy example is the Tarner Home, a Georgian house with room for sixteen patients, founded in 1935 in Brighton. The building is linked to a row of smaller Georgian houses for the use of the staff. It has only single bedrooms and, except for the nursing area, drug storage, elevator, and bath hoists, is completely residential in appearance. There is a large living room and a suite for family overnight stays. The Tarner Home is furnished with period antiques and the personal items of patients, including large pieces of furniture. There is a large garden that supplies flowers to adorn the patients' rooms. The patient's stay can extend from a few days to several years; payment is obtained from endowments as well as charities and the National Health. Each patient also receives weekly pocket money at the Tarner Home, which tries to provide compassionate care at all levels.

Another fine British hospice is the twenty-five-bed Michael Sobell House, constructed in 1977 on the campus of Oxford's Churchill Hospital. As described in the *Ohio State Medical Journal*, several design elements contribute to the hospice's homelike atmosphere:

> The walls invariably were painted white or paneled in light wood, and there were many windows to admit outdoor light. Green plants abounded; they were not "decorator perfect" but gave a feeling of things thriving and growing. The plants were in rooms, at bedsides, in halls, and other locations. We also saw many, many chairs and they were easily movable. Day rooms or sitting rooms tended to have an assortment of chairs . . . the day rooms always had a somewhat cluttered look because people were at home there and they moved things around. We particularly liked the woodburning fireplace we saw . . . all hospices had chapel facilities . . . At Michael Sobell Hospice, the large day room area had a pair of sliding doors at one end. Behind them was a simple and lovely altar for services (Rose and Pories, 1977).

There are more than thirty hospices in Great Britain, including several hospices discussed earlier in the book: St. Anne's, St. Christopher's, St. Joseph's, and the Royal South Hants continuing care unit. As pioneers in the hospice movement, the British have provided a range of quality service for the terminally ill not yet matched anywhere.

The state of the art of hospice inpatient unit design is far from realized. The units surveyed in the compendium are some of the best in the United States, England, and Canada. Still, hospice care is so new that the design problems and solutions of

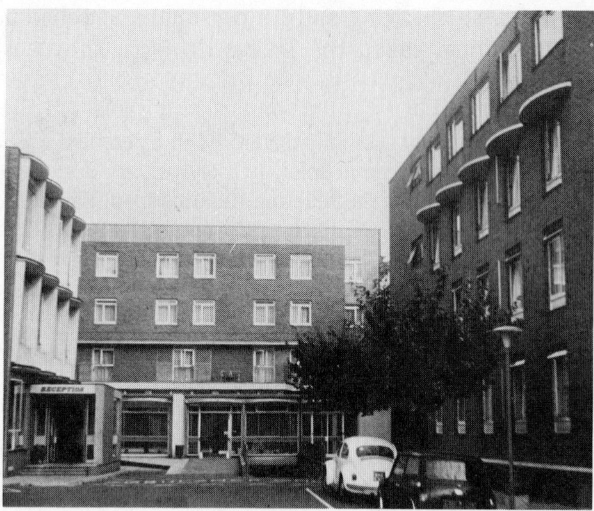

Entrance, St. Joseph's Hospice

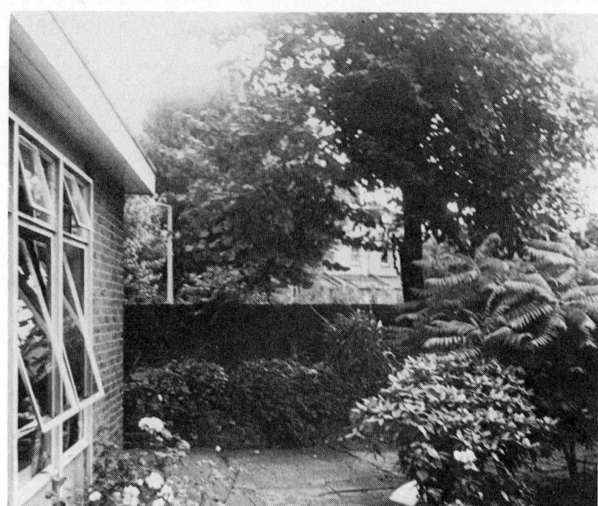

Gardens, St. Joseph's Hospice

the inpatient unit pale in comparison with the difficulties of providing any care at all. Nevertheless, some remarkably ingenious and thorough units have been created, and these should provide designers, planners, and care providers with examples of successful hospice environments, as well as common hospice problems.

Part Three

Architectural Guidelines: Hospices and Palliative-Care Units

The Bustle in a House
The Morning after Death
Is solemnest of industries
Enacted upon Earth—

The Sweeping up the Heart
and putting Love Away
We shall not want to use again
Until Eternity

—Emily Dickinson

Chapter Seven

Hospice Design Guidelines

The compendium has provided identifiable characteristics of contemporary hospice design. Now it is time to consider the range of possibilities for innovation and implementation of each of these design priorities. The potential variations on each element are, of course, limitless in the imagination, but constrained when the considerations of economics and design are added.

Design guidelines are necessary because most designers find that they have neither the time nor the money to do extensive basic research. Without research, designs can be based upon intuitive, arbitrary, or unsubstantiated judgment. This set of guidelines is presented to synthesize the compendium results and to project future hospice design. It can help the caregivers and public at large to evaluate planning and may stimulate discussion and further clarification of the aims and options of hospice care. These guidelines are intended to encourage thought and experimentation rather than provide a formula solution to very complex design issues. Palliative-care units vary so much in size, location, and care that one prescriptive program would not be helpful in discussing design considerations. Rather, a strategy that explores intent, architectural definitions, and specific design options is more suited to inform designs and users of architectural solutions to palliative-care concerns.

A word of caution on this approach, however, seems warranted. In health-care architecture, the concerns of the patients and families change over time as new people come to use the facility. Often, planners and architects consider it impossible to meet the specific and intimate needs of these users, and, in the end, design a "common denominator." This approach is particularly inappropriate for hospice design; hospices strive to meet the needs of the individual patients and families.

In addition, hospice caregivers are often the sole or primary contributors to design. They are the long-term users; they remain, as patients come and go, to answer the questionnaires. These caregivers have the difficult duty of managing the social aspects of dying for a society with ambiguous feelings about death and dying. This responsibility, combined with their continual use of the facility, gives great authority and weight to their recommendations concerning hospice design. To fulfill the philosophy of hospice care, however, caregivers and designers must be very conscious of this authority and seek to minimize its effect, to empower those around them.

As noted earlier, it was unfortunately not possible to include hospice patients and family in the compendium survey data collection. However, one such post-occupancy study was completed at Hillhaven Hospice (Lupu and Monahan 1968). The conclusions of the report help to illustrate the different viewpoints of the users and the relationships of those viewpoints to design. Overall, there was considerable unanimity in family, patient, and staff attitudes toward hospice architecture. All felt that family spaces, retreat areas, and kitchen facilities, for example, were necessary and that the chapel as well as the hospice's access to the outdoors contributed to the ambience. However, it became evident that the patients had no firm expectations of the hospice inpatient environment. Hospice palliative care was so new—the study was conducted in the late 1960s—and so radically different from that provided in hospitals and nursing homes that the patients were delighted with every attempt to enliven and comfort them. Concentration was on the positive aspects of the architecture and care, although patients, family, and staff were quick to point out their difficulties with the physical facility. This made for some interesting conclusions, among which was that patients were satisfied with single rooms if they were in single rooms, and preferred double rooms if such was their accommodation. Thus, rooming preference was not established. The greatest criticism offered concerned the size of the conference or meeting rooms, not the number of beds or the degree of privacy provided.

Designing the inpatient environment includes, among other things, establishing a sense of place. Typically, individual meaning is given to a place when territory is established and embellished with personal articles, people, and memories of past events. Because hospice care is short-term, it is often hard to encourage patients and family to personalize their space. When time is short, however, as for the dying, the smallest event can take on great meaning for the dying person, the family, even the caregivers. Glaser quotes Bernice Kavinovsky, who, dying, spoke of the heightened awareness she was experiencing:

> All week, although I teach my classes, arrange for a substitute, put dinner on, telephone my son at his apartment, shower, mark manuscripts, I perform each act almost clinically aware of the obstruction in my breast . . . assailed on every hand by beauty's endless argument—an arc of light or the curve of my husband's cheek . . . or the noise of the children's games on the roof next door (Glaser and Strauss 1968, 167).

The inpatient hospice environment takes on the qualities of the mundane and the unique; it can stimulate as well as reassure the patient, family, and caregivers. The design can encourage palliative care and the actions of choice, comfort, privacy, socialization, food, and access to diversions. It can provide quiet, private spaces for the family and staff who must deal with the dying while coming to terms with their own confusion, grief, and pain.

However, the environment is a support for this care and concern, never a substitute for it. The various ways in which the environment can aid and serve the physical and psychological functions of hospice care are only adjuncts to the caregivers.

In the compendium of existing, planned, and programmed inpatient hospice units, the intentions of the caregivers have been compared with their existing facility in order to determine whether these intentions had been carried out. In many cases, the caregivers expressed dissatisfaction with one or more aspects of the hospice. Frequently, the caregivers' expectations could not be met because of a lack of sufficient funds for renovation. In other hospices, the optimum solutions were impossible to achieve because of structural and location limitations or local restrictions. Often, the designers were hampered by inadequate information or a lack of examples of possibilities for hospice architecture.

In this chapter, each of the architectural elements of hospice inpatient design identified in the compendium will be examined, first by establishing intent, then discussing definitions, and finally illustrating choices and tradeoffs, and overall implications for design. Hospice planners and architects can use these guidelines to stimulate their own ideas; hospice caregivers and administrators can compare these same guidelines to evaluate their own intentions and the designs of those they employ. In a larger scheme, it is hoped that these guidelines will shed some light on the functional implications of certain traditional solutions in health-care architecture.

Choosing an Image for the Hospice

When considering a remodel or new construction for an inpatient hospice unit, one of the most significant decisions to be made is the hospice's appearance as well as the connotations of that appearance, or the hospice's *image*. The strongest factor in the development of the image is the life-safety codes that apply to every health-care facility and now to hospices as well. The uniform building code classifies health-care facilities as Group I occupancies and restricts them, for the most part, to buildings constructed of steel, iron, concrete, and masonry.

Other factors in this decision making process include the available budget and the hospice caregivers' philosophy of care, such as a wholehearted adoption of the British model of hospice care or more active and medical intervention. The size and location of the unit is an important element, and design solutions are also often shaped by the nature of the available resources, such as the existing structure of the building to be remodeled or the kind of items that have been donated. Idiosyncratic and personal tastes also influence the final decision, in terms of colors and materials chosen—even the overall organization and approach. Some architectural solutions will be adopted because of convenience, fear, or experimentation, some through short-sightedness or limited experience.

How can we make a hospice homelike and still meet the life-safety code requirements? How far can we go to make the institutional context homelike? Establishing a distinction between derived and designed architectural forms may help.

Thompson and Goldin introduce this distinction in *The Hospital: A Social and Architectural History*. They note that the designed form is primarily a by-product of modernism, a result of its credo, "form follows function." Consequently, the image of many buildings today reflects a series of smaller decisions about functional areas. For example, certain functional areas, such as the operating-room suite, have distinct spatial requirements. In meeting the requirements of distinct functional units, the organization and, hence, the image of the building, is evolved. Earlier in the history of building types, derived forms were far more common; a monastery, for example, would become a hospital. Sometimes one building was converted for another use; more commonly, a new building was built, in the same image, for a new function.

For hospice architecture, derived architectural forms can be used to decrease the medical institution appearance of the facility. In general, people are more comfortable with other institutions—the school, the monastery, the library, the hotel, the university, even the sanatorium. Using a form derived from a nonmedical institution can help the hospice to gain acceptance within the community and raise the expectations of the prospective users. Each part of the hospice may have a reference to a different image or building type, but one general image should predominate.

Stephen Verderber, in his study of hospice design for the New Age facility in Houston, developed a chart of seven building types to categorize different areas of the hospice (Verderber 1982, 19). His basic idea, greatly modified to represent the findings of the compendium study, is as follows:

ARCHITECTURAL REFERENCE

Elements	Hospital	Hotel	Monastery	Home	Dormitory or School	Village	Sanatorium
Patient rooms	C	A	B	A	B	D	A
Family lounge	C	A	D	A	B	D	D
Family private room	C	B	A	A	B	D	D
Sacred rooms	C	C	A	B	D	B	D
Nature (indoors)	C	B	B	A	B	D	A
Nature (outdoors)	D	B	B	A	B	B	A
Nurses' station	C	A	D	D	A	B	D
Nurses' retreat	C	B	A	A	D	D	D
Inpatient services	B	B	C	B	A	B	D
Kitchenette	C	B	D	A	B	D	D
Dining room	C	A	D	B	B	B	D
Offices	B	A	D	B	A	A	D
Main entry	C	A	B	B	A	B	B
Bed entry	C	B	D	B	D	D	A
Linen/laundry	B	A	D	B	A	D	B
Janitorial	B	A	B	B	A	D	B

Key
A   Appropriate image
B   Possible alternate image
C   Inappropriate image
D   Minimal reference

Architectural Elements of Homelike Design

The incorporation of homelike elements into the environment is a primary requirement of hospice architecture. Homelike and institutional are the extremes of a continuum, a structuralist pair. What of home and residential architecture is essential, and what is superfluous in the design of a palliative-care facility with homelike environment?

John Summerson, the architectural theorist, says that architecture today cannot be monumental. "All those things which suggested and supported monumentality are in dissolution," such as distinct and powerful social classes, and a common sense of the importance of religion (Summerson, 1963, 203). Summerson claims that "houses, blocks of flats, schools, libraries, hospitals, offices, administrative buildings—none of these in their modern form is susceptible of that grand increase of scale which is the essence of monumentality" (Summerson, 1963, 204). He believes that we must look to the private home for cultural and architectural meaning, and goes on to say that giving primacy to the individual dwelling leads to primacy in human scale of architecture. Summerson recommends that public architecture, such as hospitals, libraries, university buildings, and theaters, should be broken down to human scale, which will form the large but nonmonumental buildings of the future.

Something must be done to modify the current crop of large, amorphous, institutional buildings. Institutional buildings of the modern style, incorporating the machine aesthetic, have come to symbolize repetitive, impersonal treatment. When combined with institutionalized medicine, the institutional health-care facility can be inattentive to the needs of the individual. For hospice care, this means the inpatient unit must counteract two separate architectural messages: the first allied with the modern architectural style, the second part of a long-standing, often hidden antipathy toward those who cannot afford private care and must be "institutionalized." The spareness of the hard, shiny, economical, and streamlined machine aesthetic reinforces an economizing that surfaced as care became secular rather than religious. Some have characterized secular care as frugal when applied to the sick, poor, and weak.

Of all the building forms or archetypes presented, the image most commonly referred to in hospice literature and the most significant image for the hospice is the home. Although the model of the American home is not uniform, certain ideal home images prevail in the advertisement of houses and home appliances that suggest what a modern home ought to be.

Kent Bloomer and Charles Moore draw an analogy between the architecture of a house and the anatomy of the human body (Bloomer and Moore 1977, 50). They emphasize the human need to have examples of natural elements, such as fire, water, light, and so on, incorporated into the home setting. These examples, such as the fireplace in the American home or the fountain in the Mexican courtyard, symbolize our connection to the earth. The hearth serves as a place for social rituals, recalling and celebrating the basic life-supporting elements, and is decorated with personal items, such as photographs. Many of these associations are subconscious, yet play a large part in the meaning of the term *homelike*. These subconscious associations as well as more conscious associations with the home—personalization, territoriality, and freedom—are what give meaning to architectural form and make the house a home.

The intention of hospices in incorporating homelike elements in the hospice setting is to encourage these warm and comforting associations as well as foster the privacy, freedom, socialization, and other elements of individual choice that take place in the home.

The architectural components of the home in the United States include the following: context, massing, scale, portal, plan, detailing, surfaces, lighting, equipment, and fixtures. Each is briefly reviewed below to clarify its use and ensure common definitions. Nondesigners will find this information helpful in conversations with their planners and architects.

Context is concerned with the siting of the building, including the location of a house in a residential neighborhood with planting strips, shrubbery, open lawns, sidewalks, curb cuts, and many layers of screening between the street and front door of the building. The *massing* of a residential building involves the use of traditional shapes with roof forms and little use of boxes or rectangles with flat roofs. *Scale* for the house is generally established by breaking down any large element into smaller and smaller sizes until some reference can be drawn to a human body. Examples of scale include window panes that compose a larger operable window or a roof that has dormers repeating larger gable shapes.

Approach refers to the path leading to the portal, with a privacy gradient that may include a semipublic yard, semiprivate path, and private porch. The entry, front door, or *portal* of a house describes the private chamber; inside a house, there are few other gradations of privacy. In contrast, an institution has a semipublic entry area and many further private realms, such as offices or exam rooms. Institutions and houses differ greatly in *plan organization*, the most obvious difference being the large amount of circulation space of the institution and the specialized use of rooms. *Detailing* provides scale within the house, such as trims for the room or handrails for the stairs. *Surfaces* in homes add softness, texture, and damping qualities, and make a warm and comforting environment. In residential rooms, *lighting* tends to be natural, typically provided by windows on more than one wall; most of the artificial lighting is incandescent and task. Institutional lighting, in contrast, is usually fluorescent and overhead, and there are seldom windows on more than one side of a room. *Equipment* and *fixtures* in homes are easily controlled for multiple use. The furniture is usually of softer and natural materials and is movable and changeable (Moss 1981, 87–103).

The homelike hospice components identified in the compendium vary considerably; however, certain elements remain prevalent. These are the homelike elements that seem to translate into the institutional setting: large bedrooms with varied decor, accommodation, location, and size; family spaces; residential finishes and furniture and personal belongings; more room per patient on unit than in an SNF or acute-care facility; the location of the unit itself near, but not in, major activity; and views of nature and gardens. Nonarchitectural aspects of homelike atmosphere include privacy, security, community, and flexibility.

To explore the parameters of homelike architecture within an institutional setting, the following breakdown of architectural and other components is presented:

- privacy and community gradients
- adaptability, duplication of function, and multifunction
- finishes and furnishings
- personalization, participation, choice, and variety
- organization and quality of life

None of these elements is completely distinct; all interact to support the functions of the hospice unit within a homelike atmosphere that reinforces hospice principles. Each component has important architectural implications for the entire inpatient hospice, not all of which can be discussed here. However, taken separately, each of the above will suggest how a homelike atmosphere can be maximized in an institutional setting.

Privacy and Community Gradients

When Lo-Yi Chan designed the Connecticut Hospice, he planned transition spaces—alcoves or vestibules— as areas in which people could pause to collect their thoughts or retreat temporarily. These transition places are not rooms in the traditional sense; rather, they are analogous to airlocks in caissons. The transition spaces allow staff and visitors to adjust, for example, when passing from a patient room to the hallway. Thus, the architect was acknowledging, physically, the need for a gradient of privacy.

Instead of thinking of privacy as a wall or barrier, it is helpful to consider it a combination of social conventions and architectural obstructions. For example, a closed door functions as a barrier to a room, but the social convention of knocking on a door before entering works with the architectural barrier to provide the inhabitant of the room with privacy. Of course, social conventions vary according to geography and circumstance. We know, for example that it is possible to feel alone in a crowd because of social atmosphere. It is possible for the Japanese, with their sophisticated social culture, to feel complete privacy with a thin paper screen separating them from others. However, within the heterogeneous American society, social rules are not universal; thus, architects may turn to physical

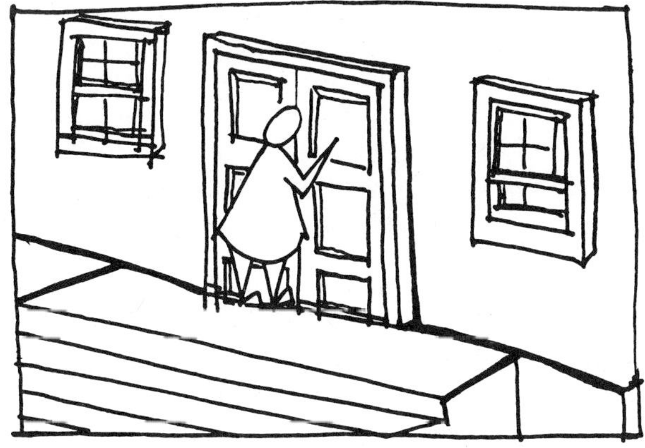

Social convention and architecture work together to form a barrier to the room.

barriers to structure relationships. This explains, in part, the predominance of single rooms as the solution to privacy problems in the hospital. Designers know, on the other hand, that they cannot substitute an architectural solution for a cultural ambiguity. In hospice care, the participation of the family and patient in giving care should promote the social homogeneity necessary to protect the rules for privacy, courtesy, and dignity.

Below is a chart that displays some of the architectural options that can be used to support a range of behaviors, from isolation to large gatherings.

Privacy	*Community*
Acoustic screens/curtains	Movable screens/curtains
Handicap access	Handicap access
Single-bed rooms, baths	Multibed rooms
Quiet rooms	Noisy rooms
Adaptable spaces	Adaptable spaces
Private areas, rooms	Group areas, rooms
Zoning and orientation	Zoning and orientation
Personalized areas	Personalized areas
Outdoor plantings	Outdoor patio space
Nooks, stopping places	Vistas, amphitheaters
Single activity rooms	Group activity areas
Transition areas	Transition areas

In addition, supplementary equipment can be used to foster privacy or community: earphones, art carts, telephones, television, bulletin boards, microphones, closed-circuit television. Some of the elements above are repeated in both columns, indicating that the same element can provide either privacy or community depending on how it is used, such as adaptable space that can be used by groups and individuals at different times. Many of the above elements are opposites, such as group and private areas: all are necessary if both privacy and community are to be achieved. Areas that are incompatible must, of course, be separated, but it is important that the full range of choices be available for patient, family, and staff in a convenient and accessible plan. This may mean some duplication of function, as well as adaptable areas.

Privacy and community are issues that touch all the other components of homelike design and examples of their architecture will be found throughout the section on guidelines. Examples of architectural components of privacy and community given here are representative rather than comprehensive. Design for this continuum can and should occur

throughout the facility in many ingenious ways. If the designer looks to maximize possibilities for privacy, interaction, and community throughout the design of the hospice, better bedrooms, nursing stations, or inpatient services can be planned.

Patient rooms are the arena for privacy, community, and interaction. Single rooms are commonly found in acute-care units; the inappropriateness of diagonal-bed placement in hospice design has already been discussed. However, single rooms are valuable for hospice patients, who may wish to be physically or sexually close to their partners, who may have large families, or who may simply desire their own room. Single patient rooms should be designed to maximize the patient's mobility. The room should be large, furniture and sinks should be out of the patient's way, and the door should be wide, to permit bed access. Adding handicap bars, nonslip surfaces, and other handicap features enables the patient to get to many places unassisted. So that the patient will not feel abandoned, views from the bed of the windows and doors are necessary.

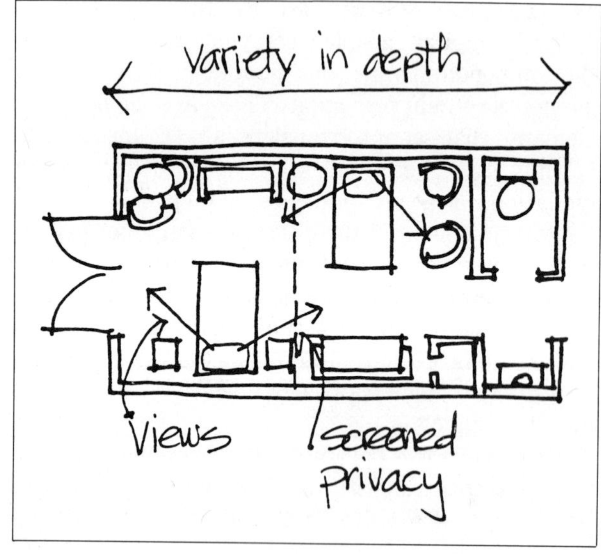

Toe-to-toe bed arrangement in double room

On the other hand, the single room is not appropriate for all hospice patients. Multibed rooms increase the patients' opportunity to interact; communication is as important as privacy. One solution is the toe-to-toe bed arrangement, which permits easy patient discourse as well as screening. Another example of architectural design for privacy as well

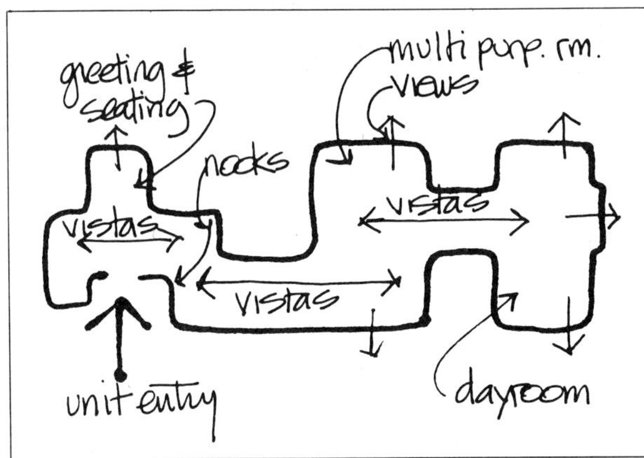

Corridor system, St. Peter's Hospice

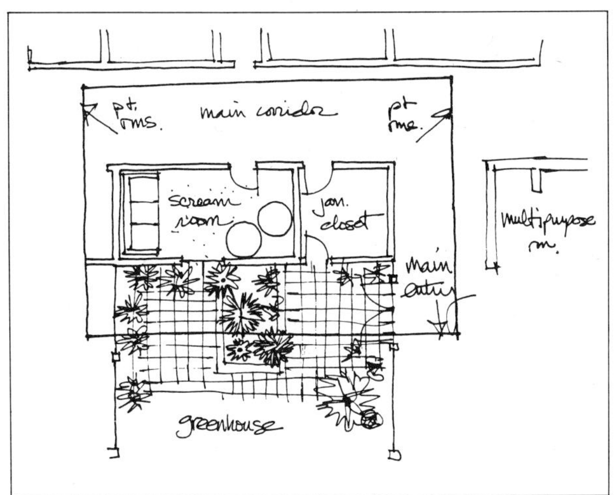

Scream room, Nathan Adelson Hospice

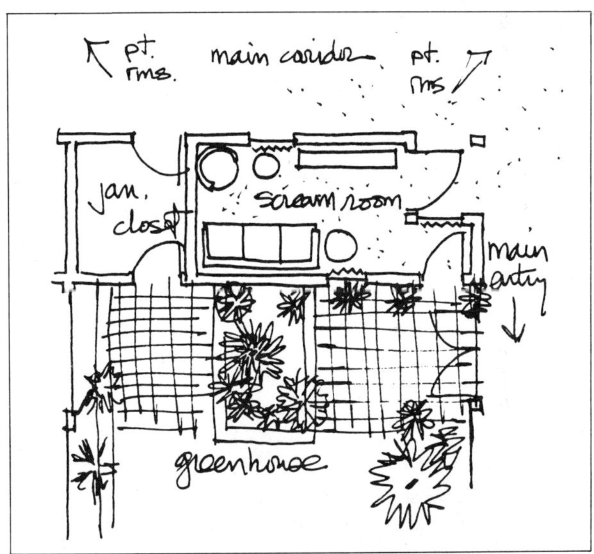

Alternate design for scream room at Nathan Adelson Hospice

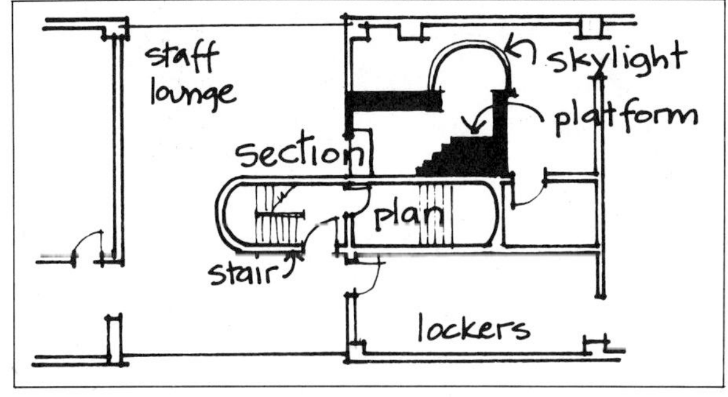

Staff "scream room," Connecticut Hospice

as community is the use of nooks and community rooms. St. Peter's Hospice's previously double-loaded hallway was modified into shorter corridors with turns and openings into family areas.

The needs for privacy and community are served as well by areas designed specifically for one or another of the extremes. Private rooms for personal introspection and emotion can be designed and located for all to use, or they can be designed for staff use only, or for a single family or family member. The staff retreat room at the Connecticut Hospice, called the scream room, is located close to the staff lounge and lockers. In addition, this section of the Connecticut Hospice houses the child-care center, so that staff may share meals or otherwise interact with their own children. Some retreat rooms should be located near the patient bed areas, so that the staff or family will not feel that they are shirking their responsibility to the patient, but they should also be located far enough away so that no one is disturbed. A concern for privacy should lead the designer to equip the private rooms with a screened entry and exit so that the use is less uncomfortable. At Nathan Adelson, the location of the scream room on a main corridor may make its use apparent to too many people, thereby hindering its purpose. The stigma of uncontrolled emotion in this society gives form to many social rules on the appropriate show of public and private grief.

Quiet rooms for the family, such as the private room, are found in most hospice facilities in the compendium. They double as conference areas or as overnight rooms in some schemes. Care should be taken that the uses differ with time so that the original use is not confounded. Noisy rooms or group activity areas are examples from the other extreme in the continuum of privacy and community. Rooms dedicated to noisy and group functions must always be large enough to incorporate patients in beds or bed-lounge chairs and also their family. The size must therefore be at least 18 square feet per patient, with additional seating areas for staff and family calculated. Of the larger facilities, Rosary Hill Home has one of the nicest group areas with an outdoor and indoor orientation, overlooking the entry and view, and with plenty of room for patients, family, and staff.

At St. Peter's Hospice, the dayroom is located farthest from the unit entry, to motivate the patients and visitors toward the activity areas and away from the bedrooms. This promotes circulation through the unit and is enhanced by the nooks and alcoves also present. Location of group areas is important in encouraging mixing of patients, family, staff, and visitors. Other units put the larger group areas in a central location, such as the outdoor patio at Calvary or the living room of the Hospice of the Good Shepherd. Activity areas can be duplicated, as at Nathan Adelson, where dining, outdoor rooms, and indoor activity rooms are located throughout the unit. Many smaller and more modest hospices have only one general gathering area.

For staff and their family, community areas such as the multipurpose rooms, dining areas, and day-rooms, can be used. These rooms need zoned furniture arrangements, in which furniture is grouped for different functions, to allow for privacy and community. The use of adaptable devices, such as movable assemblies, plants, accordian room dividers, acoustic screens, and extra unassigned space, adds to the options for privacy and community for all hospice users.

Adaptability, Duplication, and Multiple Functions

Flexibility within hospice design allows for the introduction of a homelike accommodation to uses.

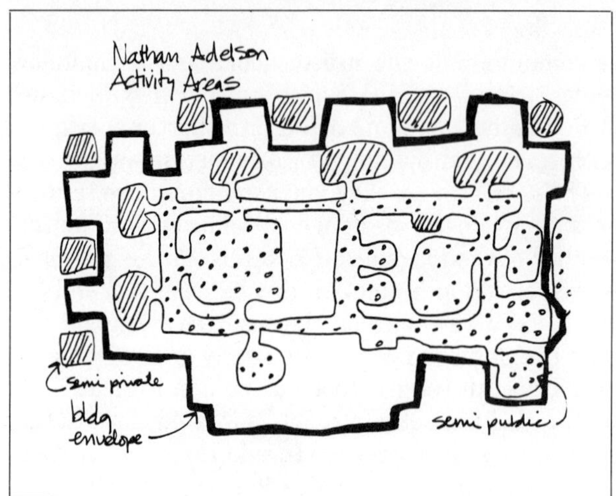

Activity rooms, Nathan Adelson Hospice

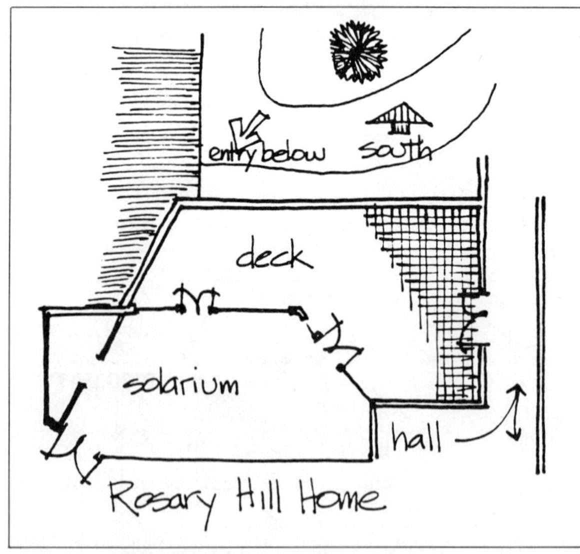

Solarium and deck, Rosary Hill Home

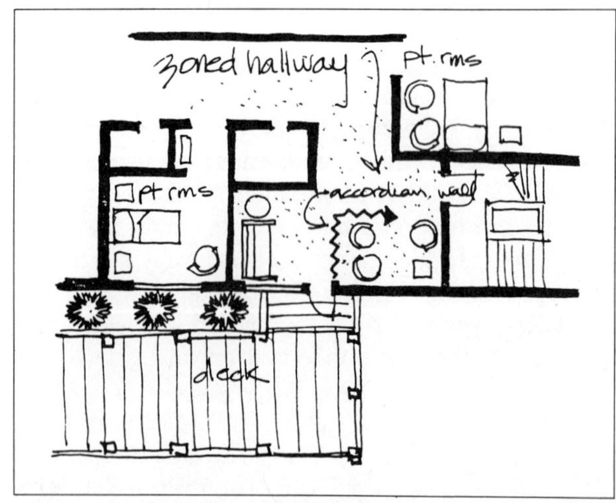

Hall plan, Hospice of the Good Shepherd

Institutional buildings have been designed after factories, with many of the areas assigned one specific function. Residences, in contrast, encourage various activities at each location. For example, the dining table is adaptable for eating, conversation, conferences, office and schoolwork, or family projects, even as a mail or supply area. Every area of the home must be able to do multiple duty, too, as the family needs change over time with new or different circumstances. This multiplicity of function is a fundamental component of the home and is part of good hospice design.

Flexibility in the design of spaces in a new kind of institution, like the hospice, where needs are not yet set, population and use patterns change over time, and ethnic backgrounds and ages vary, is only common sense. The provision of areas with unspecified uses is hard to protect, especially within the current payment procedures of United States health care, but it is essential that this concept be part of the social and physical aspect of hospice inpatient settings.

Adaptability and flexibility are part of the design of hospices at many locations, with a few basic guidelines. Uses can be combined with similar space and equipment needs, and different temporal ones, such as conference rooms that double as boardrooms and dining areas, for example. General space allocation can allow for zoning of open-plan areas for meeting, small personal discussion, or passive activities, with or without architectural barriers. Additional space allocation for changes in use over time is possible in remodeled units, whereas new facilities may be designed for expansion. In addition, certain development strategies will enhance possibilities for adaptation and flexibility, among which are adaptive reuse, stage and contingency planning,

and the use of a limited group of construction materials as well as a simple, repetitive structural system, such as post and beam on a grid.

Loose fit, the ability of a room or building to serve several different functions, allows flexibility of use. The loose fit found at the Hospice of the Good Shepherd and the Hospice of Northern Virginia is partly a result of the fact that both buildings were originally schools, now transformed into palliative-care units. The often tightly designed and "economical" areas of former acute-care wards and skilled nursing facilities are more difficult to modify for multipurpose hospice use. A loose fit suggests that the building can provide for new occupants over time and that the unit will change and grow in a flexible, undogmatic way.

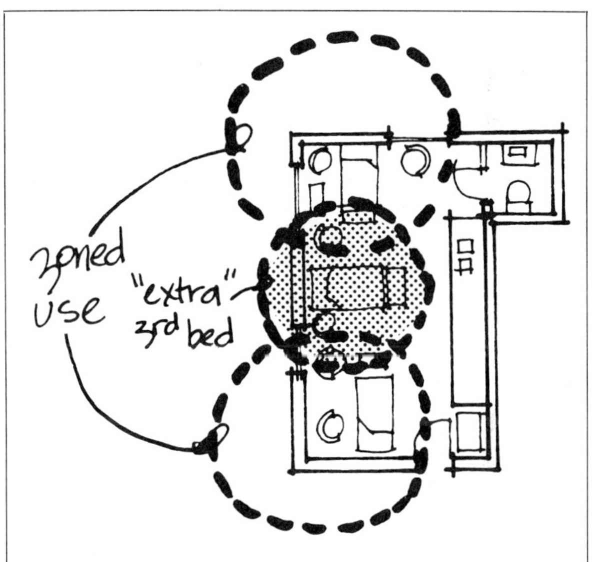

Patient room, St. Peter's Hospice

Areas of adaptable use in the hospice extend from entry to bedrooms, nursing stations, conference and physical therapy rooms, and daycare; indeed, all areas of the unit. At St. Peter's hospice, for example, the three-bed rooms are typically used as doubles, but can extend to triples, should the situation warrant. This allows more room per patient, greater family use, and extra patient space as well.

Multibed rooms can also contain chairs and tables for display of personal items, entertainment, talking, eating, and so on. Multibed rooms and private rooms in clusters can be adapted for different needs of the family, such as places for smokers, rooms for

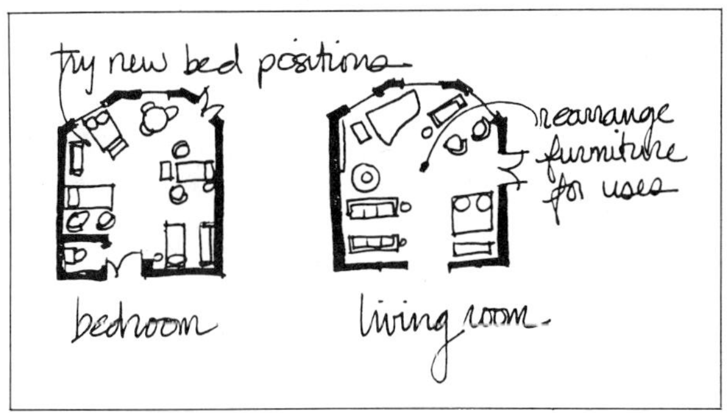

The bedroom and living room areas at the Hospice of Northern Virginia can be adapted for other uses.

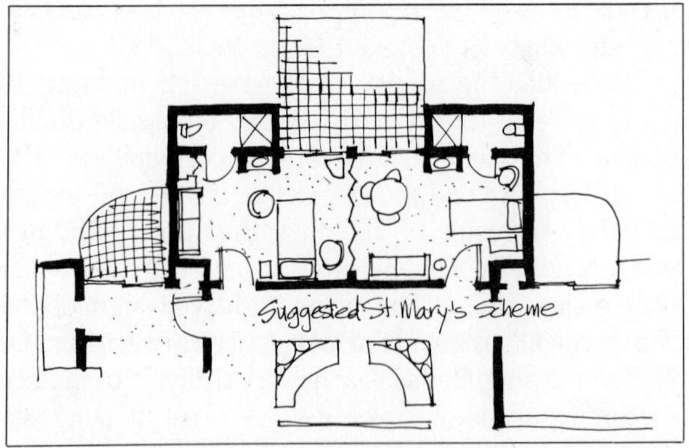

Cluster arrangement of bedrooms, suggested for St. Mary's Hospice

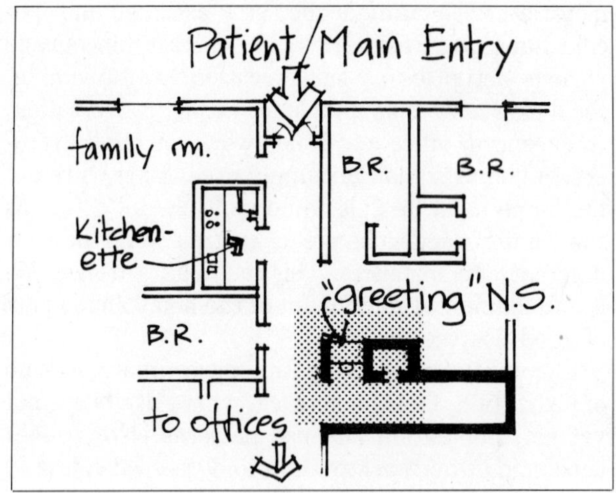

Patient entry, Hospice of Northern Virginia

physical intimacy, or space for families of different sizes. In some cases, movable partitions can be constructed between single rooms, so that the rooms can be connected or divided at need. This was the early plan at St. Mary's Hospice in Tucson.

Other areas of the hospice are likely places for multiple functions. At St. Peter's, the nursing station is located at the entrance to the patient floor, which allows nurses to greet patients, family, and visitors, and also serves to centralize typical nursing functions. This pattern is repeated at Clover Hospice. In designing such a multipurpose area, however, the designer must take care not to overwork the area, creating a nursing station too imposing in the design. At St. Peter's, Clover Hospice, and the Connecticut Hospice, administration offices are located in a different area from the nurses' station. It is also important that these greeting stations have a friendly low counter, open plan, and that they are located right at the entry, rather than viewed from a long corridor, as at Mercy Hospice.

Combined functions demand that each job be planned and designed for, so that sitting areas are adjacent to the greeting station, and that the station, itself, has adequate work space and privacy, too. At Northern Virginia, for example, although the seating area of the family room is not directly adjacent to the nursing station, the kitchenette and nurses' station surround the patient entry and welcome new arrivals. Again, the administrative and staff entry is located elsewhere at Northern Virginia, so as not to overwhelm the activity and roles of the nursing staff.

Further areas with multiple use include conference areas, which can also be used as libraries or even dining rooms. Family rooms can double as massage rooms for patients, as overnight or counseling rooms, and for personal grooming areas for visitors and others. At St. Mary's Hospital for Children, their special needs and small space have led them to consider adding an exam room that would double as a body viewing room. Here, the more sacred viewing function can soften the examination atmosphere, enhancing both uses. The extra family room with bath, added at St. Peter's, can be used for many functions, such as sleeping or retreat space. It is located near the patient rooms, but is central to the large multipurpose room and dayroom.

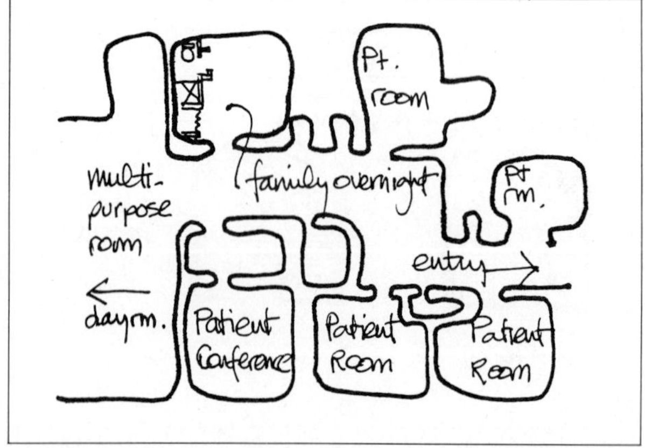

Family room, St. Peter's Hospice

Larger family rooms, to provide another example, can be used as child-care areas, for crafts, physical therapy, occupational therapy, dining, reading rooms, information meetings, and as a celebration area. The large multipurpose room at Rosary Hill Home can serve various size groups with different needs, by virtue of its proximity to the building entry and offices and its movable wall divider.

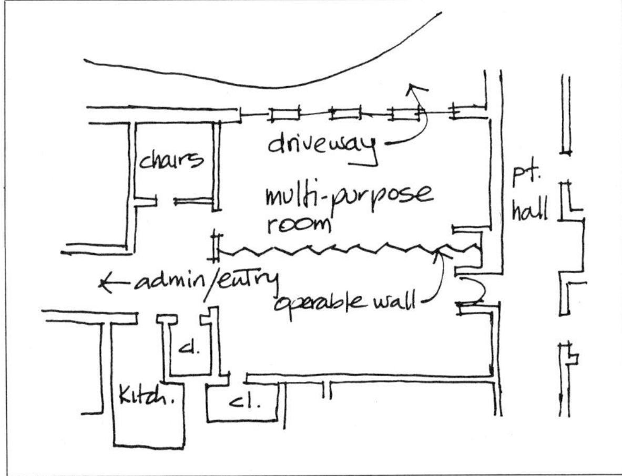

Multipurpose room, Rosary Hill Home

The multipurpose dayroom at St. Peter's Hospice has an adjoining large kitchen, as do most of the other hospices. At Mercy Hospice, the movable partitions in the family room and kitchenette can expand to encompass the chapel next door to provide room for larger celebrations and weekly or memorial services, if needed. Otherwise, the chapel remains small and intimate for quiet prayer and meditation. This technique is also used at the Connecticut Hospice to transform a small and uniquely designed meditation room into a larger area when needed.

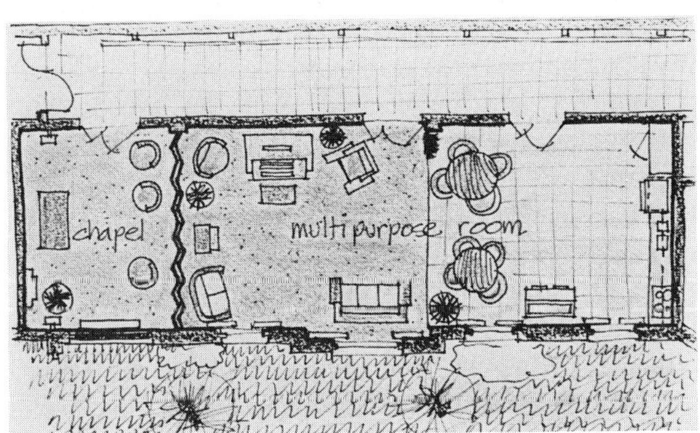

Plan, multipurpose room and chapel, Mercy Hospice

When the connection between the viewing room and chapel or family room and chapel is less flexible, adding connecting doors or placing the rooms in view of one another promotes flexibility. Garden areas can also be used in a number of ways. Nathan Adelson provides both covered and open gardens of various shapes and in different locations for a variety of uses. Flexibility is encouraged by placing outdoor patios and gardens directly outside patient and family rooms, with doors and windows that view out. Rosary Hill Home and the Hospice of the Good Shepherd also adopted this design.

The duplication of function adds flexibility to the unit as a whole. The two floors of St. Peter's and the Hospice of Cincinnati, for example, have kitchenette facilities at both levels, so that activities are accessible to all the users of the unit. This breakdown of scale provides the flexibility and duplication necessary to allow every user of the facility easy access to each area. Services provided irregularly or infrequently on the unit, such as physical or music therapy, are perfect for multiple-use rooms. A soundproof room can suffice, at different times, for meditation, music therapy, games, and reading. Even smaller details, such as corners, ceilings, and leftover areas, can take on adaptable use, for display or children's play. Especially for smaller and tighter units, the multiplicity of function and adaptability of form becomes a matter of constant finessing of ever restrictive plans. Thus, window boxes are added to patient rooms to make gardens at bed height, televisions are placed in the bar area, and mobile art carts provide new pictures for the walls. Flexibility and adaptability are part of the control by all the users of the hospice and reflect a domestic concern with the minutiae of hospice use.

Furnishings and Finishes

The third component of homelike hospice design is the contribution of furnishings and finishes. Perhaps the most frequently mentioned of the homelike qualities in hospice literature, furnishings and finishes are the easiest and cheapest modification to hospice inpatient space. Moreover, using furnishings and finishes to modify design is a typical nonprofessional experience, one that allows for personal control and individual tastes.

A quote from one of the most respected writers on hospices shows, in designer-layman terms, the homelike atmosphere that finishes and furnishings can effect:

Azaleas, ferns, chrysanthemums, cyclamens, African violets, two single rooms at the end of each hall, four beds in each large and airy bay, each with its own curtains that can be drawn shut, and each with its own furnishings around it—tables, chairs, armchairs, photographs, cards, books. Colored quilts, knitted coverlets, and plenty of down pillows on each bed. Fresh white linens, worn and soft. Letters, newspapers, cigarettes, lamps, baskets of fruit. A bottle of port and two glasses (Stoddard 1978, 103).

Sandol Stoddard contrasts this homelike atmosphere with that of the hospital, where bells, lights, buzzers, and steel machinery create a rushed, sterile atmosphere inappropriate for the dying.

Standards for residential furniture and finishes are more restrictive in an institution, as furniture and finishes must be easy to clean and fire-resistant. A review of the hospice architecture in the compendium reveals four basic approaches to the addition of homelike furnishings and finishes to a basic complement of hospital bed, overbed table (optional), and the patient lounge chair. These approaches include: the addition of donated residential furniture, plants, and new paint; contribution of the patient's own furniture to basic pieces, and paint; a plain, neutral background with designed interior furniture; and a designed interior with matching furniture, wallpaper, and paint and coordinated lighting and trim. Any hospice could incorporate a mixture of these approaches, combining, for example, the patient's own furniture with donated pieces or a designed interior. In general, basic residential furniture, such as sofas, chairs, and incandescent lamps, is added to patient and family rooms first. Later, these items may be added to staff rooms, offices, retreat rooms, and possibly to the nursing station or other inpatient service areas.

In addition to the basic bedroom furniture mentioned above, most hospices in the compendium are equipped with many different kinds of chairs, sofa beds, bedside tables, dressers, chests, bookcases, tables, lamps, and display space for possessions, plants, and pictures. The family areas often have a living and dining set, tables, children's furniture, and wall display units. The hospice unit, as a whole, generally has artwork, carpeting, new paint, incandescent lighting, window blinds, curtains, and residential details, such as wall clocks, fireplaces, and kitchenette equipment. Institutional equipment is deemphasized.

Outdoors, hospices try to provide covered and open seating, planters, terrace areas for activities, and fountains. Children's play furniture is a priority if possible, and a barbeque and games can be added to the outdoor equipment.

Most hospices are working with extremely small budgets and need to use donated furniture. This solution, although not coordinated with other aspects of design, is flexible, comfortable, and automatically provides variety. In addition, donated furniture represents less initial investment, allowing the hospice to adapt furnishings and to upgrade over time, as is typical in the home. Of course, the donated furniture may not be of a set, and may not match the building architecture. Certain types of furniture are easier to keep clean and move than others; donated pieces may also be worn or sprung. All this is less easy to control with a donated scheme.

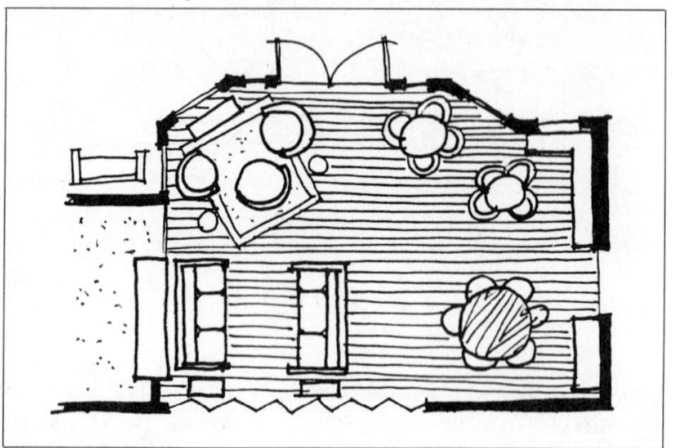

Zoned furniture

In contrast, a designed interior represents a great investment, one that provides an instant image for the hospice. A total design is less flexible to changes over time and to personal idiosyncrasy. A fully designed unit must have a planned variety rather than variety that grows or is spontaneous with use. At Nathan Adelson, variety is a planned aspect of design. The patient rooms are decorated in one of five schemes: contemporary, colonial, Victorian, provincial, and traditional. Such an approach attempts a total residential motif and a coordinated design.

The use of a neutral design that provides a uniform background for patient furniture is less appropriate here than in Great Britain, where inpatient stays are usually much longer. Here, most hospices offer short-term stays, for which the addition of patient's own furnishings may not be convenient. The bleakness of some background designs is evident in the illustration of patient rooms at Riverside Hospital;

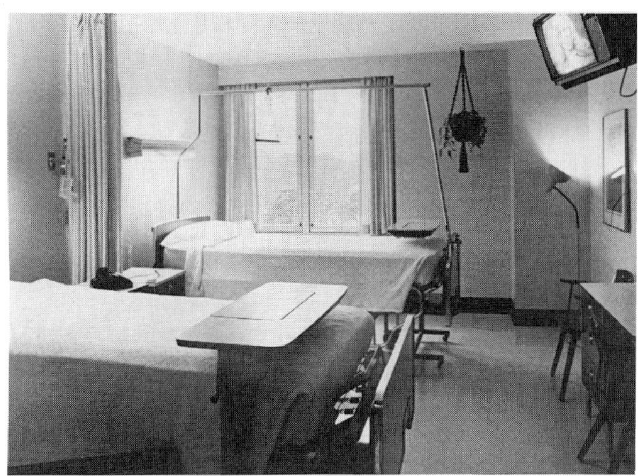

Patient bedroom, Riverside Hospice

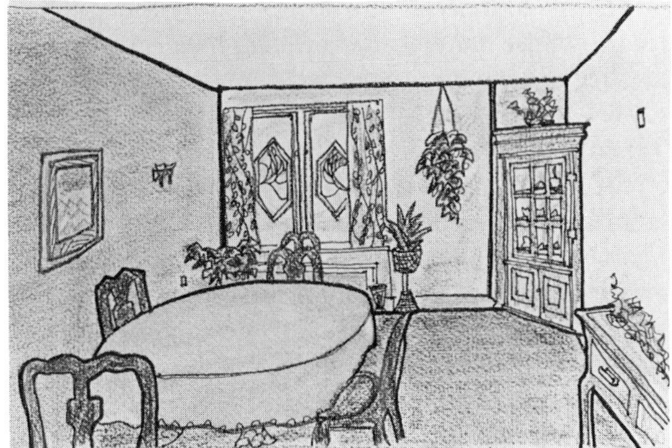

Some hospice facilities have a formal dining room set, complete with sideboard and china cabinet.

however, it is obvious that such bleakness should encourage patient and family involvement with the room decoration when the patient is admitted.

In general, hospice furniture must be sturdy, to prevent falls, and serviceable; it must allow for group and individual comfort. Chairs for visiting, reading, handholding, and so on, are most important, as are overnight sleeping arrangements and storage space. The residential furniture used at hospices is often made of natural materials, including wood, warm twill, or cotton-like fabrics. Additional equipment is often made of functional material: blinds are often metal; shutters, cabinets, and counter tops are wood or plastic laminate; carpeting is usually a low-nap, fire-resistant material. Hospices often have special areas decorated in another style, such as the sunroom with patio furniture at the Cincinnati Hospice, for example.

Hospices have been able to deinstitutionalize some of their bathrooms by adding chairs, vanity areas, and pretty touches such as plants and other decorative items. Nurses' stations and inpatient services often have built-in cabinets; other custom furniture used in hospices are room dividers, kitchenettes, and the chapel dais. Bookcases, magazine racks, and desks are all important. Some facilities have a formal dining room set, complete with sideboard and china cabinet. Towel racks and other smaller elements can add a personal touch. Hallways with furniture, residential detailing, and incandescent lighting need not look quite so institutional.

A word here on paint colors and wall and ceiling finishes. New fire-resistant materials for wainscots and walls are being introduced on the market every year. No unanimity on the selection of appropriate hospice colors was discovered in the survey, but textures were considered important and many units had wallpaper and wood trim in at least a few rooms. Proper colors for hospice use may simply be those not usually associated with traditional hospital interiors, such as deep greens, dark blues, strong peaches, and so on. Institutional pale green should be avoided. Some patients will have mental confusion and resulting perceptual difficulties; busy patterns in the wallpaper, and dark reds and purples, which are often the first colors to become indistinguishable with darkness, should probably be avoided as well.

Providing a variety of colors and decoration can alleviate such discomfort or even a patient's hearty dislike of a color or scheme. The greatest difficulty may occur as a particular decorative scheme triggers an unpleasant association in the patient's mind, rather than physical or perceptual difficulties the patient may have. For the designer, the most important thing to know about hospice colors is that there is still disagreement and that neither "neutral" white and beige nor very brilliant and saturated hues is appropriate. Moderation and a willingness to change colors should they not be acceptable may be the best strategy. Hospices have called every color from palest yellow to deep green homelike; judging from the survey, reds, grays, and blues are also quite popular. The more somber and tranquil atmosphere of the hospice chapel should be contrasted with light and airy views of the outdoors.

Personalization, Participation, Choice, and Variety

Personalization, participation, choice, and variety are not architectural elements of homelike design, but behavior that can be encouraged by thoughtful design. These four characteristics have great significance for hospice care, as they represent the antithesis of behavior found in institutions, which often discourage individualization. Hospices very definitely designate these characteristics as being essential to care in a palliative unit or at home.

Participation, personalization, and choice are the most active results of homelike design. They imply the involvement of all hospice users in the running of the hospice. The hospice environment then reflects the needs of the users, unlike the institution, which typically imposes a finished environment on its users. Hospice care depends on a continual dialogue among all users, in an atmosphere where every individual is respected. The empowerment of the individual is necessary for all involved—staff, nurses, volunteers, friends, family, and the dying one at the center of care. Thus, this activity represents the dynamic function of the facility in all respects and among all participants.

The importance of this dynamic interaction in the institution is very great. As Kevin Lynch, a planner, comments, interaction is necessary in order to inculcate a sense of place (Lynch 1976, 21–30). The home itself can be seen as a worldly retreat in which optimal freedom exists for the individual in a microcosm. Within the home, the qualities of participation, personalization, variety, and choice are maximized. These activities are the dynamic of the individual in the home and, therefore, represent that dynamic element of home in an institution.

Personalization, participation, choice, and variety have many architectural ramifications. Personalization, for example, is aided in an institution when places are set aside for pictures, displays, plants, even fish tanks and bird cages, and storage for the displaced hospice items is programmed. For example, should patients want to bring their own dressers, storage of the hospice dressers should be available and the move easy to accomplish. Placing bulletin boards in elevators, halls, and in rooms can discourage people from taping things to the wall and chipping the paint, although regular repainting instead of cleaning is another answer. At bedside, personalization can be encouraged with human scale, zoning, and the establishment of individual territory. Bedside tables and windowsills should have plenty of room for personal items. The foot of the bed can have a display board or trunk with room for items. In addition, bedroom and bathroom areas should have vanity details, including places for personal

soaps, hair brushes, colognes, and similar items. The hospice may encourage display of family pictures of staff and volunteers, greeting cards and notes, festivity photographs, artwork, flowers and mementos, as well as such handmade items as quilts and crafts, decorated sheets, and pillowcases. Many items, such as flower vases and planting equipment, need additional storage places to encourage decoration with growing and cut flowers and plants.

Participation in the initial design involves all members of the hospice community in the architectural process. Community, staff, volunteers, home-care patients and families can be encouraged to participate when viewed as codesigners of the hospice. One common system is to set aside a planning room with a bulletin board, to be used during the planning process. A large bulletin board with columns for idea cards is also commonly used, to display concerns, concepts, and architectural designs developed during various discussions with the codesigners. Such a method works well to itemize the issues brought up by users and architects. Later, as the facility is completed and functioning, design changes will undoubtedly occur over time. Some of the changes suggested by the hospice staff members during compendium research were often difficult to add to a completed unit, such as sun porches; however, other changes were more easy to implement.

Change is unavoidable in hospice care. Some time should pass before revisions are undertaken to make sure of their necessity. At the Connecticut Hospice, hall closets were recently added in order to shorten the distance to fresh linen storage. These modifications to the original design were not considered oversights in the original design so much as changes needed as use patterns were established. At Calvary Hospital, the increased participation of families in care strained existing training and outpatient areas. New construction is being planned to accommodate these changes. Other facilities have found initial planning unable to foresee changes in ethnic base, age of the dying, even in interior use and locations of kitchenettes, nursing stations, and so on. Such changes should be viewed as part of the users' participation in the design process, which cannot cease if a building is to adapt to its users.

The third element, choice, is a basic concern of the patient, caregivers, family, volunteers, and hospice proponents. It is a factor in the concept of family and patient as the unit of care, taking into account the palliative needs of the dying and their loved ones. It is also necessary to any building of community in the hospice. There is a need for a wide range of choices within the activities of hospice caring. For example, it is the patient's and family's choice to enter the hospice and decide how long the stay should last. The architecture can ease and dignify that entrance and exit by placing bed-patient entry with the formal ambulatory entry, instead of a back-door ambulance platform. Choice in bedroom accommodation is provided by variety of room types, from single to multibed rooms. Choice is encouraged when variety is evident, too, in view and exposure, for smokers and nonsmokers, and for those with a small or a large family.

The hospice inpatient setting allows for more choice when task lamps at bedside have easily accessible switches, when the operable windows have blinds and curtains for the regulation of light and view, and when rooms have fan coil units for individual control of heating. Handicap accessibility increases choices for the patient, as does convenient access to the out of doors and interior activities. In some units, oxygen and suction in the walls of dayrooms, chapel, and other rooms make patients far more comfortable about venturing outside their bedrooms.

Choice, therefore, is an enhancement of mobility and access to entertainment, food, comfort and control, at any hour of the day or night. It is aided by telephones at the bedside, by nonabandonment views for security, and by variety and ease. For the family, choices are supported when their own retreat is placed near patient bedrooms, but far enough away to be private. Access to many areas of the unit, including bathing areas, kitchenette, the outdoors, dayrooms, dining areas, laundry facilities and more can help the family to cope and help to care for their loved one. Choices for parents are increased when there are places for children to play and where supervision might be provided. Visiting is facilitated when the hospice has adequate parking, easy entry, is centrally located for public transportation and airports, and provides overnight sleeping arrangements.

For staff, choice is supported when necessary facilities are provided: a convenient staff retreat, comfortable changing and personal grooming facilities, and places for resting and reading. Staff needs easy access to the outdoors, including a thoughtful connection from parking to their unit. They need adequate space for nursing and maintenance functions too. Volunteers need their own space for projects and conveniently placed respite and contem-plation areas. Childcare allows the staff and volunteers greater convenience and opportunity. In addition, transition areas add to choice by making changes more manageable for all members of the hospice community. Good design makes privacy and socialization, personalization and participation possible and ultimately enhances individual choice. There will be conflicts in an architecture that maximizes choice, but the alternative is an architecture that imposes control, totally inappropriate for a kind of caregiving that emphasizes personal freedom.

In hospice design, variety is more than the different bedroom finishes at St. Peter's Hospice, more than the disparate pathways at the Connecticut Hospice, or the varied kinds of outdoor and family spaces evident at Nathan Adelson. Variety is the result of a change in perspective, from that of an overview of the hospice facility to that of the stationary or moving person within the walls of the hospice, looking, feeling, hearing, touching, and thinking about the mundane, emotional, and deeply philosophical issues of his or her life.

Hospice users will be in beds, in lounge or wheelchairs, using walkers or walking slowly; they will also be little children, teenagers, elderly, or middle-aged family members, friends, or volunteers. The points of view of all these users are extremely diverse and challenge the best design. The designer should contemplate the point of view of the bedridden patient, for instance, and provide an interesting ceiling design, perhaps stencils on a band of trim, skylights, or hanging plants, rather than repetitive acoustic tile. The wheelchair patient has another vantage point and needs lower window sills in order to admire an outdoor view and vanity and activity areas built for the handicapped. For visiting children, a sandbox or messy drawing area permits varied activities.

Variety results from the designer's attention to a small growing tree visible from a new corridor window, from the placement of birdfeeders and fountains, of greenhouses and stained glass; it is part of a southern orientation for the dining room, and ceilings that vary in a building to accommodate intimacy one place and a 15-foot Christmas tree in another. A variety of celebrations and festivities are made possible when storage space for firewood, seasonal displays, crafts, and choral music is designed. Variety is enhanced by flowers on the food carts, by art carts for selection of pictures, and by a piano in the living room.

In hospice care, a basic element of variety is the provision of kitchenette facilities, dining areas and nutrition stations for the preparation of customized patient meals. Eating together and encouraging families to prepare the patient's favorite meals is a pleasure for the dying and their families.

At one hospice, variety was enhanced by deep woods on one side of the unit and a busy street on the other. At another, variety was emphasized by a special entry with a carved door. The enhancement of variety for the individual is a result of the imaginative efforts of the designer, caregivers, and participants.

Variety in room shapes, decorative schemes, and orientation must never be different simply for the sake of difference. Variety should enhance choices for the individuals, spark memories, and decrease boredom, but it is not a panacea for the users. In addition, too much variety is confusing, more like an amusement park than the home. The homelike variety sought in inpatient hospice design is one that reminds us of our home but does not mimic the home inappropriately.

Overall Organization

There are limits to the infusion of home architecture into any institutional setting. However, hospice caregivers and proponents are clearly committed to deinstitutionalizing the hospice environment. Homelike modifications enhance care by developing, in Izumi's sense, a meaningful rather than a purposeful environment and by comforting with the symbolic elements of this culture's archetypal home (Izumi 1978).

The size of the hospice unit is very important, for the American ideal of the single-family home is collective living for a small unit, certainly not more than fifteen people and probably four or less. If hospice nursing units are organized with this end in mind, the match of personalized care and homelike scale will be maintained.

Extending the analogy of the hospice to the home, a multibed room becomes, in effect, a family unit, needing some community and some privately zoned areas—a central table and chairs as well as screened bed areas. A cluster grouping of various bedroom accommodations, under the supervision of one nursing unit, becomes the extended family of patients, families, and staff. This cluster needs a full set of family rooms, kitchenettes, retreat spaces, and outdoor facilities. This approach should result in a duplication of services throughout the facility;

duplication is necessary to establish homelike accessibility and scale.

Compendium research revealed that the manageable size for one nursing unit is approximately fifteen beds. Especially with active family and volunteer involvement, the hospice unit should not grow beyond this size. At several hospices with a larger unit of scale, a breakdown has been accomplished with subsidiary nursing desks, such as at Nathan Adelson, where each four-bed cluster has its own desk supervisor and living room. Many hospices are content to manage an inpatient unit with no more than fifteen patient beds and quite a few of the parent-based units are smaller. Fifteen patients was the designed size for the two remodeled school facilities, Hospice of Northern Virginia and Good Shepherd. It is apparently the smallest complement that can support an institutional kitchen with a minimum capacity of 100 meals a day. Small units with duplicated services are the basic building blocks of homelike hospice organization. These extended family units can be planned to maximize homelike relationships within an institutional setting. Any plans for new hospice units or plans for the remodeling of institutional space for hospice use should be based on the fifteen-bed unit and incorporate the following modifications: deinstitutionalized corridors and rooms; unspecified space; clustered areas; carefully designed entrances and exits; consistency of hospice size, image, and use; and nature and spiritual connections.

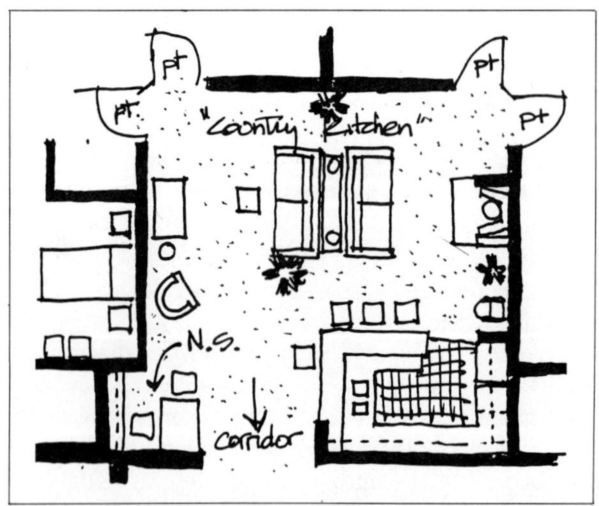

Cluster arrangement of patient rooms, country kitchen, and nurses' station, Nathan Adelson Hospice

Deinstitutionalized Corridors

The long double-loaded corridor that is so often the solution to medical and nonmedical institutions should be avoided or modified. Although a double-loaded hall may occur in the home, it is usually short, has intervening rooms, alternate uses, changes in levels, and incandescent and natural lighting. Corridors in existing buildings to be remodeled for hospice use can be turned, shortened, given viewpoints and vistas, and residentially decorated, as was done at St. Peter's Hospice. Small nodes of transverse circulation can also be used to shorten the hallways psychologically, as can changes in ceiling height, doorways, and their spacing along the route. Different uses along the hall will also promote interest and shorten distances visually.

Deinstitutionalized Rooms

Typically, residential rooms have windows on more than one wall. Windows are often placed carefully in the walls to provide certain views and kinds of light and privacy. In the home, rooms are usually not strung along on a corridor, but are more likely to provide access through other areas or a connection to the outdoors. Residential kitchens and living rooms are of different sizes, not some universal norm. Most houses, in addition, have little equipment and lots of storage space for maintenance supplies. For example, sinks are usually in countertops with personal storage for supplies and amenities below. Other homelike modifications can include the addition of relights for the remodeling of double-loaded rooms. New design should emphasize rooms with a variety of shapes, sizes, uses, storage, and ground-floor location to maximize the homelike atmosphere.

Unspecified Space

Although there may be extra room in current medical institutions, it is not judged economically viable to design unspecified spaces. Institutional designs,

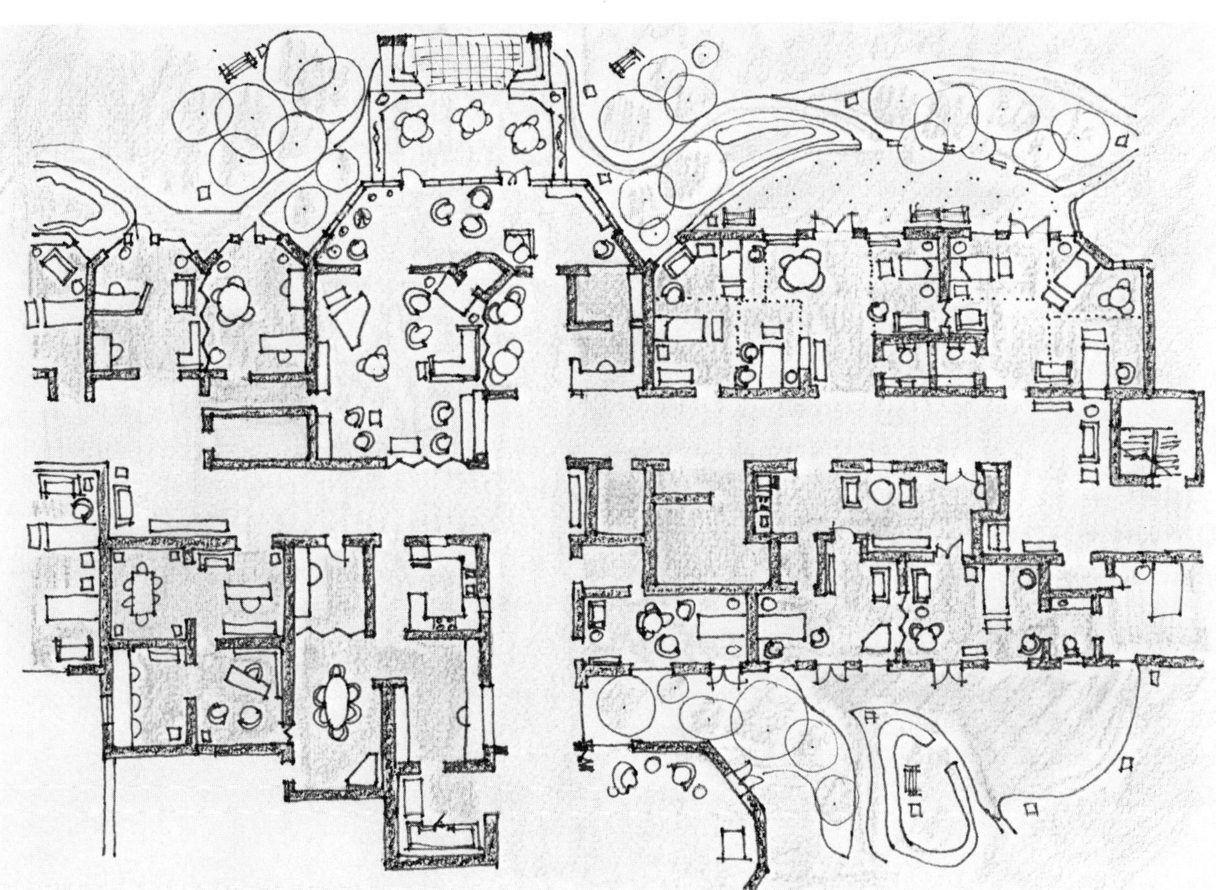

Deinstitutionalized corridors

therefore, emphasize minimal sizes and configurations. One of the best ways to deinstitutionalize such buildings is to allocate generous amounts of space for rest, dawdling, comfort, and decoration. Such space is part of the larger square footage per person in hospice bedrooms. Corners, nooks, stair landings, antechambers, and outdoor areas are additional examples of unspecified space. This extra spaciousness must be usable, but it should entail no specific economy, representing a homelike loose fit and concern for detail.

Clustered Areas

Hospice family units need duplicated services. Thus, bedroom groups will cluster with living rooms, kitchenette facilities, family private rooms, retreats, and the outdoors. The larger-scale elements of hospice units, such as the collectively used kitchen, offices, dining areas, multipurpose rooms, chapel, and outpatient clinics could become segregated from the bedroom-living room clusters. However, as much as possible, given code restrictions, the uses should be designed to complement each other and placed in some close connection. Designing clustered areas supports the basic philosophy of hospice care by combining people with different skills, backgrounds, and experience in the real work of the hospice. Patients and families benefit enormously from feeling connected to the daily life of the hospice, a structure that sustains them and will continue to sustain others. Workers and volunteers can see and understand one another's particular skills and the community that unites their efforts. Personal example sets the standard instead of the less satisfying memo. Institutions that grow too large and in which separation of areas is great often have difficulty maintaining a community standard. Mixing uses in a facility contributes to a homelike organization and, therefore, to a community involvement in care.

Carefully Designed Entrances and Exits

First impressions are often made from the portal and approach of the building. Hospice entrances for the ambulatory and bedridden should be designed much like residences, if the facility is small enough to support this scale. Larger facilities can make use of the hotel lobby image to handle seating, greeting, and the volume of usage, such as at Rosary Hill Home. Hotel lobbies often have mixed use, supporting shops, tearooms, or meeting and infor-

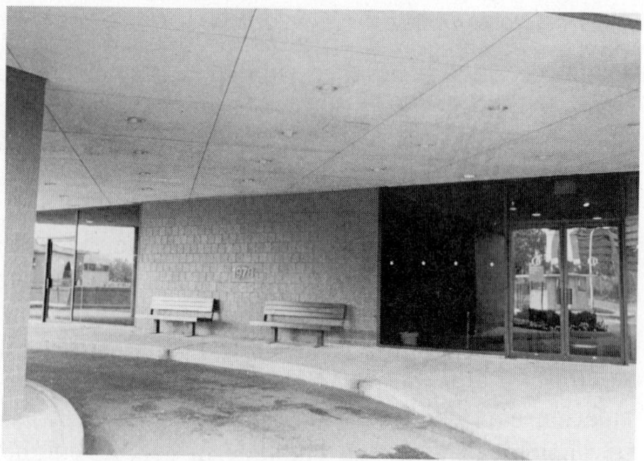

Combined bed and ambulatory entrances, Calvary Hospital

mation areas. At the Hospice of the Good Shepherd, the formal entry will have a staircase to the upper story and residences next door, and a large meeting room directly off the main entry and seating area. Indoor gardening with skylights and fountains is also reminiscent of the hotel and can mark an entry with distinction and dignity.

The patient bed entry into a hotel-like lobby should be organized to give the patient some privacy, but still allow the patient's family and friends to walk alongside the bed. At Calvary Hospital, the main bed and ambulatory entries are contiguous; inside, there is a convenient elevator to take the bedded patient to the bedroom. One alternate solution was adopted at the Hospice of Northern Virginia, where there are two main entrances, one for patients at the building's formal entry, another for staff, family, and visitors, near parking. Here, the building's existing architecture was put to use to dignify the ambulance and ambulatory patient entry, while keeping it private and convenient to bedroom and living rooms. Such a design also allows for the dead to be transferred out of the hospice with dignity through the ambulance and ambulatory patient entry.

The other users of the facility—administrators, nurses, and support staff—often find convenient alternate pathways to the entrances and exits, such as emergency exits and underground routes. Whichever pathways are commonly used should be designed with coverings, windows, and decorations to enliven their daily journeys.

At many parent-based hospices, especially those located above the ground floor, the hospice entry is located at the end of a long corridor that leads through the hospital or skilled nursing facility. This long walk through institutional pathways does little to deinstitutionalize the hospice portal, although the contrast between the institutional corridor and the modified corridors of the hospice does provide a favorable image for the hospice, as a home in the midst of an institution. At the Hospice of Cincinnati, a new stairwell was added to connect the unit to the ground floor. This is the hospice's main entrance. It is not much of an amenity, however, especially with the necessary security system. Most of the parent institutions have separated ambulatory and ambulance entries; the bedded hospice patient arrives at the loading dock and is admitted through the emergency entrance. This approach is detrimental to hospice care and contrary to stated hospice principles.

The parent-based hospice units are quiet havens once their doors are passed, however. It is important for hospices to have a greeting station close to the unit entrance. Usually, offices or nurses' stations are located right at the entry, which permits staff to monitor for security purposes as well as greet new arrivals. Placing the greeting station at the end of a long hallway, such as at Mercy Hospice, offers a less inviting welcome. Integrating the entry with other functions, such as admitting, examining, or monitoring the area for security, seems to make the greeting informal for visitors and patients. Families and volunteers may need a more formal greeting area, with meeting and administration desks and office space. Thus, those hospices with two entries seem to respond to these two needs: the first, for a formal entry for new visitors, families, staff, and volunteers; the second, for an informal entry for all patients as well as visitors and staff familiar with the unit.

Consistency of Size, Image, and Use

Smaller inpatient units, those with fewer than ten patients, can use an image that resembles a large house in the neighborhood for their new construction. In some cases an existing house can be remodeled, although bringing the house up to life-safety code requirements must be taken into account, as it may affect the appearance of the building. Hospices with larger inpatient populations often adopt a school or monastery building form. Both the Hospice of the Good Shepherd and the Hospice of Northern Virginia are remodeled schools, and the Connecticut Hospice resembles the suburban school across the street

from the hospice. The newer hospice at Las Vegas, Nathan Adelson, is reminiscent of a monastery and is quite appropriate for its desert location.

Size and image must be consistent in hospice design. Too large a hospice cannot be homelike on the outside, but must borrow from another institutional building type. Designers can adopt the form of other institutional buildings, such as the university, library, and hotel, to help in the image of hospice as a nonmedical institution.

Nature and Spiritual Connections

Human beings are intimately tied up with nature. The biological processes that create us ultimately kill us; part of circumstances and cycles we are just beginning to define. Humans have been examining their place upon the earth and in the spiritual realm throughout history. As hard as we may try to transcend or control our earthly selves, we find it necessary to bend to nature within and without; a nature that instructs, delights, and terrifies us still.

In the Judaic, Christian, and Islamic religions, paradise is symbolized by the garden. The Book of Genesis relates how mankind, through sin, was cast out of the Garden of Eden and earned the punishment of death. Whether one accepts religious dogma or views it anthropologically, religion, nature, and spirituality are fundamentally bound.

Modern American culture is not united in its acceptance of religious dogma. It is far more unified in its acceptance of and devotion to the value of nature and natural beauty, however contradictory the display. National parks are dutifully visited each summer; pilgrimages to the wilderness and parks are a long-standing element of national heritage and pride. Our connection to nature is far deeper than one might suppose from such visits, however. Our food, clothing, and shelter have traditionally come directly from our environments, although the industrial nature of modern society obscures our basic connection to the earth. We feel this connection when we insist on cotton and wool for clothing or natural materials for our furniture and walls. The charm of a fireplace or sparkle of a fountain are other manifestations of our delight in nature and the natural order.

Physical death summons up these connections, as we struggle to understand our lives and the purpose of existence. An individual's death is a point of contemplation and crisis for that person and his or her circle of family and friends. Especially in a culture in which dying is hidden and viewed as a failure of science and rationality, death is a shocking inevitability.

The connection with nature and spirituality in the hospice is basic to the hospice's role in affirming life and providing succor for the dying. The natural raw material for symbolic associations is ecumenical; whatever the religious underpinning, the garden and wilderness appeal to our senses and spirit. For the pantheist, monotheist, or existentialist, nature provides a symbolic realm for reflection upon beauty, eternity, timelessness, and the mutability of existence (Leopold 1981). Open space means freedom, adventure, light, public ceremony, formal structure, and idealized beauty, whereas closed space signifies the womb, security, darkness, and biological connection. Certain shapes are derived, through culture and over time, with a motion and meaning from natural rhythm, scale, and form (Tuan 1974, 27–29).

In the hospice, nature is represented in its beneficence and transition, with architectural reference to the primal elements of fire, water, air, and earth. It is found at the fireplace and bonfire, at the fountain and pond, and in operable windows that connect to the outdoors. The architectural use of natural materials—wood, stone, brick, adobe—and the presence of growing life, like children, pets, and plants, exhibit the diversity and charm of nature within the hospice. Providing a garden of any form (Oriental, kitchen, formal, landscape, or orchard) on hospice grounds serves as a reminder of the gardens of legend and the timeless seasonal cycles. Within the hospice, artwork of representational and nature scenes reminds us of the human connection of nature with beauty; places for plants and other growing things bring the tended garden indoors.

The spiritual element of nature is often connected to the quality of light, as well as seasonal celebration. Thus, hospice chapels have opaque stained glass and rheostatted lighting for serenity. The quality of light is a concern throughout the facility, with window and incandescent lighting predominating and skylights, high ceilings, operable doors, and windows providing air and a link to the outside. Nature and spirit are cyclical: sunrise and sunset, moon and sunshine, spring and fall, birth and death. These are represented in the hospice by connections to gardens, street life, childcare, orientations to the sky, and east and west views.

Nature and the spiritual are also part of the hospice emphasis on homelike architecture, as the home is a center for personal contemplation and the natural daily activities of bathing, sleeping, eating, and sex. These activities are the domestic and personal expression of our natural selves. They bond us to nature and the cycles of life and death. The hospice celebrates these domestic rituals and concerns with a homelike context. It includes the larger spiritual sphere too, with nature and the chapel, artwork and light.

In hospice inpatient design, connections to nature and spirituality can be divided into the following categories:

- chapel, meditation room, and viewing room
- artwork and lighting
- interior gardens
- exterior gardens
- connections to life and light

Chapel, Meditation Room, and Viewing Room. Compendium research has divulged a variety of examples of spiritual and natural elements in hospice inpatient architecture. The most obvious and controversial element is the inclusion of a chapel. In some cases, a desire to provide a nondogmatic and ecumenical hospice image has brought about the design of so-called meditation rooms, rather than traditional chapels. However, the sacred atmosphere is quite similar in either case. The use of subdued rheostatted lighting in ornamental wall fixtures and opaque stained glass is common, as are carpeting and acoustical quiet.

At Northern Virginia, the meditation room is furnished with a dark green carpet, rheostatted lighting, and a cabinet for religious articles and storage. In addition, walls are painted a beige/ochre color, and the room is furnished with colonial wooden furniture. The meditation room is located at the approximate center of the facility, near conference and library room and the nursing director's office. It views the landscaped garden and has a seating alcove off the main corridor to create a small antechamber and congregation area.

Some units do not have a chapel or meditation room, but do provide a quiet room that can be adapted for many functions. Clover Hospice is one example. Riverside Hospice has decorated the dining room with stained glass and rheostatted lighting; St. Peter's Hospice has planned to add a stained-glass window in the multipurpose room to make the room suitable for chapel functions. The Hospice

St. Paul has a stained-glass panel at the end of the corridor. Such spiritual decorations work with homelike elements to reflect the serious, yet comforting, atmosphere of the hospice. Larger facilities have chapels too, but off the unit, such as those at Calvary and Rosary Hill Home. Calvary is planning to expand its chapel in the remodel to provide for more bedded patients and families, although its services are also available through closed-circuit television.

The viewing or transition function at hospice inpatient units usually takes place in the bedrooms. In most cases, the single-bed rooms are appropriate locations for privacy in grief. However, some facilities with multibed rooms may plan an alternative area for this time after death. The Connecticut Hospice has a transition room with additional sitting area attached for this purpose. It is a linear arrangement, with no windows. There has been some criticism of this organization, because of the narrow plan and because the absence of windows severs any connection with life and the outdoors. Most transition or viewing areas are decorated differently from that at the Connecticut Hospice, however, and emphasize a natural and homelike quality. Homelike planning and decor seem more appropriate to transition rooms than an extensive "spiritual" decor. Juxtaposing the viewing room with a chapel allows a natural flow from attention to the body to spiritual concerns. Kaiser Norwalk is an example of this plan organization. In general, the caregivers must decide their protocol when dealing with the actual death and grieving and be aware of the laws concerning disposition of the body. To a large extent their decisions will determine the location and type of the viewing room.

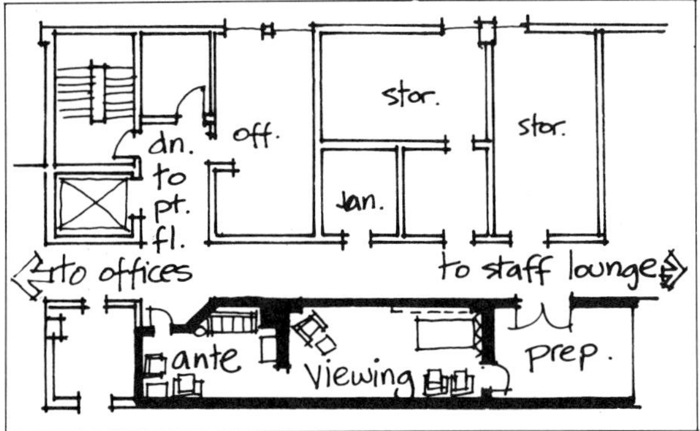

Viewing and transition areas, Connecticut Hospice

Artwork and Lighting. An overwhelming majority of artwork on the walls at hospice inpatient units consists of human and nature representational scenes. Spiritual designs are more common at religious-sponsored facilities than elsewhere, although abstract stained glass or woven or appliqué panels are commonly favored over more traditional symbols representing Christianity or Judaism. Where traditional symbols are used, such as at Cabrini or Mercy Hospice, they are background pieces, rather than large focal points. The religious-sponsored institutions seem to feel more at ease with their traditional decor, and private hospices, such as North-

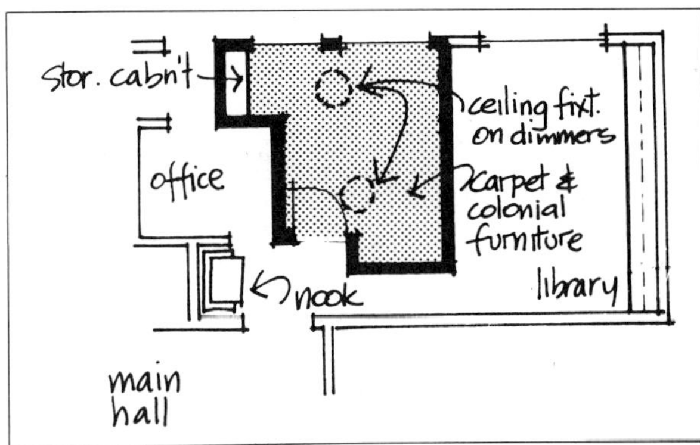

Meditation room and hall, Hospice of Northern Virginia

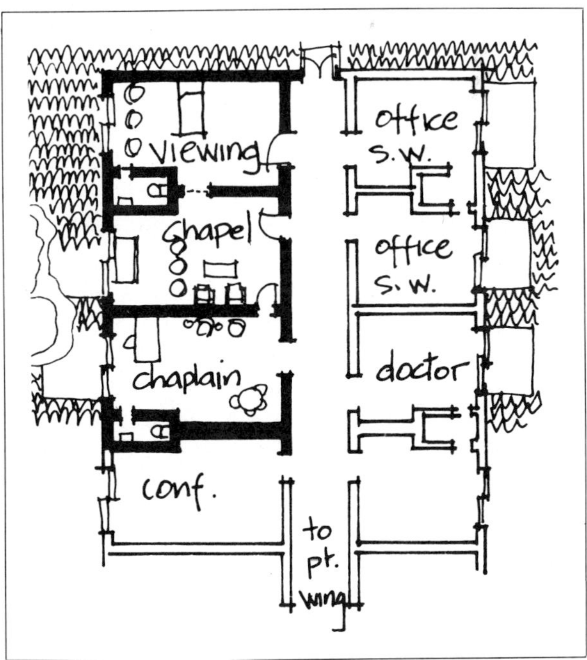

At the Kaiser Permanente Hospice, the viewing room is adjacent to the chapel.

ern Virginia, stress a meditation image without any obvious religious symbols. Nature representations in artwork provide a link between the homelike and the spiritual.

Realist pictures with human subjects or landscapes predominated in hospice art. Stark and chaotic scenes were avoided, although the art displayed was typically neither simple nor merely decorative. It is one thing for the well person to view the abyss in art and modern life; quite another to assail the dying with such imagery.

Hospice lighting differs greating from lighting typically provided in acute-care settings. Most hospices have replaced fluorescent lights with incandescent task fixtures or indirect lighting. Wall washers seem typical for corridor remodels. At St. Peter's, the remodeling has included windows on corridors to emphasize natural lighting, which, in turn, allows staff to turn off corridor lights during the day.

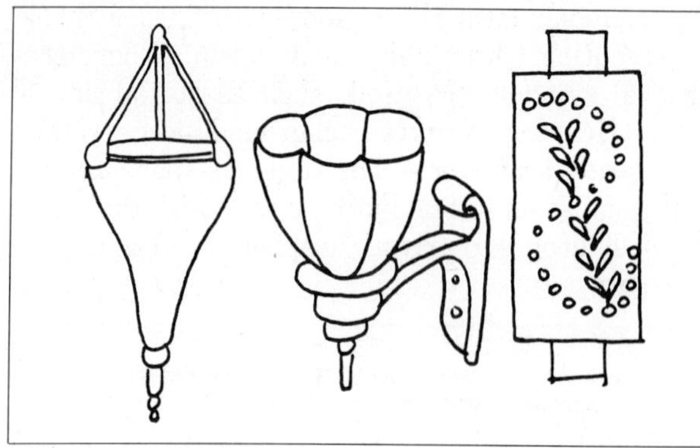

Meditation room lights

The use of spiritual lighting—opaque panels and rheostatted incandescent fixtures—is very important in the chapel and meditation areas. The incandescent fixtures commonly used in hospices are decorative wall lights, often in pairs, that produce a soft glow on the surrounding walls. Opaque panels of stained glass provide a subdued light in chapel and meditation areas, as well as privacy from the outside. In surveyed hospices, where translucent windows were used, the interior viewed to a garden or treetops, but was not easily visible from outside. Nathan Adelson's meditation room is an example of screened privacy in a chapel design.

Variety and personalization of artwork were stressed by many hospices in the compendium sampling. Art carts displaying local art, handmade crafts, and drawings help to support these goals. While

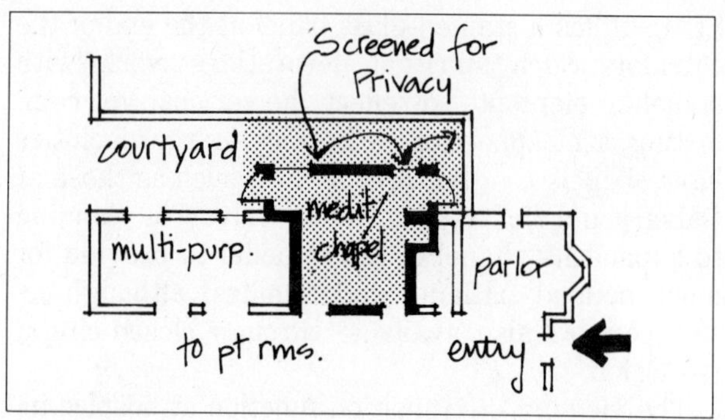

Meditation room and chapel, Nathan Adelson Hospice. These areas are screened from the courtyard, to ensure privacy.

spiritual decoration was more permanent, artwork was occasionally changed at St. Peter's and Calvary.

Indoor Gardens. Hospices were unanimous in their inclusion of plants and gardening. Many units also encouraged families to bring children and pets. The Connecticut Hospice has adopted a caged bird for the delight of the users and incorporated a daycare facility for children. Plans at St. Mary's Hospice in Tucson and Nathan Adelson call for a daycare unit; however, childcare was not provided in most compendium hospices.

Pets have recently been recognized as stress reducers and, therefore, life extenders, especially those that can be held and stroked. Given responsible maintenance, pets would be a desirable addition to palliative care. Birds or fish represent a connection with other life and are easier to care for than dogs or cats. Wild animals can be made visible and accessible to patients with the provision of window feeders.

Indoor gardening at hospice units was a major design element. In units where windows were not remodeled, planters were added. Plants were donated and tended by family, volunteers, staff, and patients. Flowering plants, evergreens, or leafy house plants were typical, as were cut flowers and dried arrangements. Where windows were remodeled, or in new facilities, greenhouse windows were added in bedroom, living room, dining room and hall areas. St. Peter's, for example, has greenhouse windows in the dayroom, whereas Calvary and Rosary Hill have windows throughout for greenhouse lighting and plants. The Hospice of the Good Shepherd is planning to add an extensive greenhouse area off the main living room and deck. At Nathan Adelson, the greenhouse is a separate interior court,

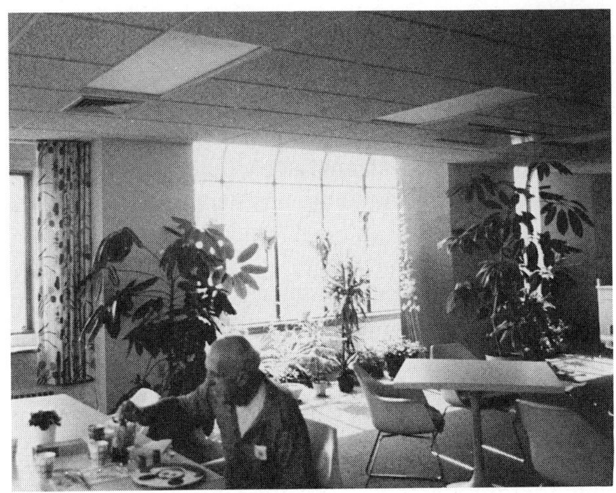

Dayroom with greenhouse windows, St. Peter's Hospice

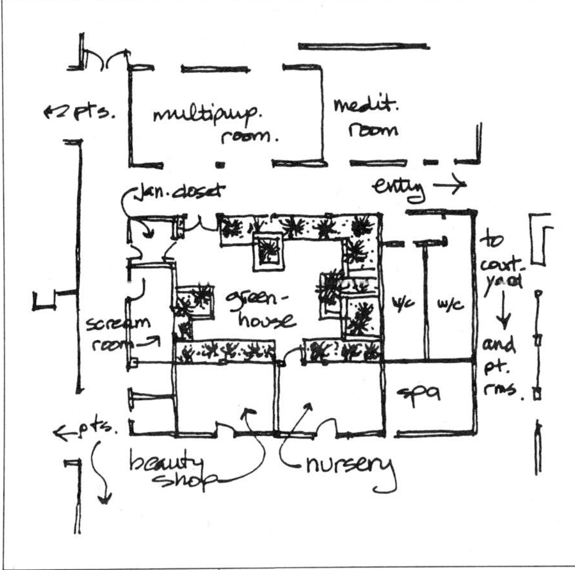

Greenhouse, Nathan Adelson Hospice

used for various activities and to allow internal relights to inpatient services.

In many cases, a room with southern exposure and many windows was selected for the dayroom. At Cabrini, the dayroom views out to a roof garden below and is the preexisting solarium. At Deer's Head Center, extensive use is made of the existing solarium in combined use with nursing facility patients. The use of solariums is typical at older institutions such as St. Rose's Home, where the rooms

view to outdoor gardens or chapel areas. The Hospice of Cincinnati has decorated a south-facing sunroom with patio furniture to increase the feeling of being outdoors.

At urban hospices, the need to bring the outdoors inside is greater than when the unit is surrounded by residential parks, or parklike grounds. A unit such as Kaiser Norwalk, with its ground-floor patios, can depend on exterior greenery to a greater extent than Cabrini Hospice, located in Manhattan. The small urban units that are situated on above-ground floors need to devote the most effort to growing indoor plants and providing connections to nature.

With its emphasis on life, nature, and light, the hospice lends itself to solar design. Operable windows, designed for a direct link to nature as well as patient controls, make design for solar heat more appropriate for hospice care than for other types of health-care architecture. No hospice has been designed strictly with passive solar heating and cooling, although the architecture of Nathan Adelson Hospice, with its interior solar court and earth-bermed exterior, is solar-tempered. A solar design based on clerestories would also be appropriate for hospice design and even make fresh food production possible in the hospice.

No matter what its size, location, or configuration, the indoor garden is fundamental to hospice design. Nature is representative of both primary design concerns of the hospice: those of homelike additions and spiritual connections. Interior gardens are a basic strategy for incorporating nature into design. No policy for energy conservation should restrict hospice units from their necessary garden connections.

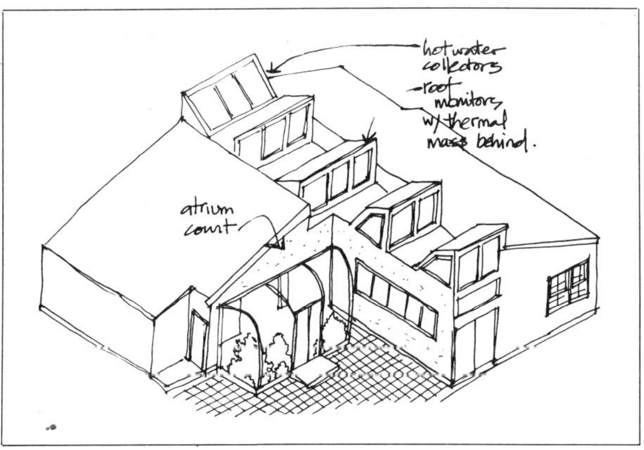

Suggested passive solar design for hospices

Exterior Gardens. Hospice and palliative-care facilities recognize the need for a link from unit rooms to the outside. Unfortunately, because of economy or practicality, some small units are placed above the ground floor. This is not recommended practice, except in built-up urban areas, where a roof garden and higher location will allow more light. Large units, such as the Rosary Hill Home, may have problems of scale that necessitate designing above-ground patios.

Usually, any above-ground deck is an extension of the communal family areas, such as at the Hospice of the Good Shepherd, Lutheran Hospital Hospice, and Rogers Memorial, for example. Small, individual patios connected to ground-floor patient rooms were designed at Nathan Adelson, Kaiser Norwalk, and St. Mary's Tucson. Other ground-floor units, such as Clover and Pinecrest, have one outdoor patio for the use of all patients. As landscaping is seldom undertaken first and may be largely a volunteer effort, it is important to have a planned design that can be implemented in stages by nonprofessionals, if necessary. The landscape design at the Hospice of Northern Virginia is not only a fine example of privacy/community outdoor design, but also illustrates a comprehensive plan for hospice use. Northern Virginia is planning formal, kitchen, and landscape gardens as well as outdoor play areas. Orchards, too, would be suitable for hospice design.

Connecting the hospice with life and activity around the facility has been the subject of some controversy, because it touches upon the question of community acceptance of the hospice. The problem of integrating the hospice into the community is twofold. The first difficulty, that the hospice is a medical building type, can be addressed by adopting a derived architectural form, such as a school, for the hospice building. The second is the stigma associated with dying and death, a problem that is not so easily addressed. The stigma of death is sometimes extended to the hospice building itself because the hospice is a place where people deal with death and dying. It can be very difficult for the dying, their families, and hospice staff to be connected to the world around them.

At some hospices, this stigma is acknowledged through the absence of any external signs indicating that there is a hospice within. The Connecticut Hospice has attempted to integrate the hospice within the larger community by providing a children's daycare center in the hospice building. This approach was taken from St. Christopher's Hospice, which has its own children's daycare center. At St. Peter's Hospital Hospice, a barber and beauty shop was located in the hospice unit for the use of everyone in the hospital. A planned hospice in Dallas will have a large educational area that will be used to train hospice nurses and physicians from all over the state in pain-control techniques.

Some hospices have decided to locate near related community services. At the Hospice of the Good Shepherd, the hospice is part of a larger building that includes doctors' offices and apartments with contracted services for the elderly. A hospice planned for West Covina, California, the Sunkist Plaza Health and Living Center, will have a ten-bed hospice building on a campus that includes medical offices, senior citizen housing, and a skilled nursing facility.

Each hospice must make up its own mind about its connection to the community, weighing such factors as existing community acceptance of the hospice program, the hospice's particular philosophy of care, and the need for other services in conjunction with hospice.

However, the needs of the patient, family, and staff to be connected to the community dictate hospice visibility to playgrounds or the street. At St. John's Hospice at Southern Illinois University, design for light and activity was judged so important that the unit was planned to overlook the busy hospital rather than the garden and woods on the other side. Too much activity too near the patient areas would be inappropriate, however. At Pinecrest, the palliative-care unit was located near the hospital entrance, directly off the parking area, and half of the patient rooms overlook this busy noisy area. A balance between activity and peace is a moderate approach that best meets hospice philosophy.

Design Guidelines: Small to Medium Parent-Based Hospice Units

Rather than present a prototypical design for a range of hospices with different needs, the following material is based upon one size and kind of hospice, the small to medium parent-based unit with a population of five to fifteen patients. Designers who have another size or kind of hospice in mind should review representative examples in the compendium for basic data on existing facility types and previous choices for architectural design. However, many of the design recommendations that follow would also apply to larger hospices that use the cluster approach to design.

In general, these smaller remodeled units are part of an existing hospital or nursing facility, have limited funds for capital improvements, and must rely upon the services of an inhouse designer. As they are far more common than larger or freestanding hospices, they are an important element of hospice care. However, these smaller units have not received much publicity, which has instead been reserved for larger, new, or freestanding facilities, such as the Connecticut Hospice.

Smaller parent-based hospices must frequently surmount difficult design problems. Often located in older buildings, the units may need extensive revision to meet fire-code standards and will usually require significant modification to make the surroundings homelike. The presence of load-bearing walls or restrictive column spacing may hamper attempts to remodel double-loaded corridors or to enlarge rooms. In most cases, the hospice is above ground and must be reached through the parent facility, rather than through its own entrance.

These architecturally distinct units, defined as having, at minimum, patient beds, family space, and a nursing station dedicated for hospice care only, are not the most common way of providing inpatient space. The scatterbed approach, in which beds are provided on a space-available basis in regular hospital wards, is the most prevalent, used by about half of the inpatient hospice facilities.

Dedicated beds, where bedrooms, usually at the end of a ward in an oncology or general medical unit, are reserved for hospice patients, are the second most prevalent type of inpatient setting. These bedrooms are often decorated with homelike furniture and finishes; sometimes a family room is provided. However, the hospice unit itself is usually not identified and remodeling is limited to this stage.

The remodeled, parent-based, architecturally distinct units, which comprise approximately 20 percent of all inpatient hospice beds, represent a more ambitious remodeling effort. Although they are remodeled units, they can provide many of the qualities that hospices seek to provide in their inpatient settings. In addition, these small to medium units of five to fifteen beds are approximately the size of a nursing unit of a larger hospice facility, an "extended family" cluster. Many of the design recommendations for these units could also be used in the planning of a larger hospice facility, using repeated clusters.

Home-care hospices considering their own inpatient unit should experiment first with a small inpatient hospice with its own nursing station. Many home-care hospices have little experience running an inpatient setting and need to establish policies. Staffing requirements, for example, are often much greater at night than in traditional hospitals or nursing homes, because people often die at night. In addition, experience with an inpatient hospice setting will be very valuable for the caregivers, should they decide to go on to a more ambitious design project. A small remodeled unit is a good place to try out different designs, such as different uses of family spaces, staff retreat areas, storage, death procedures, and so on. This information can be invaluable later on.

Patient Rooms

Assuming a patient population of five to fifteen, the inpatient bedrooms of a small parent-based unit can easily vary in size and number of beds. The smaller-size units can manage triples, doubles, and singles, and the larger units will support four-bed rooms. Maintaining a *floating bed*, a donation-supported bed located on the unit for longer-term respite stays (developed in Great Britain), can help to manage occupancies.

Recently, a formula for establishing the number of inpatient beds needed to accommodate the hospice service area has been devised by the Metropolitan Health Planning Corporation Hospice System of Care in Cleveland. This formula will work for any type of hospice inpatient unit, including the small to medium parent-based units. Essentially, the number of beds is equal to the hospice utilization percentage multiplied by the number of total deaths by cancer multiplied by a common factor of .000316. The common factor is derived in the following way: it is assumed that 60 percent of hospice patients die at home, and 40 percent at the hospice; that the average number of inpatient days for each patient who subsequently dies at home is 5, and the average number of inpatient days for the patient who dies at the hospice is 17; and that the annual occupancy rate will be 85 percent (310 out of 365 days in a year). The common factor could be adjusted to meet individual hospice conditions. Therefore:

$$.000316 = \frac{(.4 \times 17) + (.6 \times 5)}{310} \times \frac{1}{100}.$$

For example, if 500 total cancer deaths occur in

the service area and the hospice cares for 100 patients per year, the hospice utilization rate would be .20 × 500 × .000316 = 3 beds.

Patient rooms need standard equipment and furnishings, including the following: beds, tables, recliner chairs, hard and soft chairs, sofa beds, closets, space for patient furnishings, bathrooms, and a connection to the outdoors. Other elements include overbed tables, a sink, kitchen table and chairs, storage for medical and personal equipment, and lamps and task lighting. In addition, space or storage may be needed for bedpans, oxygen and suction, garbage cans, linen supplies, and so on. Medical equipment is minimized and deemphasized; charts, for example, are not usually stored in patient rooms. Screens and track curtains for privacy are typical in the larger bedrooms, with colorful curtains that match the decor or bed sheets. Quilts and pillows, carpeting, blinds, curtains, draperies, and other homelike elements are very important, as are plants and operable windows. A room-controlled heating element permits patient and family to regulate room temperature.

In general, design of patient rooms should include the elements already discussed in the sections on homelike architecture. Within these guidelines, specific requirements include the following:

- generous space allowance around the bed (especially the head) and movable chairs and tables elsewhere in the room, for visiting and comforting
- zoning the beds for privacy and community; display areas for personal items, within reach of the bed
- visibility to the outdoors and the nursing station or hallway, for nonabandonment
- connection to the outdoors with operable windows, skylights, or greenhouse areas
- convenient sink and generous storage spaces for personal items and all equipment.

Family Rooms

Family rooms are of two basic types: the community room, which has a variety of functions including greeting, daycare, celebrations, services, passive activities, eating, active recreation, and gathering; and the private family room, which can be used for family sleeping, personal grooming, grieving, and similar private family functions. The small room may also be used for body viewing and grieving, although a conference room, dining room, or other general-purpose room would also serve this semi-private function.

Hospice community rooms will vary depending on the kind of bedrooms in the particular scheme. Single bedrooms can use a small common family area in an alcove off the corridors. Multibed rooms will have a family table and chairs for gathering within the room. As a whole, the facility should have at least one large communal room for celebrations and group activities. Thus, there is a duplication of community areas, from the smaller ones serving the bedrooms to those accommodating the whole hospice community.

These community rooms have need of symbolic architecture; references to nature and the home. Fireplaces, pianos, bookcases, grandfather clocks, and dining or game tables are appropriate, as are plants and French doors leading to terraces. Com-

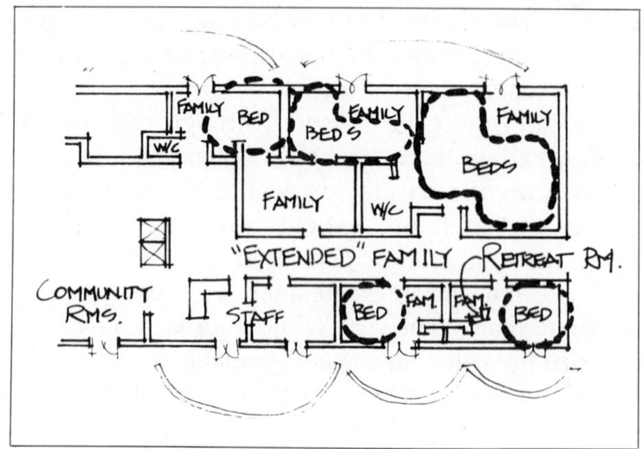

Alternative design of patient and family rooms

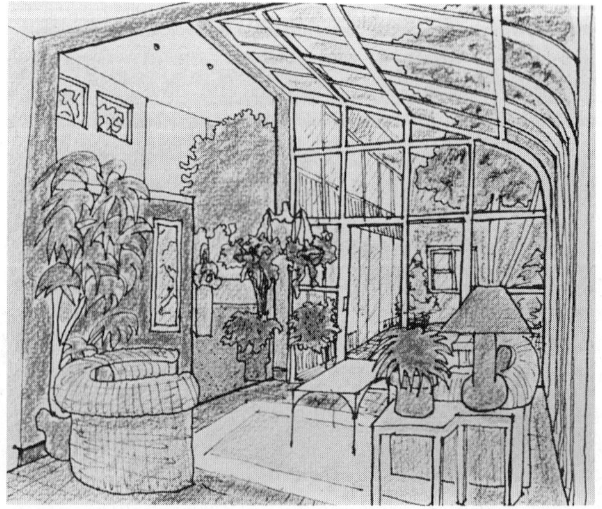

Family room with connections to nature: plants, greenery, and greenhouse windows.

munity rooms may have a combination of equipment and furnishings, including desks, chairs, sofas, tables, lamps, and other residential furniture. Space must be provided for patients in beds or lounge chairs and a connection to the outdoors must be maintained. Nursing stations may be nearby, but they should not dominate the area. Kitchenettes can be part of the smaller community rooms, and larger kitchens and laundry areas should be adjacent to the larger community areas. A television area and oxygen and/or suction may also be necessary; caregivers differ in their approach to these issues.

Smaller private family rooms are intended for intimate family activities and as a retreat from the patient areas. These rooms may be located away from the main activity of the unit, but should not be so far away as to suggest family abandonment of the patient. Private family rooms can be designed like bedrooms, with a mix of seating and sleep furnishings as well as bathrooms. Thus, they are also appropriate for massage, counseling, and staff retreat, but only on an informal basis; no scheduling should deprive a family of access to their retreat whenever it is necessary.

An example of the disposition and design of these rooms is suggested in the following scheme. Note that the basic difference between the illustrations is the location of the larger community room. In the first scheme, the community room serves to greet the family. In the second scheme, this larger living room is placed in a more private location, encouraging semipublic movement throughout the unit. These two approaches are similar to the alternate organizations in housing, where living rooms may be formal or private.

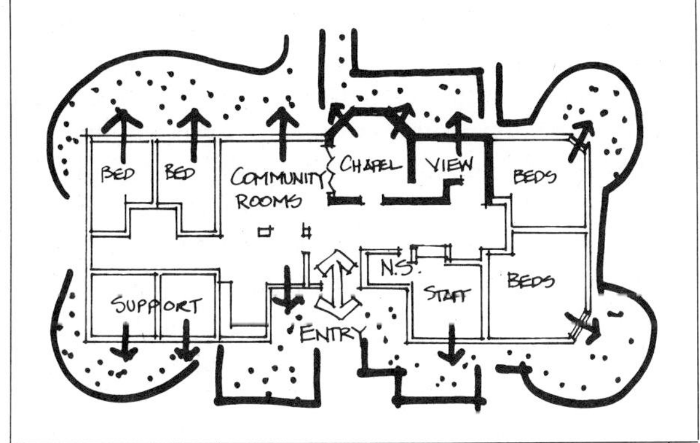

One design approach is to locate main family rooms at the unit entrance, to "greet" family and other hospice visitors.

Nature and Spiritual Concerns

General design guidelines for nature and spiritual concerns, discussed at length earlier in the book, also apply to smaller, parent-based hospice units. However, these smaller facilities often have more difficulty in designing connections to the outdoors or providing suitable chapel or meditation space than do larger facilities, for several reasons:

- The units are usually located above the ground floor, far from gardens;
- they generally have a limited budget for exterior modifications or blanket changes;
- because of tight space, smaller units must sometimes resort to a multipurpose design of spiritual space; and
- they are most often hampered by a general institutional ambience that must be modified rather than eliminated.

Some may consider a connection to the outdoors to be an amenity; it is a necessity. Every attempt should be made to maximize light and nature. Above-ground hospices could use the rooftop for a connection to nature, or might construct a covered deck. Using greenhouse windows or skylights in conjunction with indoor plants is another recommended solution. Operable windows are also recommended, especially when designed for patient safety. Parent-based hospices that intend to use an existing off-unit garden or chapel should consider the pathway that connects to these. Convenience will encourage use; otherwise, an on-unit chapel or garden is more appropriate.

Spiritual architecture includes references to specific religions as well as general spiritual elements, such as opaque lighting, quiet, natural materials, and gathering and speaking places. The rituals of a particular religion may take place in an ecumenical atmosphere, provided that storage for appropriate religious articles is available. The spiritual area must be able to accommodate a variety of groups, from small families to larger community services, so an adaptable design is desirable. A small, quiet room that can be joined with a family room is one flexible design appropriate for parent-based units pressed for space.

Viewing or transition rooms also have a spiritual element, but their architecture employs a homelike atmosphere, in most cases. A single-bed room with seating in a private, soundproof area as well as a connection to the outdoors is typical; it provides an atmosphere in which grief and attention can move slowly from the body to spirit and nature. Rushing a family into a recognizable spiritual situation deprives them of the necessary time to come to grips with the reality of death.

Nursing and Staff Space

Areas for nursing and other staff members include the nursing station, a nurses' retreat room, offices for the director of nursing and the administrator, and a staff lounge with lockers and a shower. The hospice must select the type of nursing station(s) that it wants, based on the setting to be remodeled, the experience of its nursing staff, and the hospice's philosophy of care. There are three models for the nursing station. The greeting or entry type, at which the dual functions of greeting and nursing occur, is the first discussed. Advantages to this type include easy access for the staff, centralized location for patients and families and caregivers, possibility for

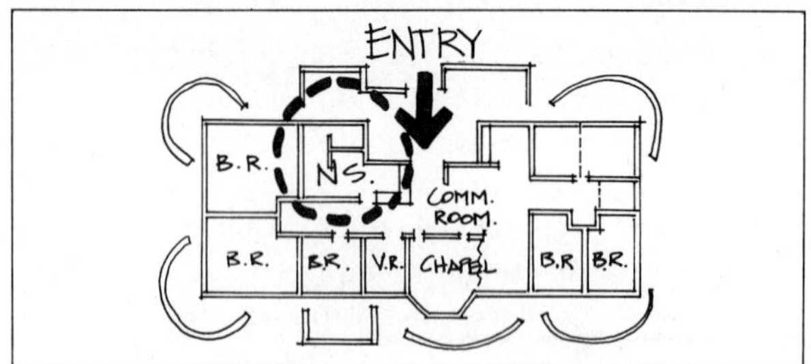

Locating the nurses' station at the entrance to the hospice is fine for greeting purposes, but can make the station institutionally imposing.

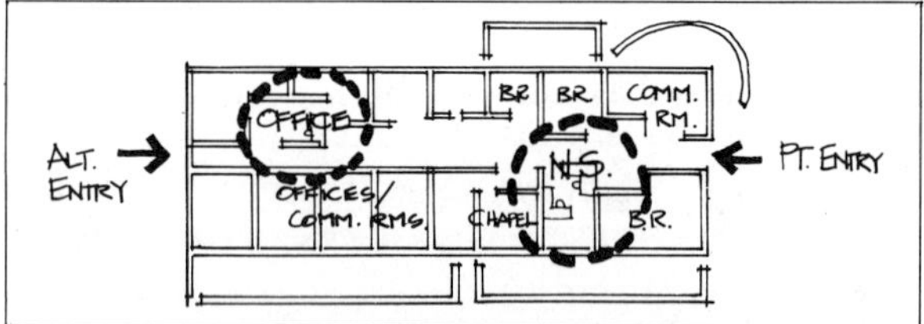

To deemphasize their function, nurses' stations may be located throughout the unit, in smaller service centers.

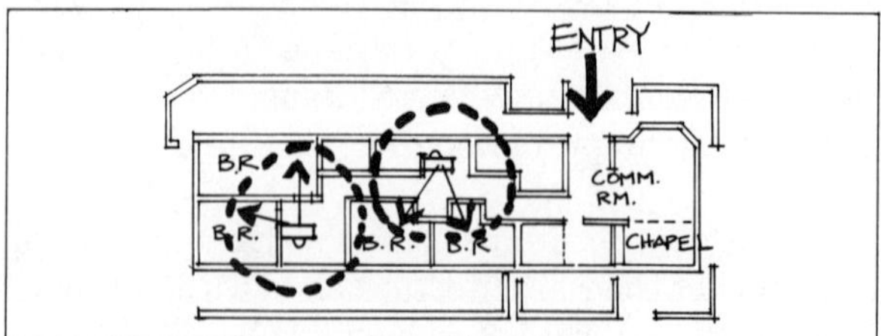

Decentralized nurses' stations

a friendly image for visitors and families, and maximized security for the unit. The disadvantages are that the central location makes the nursing station very prominent in the unit, which does not increase the homelike image of the hospice. The addition of any administrative or bookkeeping areas near the central nursing station can overwhelm the unit.

The deemphasized nursing station is a second option. Here, the nursing station is located away from the main entry, with an optional second station for greeting. The main station can be smaller, and administrative and recordkeeping areas may then be located near the nursing station without dominating the rest of the unit. In addition, all hospice staff activities can take place in the same location. One disadvantage with this type of unit is that two stations may be built, the greeting station must be manned for visitors and family, and security may be compromised.

The final option for the nursing station is that of decentralized nursing stations. In this case, at least two nursing stations are built, both of which are quite small, and administrative and recordkeeping offices are located elsewhere. These units are an advantage in that they further deinstitutionalize the hospice, but they are appropriate only for staff used to this kind of approach.

All nursing stations, of whatever kind, should be designed so that patients in beds or wheelchairs can see the nurses. The stations should have a low profile so that they do not dominate the unit. Staff and nursing rooms should have a connection to the outdoors, through windows and a terrace, if possible. The retreat space for the staff should be on the unit, but away from patient rooms.

Equipment at nursing stations and retreat rooms varies. Some institutions install silent-call devices and call lights; this choice will vary with experience, policies of nonabandonment, openness of design, and patient needs. Intercom systems and pagers are not recommended because of their institutional nature. Nursing stations in the compendium had telephones, lamps and desk equipment, bulletin boards and storage, including medicine and locked drug cabinets, as well as a sink. Retreat areas were furnished with couches and chairs, daybeds, and other homelike items, and supplied with a convenient toilet and shower unit, plants, a telephone, and so on. Some staff retreat areas, such as that at Nathan Adelson and Connecticut were called "scream rooms" and designed in unusual configurations. Connecticut's scream room has a high platform with a bubble skylight and cavelike shape; both have bean-bag chairs and carpeting. Staff may prefer this situation or find it constricting.

Inpatient, Outpatient, and Home-care Services

Small to medium parent-based remodeled inpatient hospices will vary in the provision of these services on the unit. Some may locate their home-care department elsewhere in the parent facility. Physical and occupational therapy will probably be conducted in the parent facility's own physical therapy department. Should space in the hospice permit, there are specific suggestions for these inpatient, outpatient, and home-care divisions.

In the hospice, passive, homelike activities are favored over more active therapies for the patient. These passive activities include watching others, listening to music, reading, tending plants and animals, interacting with friends and family. The design of the environment should maximize the opportunity for these activities to take place.

Active therapies can include massage and bathing, craft and other daycare programs, and celebrations of various events. Providing the hospice with a large bathroom with a sitz bath, a separate multipurpose room for massage, and a larger multipurpose room with storage can contribute to these functions. The home-care division should have an exam room, a meeting room, and office space for staff and volunteers. These, too, should have homelike and natural components in the design. Most important in the design of inpatient, outpatient and home-care services is the development of an atmosphere of trust that all that can be done is being taken care of, by staff, volunteers, and family for the good of the dying, and community at large.

Kitchenette and Dining Facilities

Small to medium parent-based remodeled hospice units do not usually have their own kitchen facilities. Meals come from the central kitchen of the parent facility. However, the smaller hospices should have kitchenettes, where family and patient can prepare or reheat favorite foods. Nutrition stations, for popsicles, fruit juices, medications that need refrigeration, and so on are also necessary. Nutrition stations should be located adjacent to the nursing areas, so that nurses can dispense these items easily. Small hospices also need a place to store meal carts

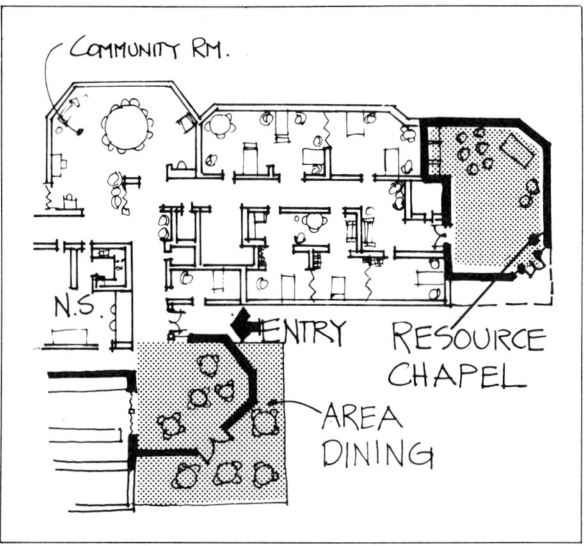

Shared services are integrated throughout the hospice

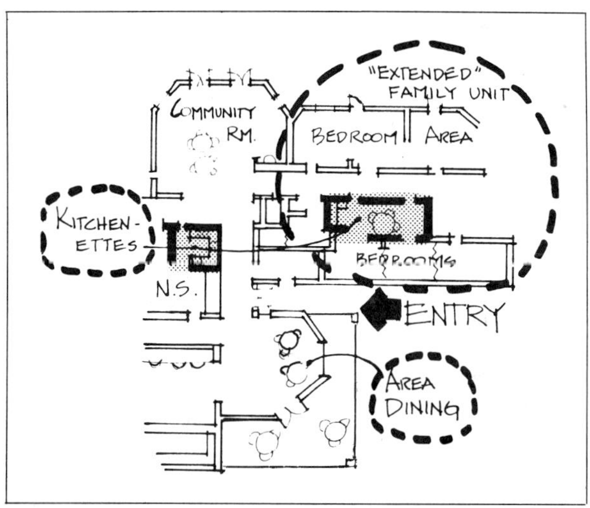

A centralized kitchen and several independent kitchenettes are desirable

from the parent facility kitchen; hallway alcoves or a special nook off the nursing station could be suitable. The hospice unit itself should be located near the central kitchen so that meals arrive hot. Breakfast foods can be prepared in the unit kitchenette, or in a pantry area, with a toaster and a microwave as minimum equipment. Meals should be provided in separate courses, with festive decorations, linens, and silverware. The inpatient unit will need a place to store hot food while the patient takes his time with each course.

Patients may eat in their beds, in their rooms

at a table with a nurse, volunteers, or family members, or in a dining room, with other patients. Providing zoned areas of various size with tables and chairs promotes this option.

Offices

Most small to medium parent-based units have a minimum of two offices, one for the director of nursing and the other for a hospice coordinator and general business functions. Offices for an administrator, medical director, secretarial and business staff, volunteer coordinator, bereavement coordinator, counselor, social worker, dietician, pharmacist, grounds and maintenance staff may also be needed. Many smaller units have two or three additional offices for other staff and share rooms for less than full-time positions.

Offices can be grouped together in the unit or spread out. If grouped together, adjacent offices can encourage communication among users, but locating some offices, such as the administrator or hospice coordinator, near the unit entrance, and others, such as the director of nursing, nearer the patient rooms can also be advantageous for patient and family care. Most meeting rooms are not used constantly, and can share such functions as dining. Task lighting should be used in these office and meeting rooms rather than the more typical overhead fluorescent lighting. Designing adequate support space, including a business machine area, an audiovisual center, and storage for paper and office supplies, is important. In addition, functions shared with the parent facility should have a convenient pathway with homelike and natural modifications, if possible.

Entry, Exit, and Corridor Design

Small to medium parent-based inpatient hospice units are usually located in institutional spaces with double-loaded corridors and a limited potential for changes to the inside or outside of the building. Homelike design and natural connections are the basic modifications necessary for the remodeling.

If possible, the hospice should be located on the ground floor; a combined ambulance/bed entry and pedestrian entry is preferred. Of course, a ground-floor location may not be possible. In a dense urban setting, such as New York City, a location that provides light, air, and views can be the next best

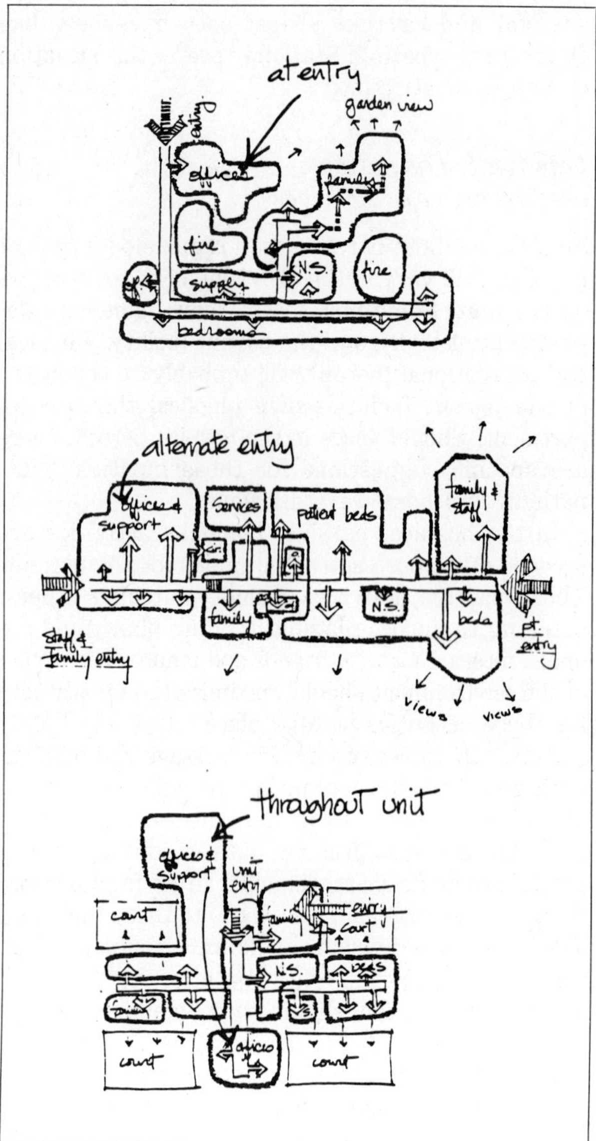

Offices may be located at the main hospice entrance (top); at the staff/family entry (middle); or offices may be located throughout the hospice (below).

thing. An outside entry to the unit when the unit is located above ground level, as at Hospice of Cincinnati, can encourage easy access, but that entrance must be as deinstitutionalized as possible. Otherwise, a modified pathway within the parent institution to the pavilion or wing where the hospice unit is located is recommended. The corridors chosen for the pathway should be remodeled with homelike and natural elements, have good signs, and be as short as possible.

The hospice unit corridor should be modified, if at all possible, with short and turned corridors, relights, furniture nooks, and circulation passing through family rooms, much like the hospice at St. Peter's Hospital. Entry at the middle of the unit can encourage transverse circulation, but this may not be possible. A special unit entry, with a greeting nurses' station or office, designed with a hotel ambience, is recommended. Double fire doors provide acoustical separation from the intercom system in the main hospital.

The hospice should establish its particular protocol for body exit from the unit to the parent unit, involving a direct horizontal or elevator connection to the morgue, and funeral arrangements. This route, too, should be modified with homelike and natural components, as the family may wish to go with the body to the funeral home.

Parking and Connections to the Community

The small to medium parent-based remodeled unit usually uses the landscape and parking lots of the parent facility. Many hospice users, especially family members, may be older and somewhat frail, so that a covered hospice entry and ample, convenient parking are appropriate. The family member or volunteer may bring favorite dishes, so an icy path from the car to the hospice unit is very inconvenient. Any hospice unit with significant educational activities or bereavement services will need extra parking, as will the home-care division.

In urban areas, the small to medium hospice unit should have convenient bus, taxi, or train connections. Sometimes the choice of a parent institution in which to place an inpatient setting for hospice can hinge on the availability of good public transportation.

Services and Miscellaneous

The remodeled parent-based hospice unit usually has a formal arrangement with the parent facility to provide laundry service, laboratory facilities, and a pharmacy. Laundry service may be contracted out to a laundry company, especially if the hospice uses colored linens of natural materials. Using an outside company keeps these linens separate from those used in a hospital or nursing facility. The unit itself will need a clean and dirty linen storage area, and a small washer/dryer set is recommended for the personal use of the patients, family members, and even staff. The unit will need a locked narcotics cabinet and ample room for supplies and deliveries. Additional storage for seasonal displays, artwork, plants, decoration supplies, kitchen equipment, and food will also be necessary. Extra storage for the patient's personal items or for unused hospice furniture is also suggested. Outdoor storage for gardening equipment, too, is a very useful addition. Wall vacuum systems, or other means for cleaning including maintenance closets, alcoves for temporary or permanent storage of cleaning equipment, cleaning supplies, paint, and repair tools are all recommended items in design.

Service pathways and connections to other parent-operated medical therapies, such as chemotherapy, operating theaters, or radiation for palliative reasons, should be modified with homelike and natural additions, if possible.

Institutional Elements of Hospice Architecture

As a health-care facility, the hospice must meet prescribed fire safety and health regulations and make use of certain functional aspects of institutional

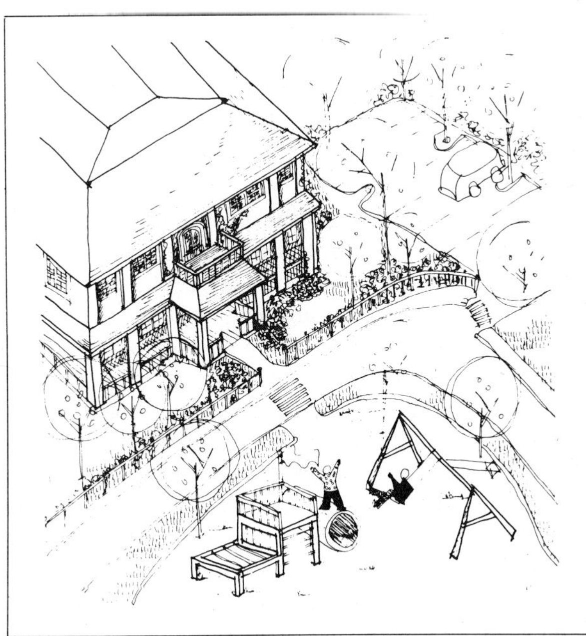

Locating the hospice adjacent to community resources, such as playgrounds, helps to weave the hospice into the local community.

design. Briefly, the institutional elements of hospice design are as follows:

- laundry, pharmacy, and laboratory facilities
- kitchen facilities
- supplies, materials handling, and routing
- building materials: fire safety, cleanliness, and durability
- climate control: heating, ventilation, and air conditioning

In this section, the specific functional requirements of institutional design will be examined. Although specific solutions will not be proposed, successful examples of design solutions, drawn from the hospices in the compendium, will be given. (In addition, see the bibliography for recent references on nursing facilities, birth centers, dormitories, and hospitals that have sought to incorporate homelike and natural elements into institutional design.)

Laundry, Pharmacy, and Laboratory

The laundries, pharmacies, and laboratories of hospice and palliative-care facilities are generally regulated under the state licensure of the facility. Since most inpatient architecturally distinct hospice units are in parent facilities, the hospices will contract with their parent facilities for these services. Thus, the licensure of the parent facility will establish the characteristics of these facilities. A hospice's special demand upon these services is not easy to separate from the demands of the parent institution.

If a hospice has elected to receive Medicare reimbursement from the federal government, that law takes precedence over other licensure. Of course, a hospice may also apply for a special hospital license or skilled nursing license, depending on the rules of its state. In any case, all health-care licensure standards for these services are somewhat similar.

In all three facilities—pharmacy, laundry, and laboratory—any areas visible to the patient or visitors should be deinstitutionalized, including machinery, signs, and carts. A small laundry area on the hospice unit should be provided for family and patient use. Where the parent facility gives laundry service, the hospice items should be segregated from those of the parent facility. These items often include colorful sheets, and quilts. Down pillows may need dry cleaning; cotton-blend or natural-fiber linens may also require gentle handling. The need to change bed linens frequently because of patient discomfort or incontinence will also put a greater demand than usual on laundry service.

In general, smaller laboratory facilities and fewer technicians will be necessary. Hospice laboratory tests are most often simple and repetitive, such as blood tests to determine medication levels. Pharmacy requirements will be part of hospice guidelines. Locked storage and storage carts are typically necessary for narcotics—increased security is also important.

Kitchen Facilities

Diet is a fundamental concern of hospice care. Dying patients often have poor appetites and difficulty eating. Meals are a fundamental element of palliation and social ritual: more than just provision of food, hospice meals are a source of comfort and pleasure for the dying and the staff, volunteers, and family who make up the community.

Breakfast is a popular meal for hospice patients, when supplied in a personal way. The long duration between dinner and breakfast has stimulated appetite, and the eggs, toast, and cereals of breakfast are simple and palatable. However, breakfast is not an easy meal to serve in an institutional setting. Eggs and buttered toast must be served immediately to be appetizing; they will not be eaten if they arrive steamed, overcooked, soggy, or cold. Inpatient hospices should consider copying the Calvary model by preparing pantry breakfasts on the unit. On-unit pantries are then available for other meals and between-meal snacks.

In large institutions, the need to plan meals in advance often supersedes the wishes of the patient. Parent-based hospices should not let this occur, but instead develop a program to allow choice for patient meals. Meals should be supplemented by particular favorites brought from home or prepared in the kitchenettes. Institutions that prepare meals in one central kitchen often serve meals on standard plastic trays with disposable silverware. This approach is not beneficial to the dying patient and should be revised or modified. Hospice meals are occasions marked by small individual portions, linens, silverware, flowers, and personal attention. Some facilities have food carts that bring a family-style selection of courses. Family and staff eat with patients in bedrooms, dining and living rooms, and outdoors. Visitors, families, and volunteers must be able to eat on a flexible schedule that accommodates the personal strains of attending to the dying.

As a result, hospice kitchens must be larger than those designed for similar bed populations in other institutions. As hospices seek to provide many dietary options, they need qualified dieticians; hospice planners, thus, should set aside convenient and large office space for them. Minimum storage requirements will vary from state to state, but hospices providing patients with ethnic favorites and a variety of foods will generally need more generous storage space. In addition, meals for family, staff, and volunteers will be necessary, and provision should be made for a separate kitchen, cafeteria, or restaurant for this function. Chits for staff and workers could allow them to use a communal dining facility, and mix with family, patients, and volunteers.

A communal dining facility for all hospice users exists used at Nathan Adelson Hospice, with additional dining made available at cluster locations. The Hospice of the Good Shepherd designed a community dining room and a large kitchen to accommodate the many daily meals a hospice needs to prepare. Good Shepherd's kitchen is also sized for potential use by the apartments with contracted services, which are next door to the hospice.

*Supplies, Materials Handling,
and Wayfinding*

Delivery of supplies and removal of waste and other products is part of any institutional function. In parent-based hospice units, most supply routes have already been established by the larger institution. Hospice can expedite the service connections by designing space for delivery and storage of supplies and waste, temporary and permanent equipment storage, alternate service pathways, and maintenance activities and cleaning closets.

Wayfinding is a term that defines a system of signs, colors, maps, flooring changes, and other devices designed to direct a person who is unfamiliar with the institution. Large hospitals are often built in stages by different architects; they can be very confusing. A consistent system of signs should lead to the hospice unit. The compendium showed that many hospices used few signs at the parent facility entry or farther outside the unit. Instead, they depended upon patients, families, volunteers, and friends becoming familiar with the location of the unit over time. This may not be the most appropriate solution to the problem of wayfinding in these larger institutions. Within the hospice unit, wayfinding should be a function of a homelike organization, rather than signs or a color system.

*Building Materials, Fire Safety, Cleanliness
and Durability*

Hospices in parent-based units will have overriding hospital life- and fire-safety codes to meet. Other units will have life- and fire-safety codes similar to those at skilled nursing facilities, intermediate care facilities, and acute-care facilities. Thus, exit signs and fire ratings will be maintained and distances to firestairs and so on established. Signs should be clear, but not overwhelming.

The introduction of homelike materials into an institutional environment will entail some modifications for these codes. Materials are rated for combustibility, so noncombustible materials must be used for wall surfaces, curtains, and carpet. Wireglass in interior windows may be necessary as well to meet fire codes. However, many new materials with good fire ratings do exist. Although it is often more expensive to do so, selective use of these new materials to provide variety and interest should be encouraged.

The cleanliness and durability of building materials is part of hospice design. However, homelike and natural concerns supersede a tight budget. The institutional quality of many durable and easily cleaned finishes, such as linoleum, makes them inappropriate for hospice use, except in kitchens or bathrooms, where they would normally be found in homes. Use of donated items, which lowers capital expenditures, can allow natural materials to take precedence over more durable, but more institutional finishes and furnishings.

*Climate Control: Heating, Ventilation, and
Air Conditioning*

Homelike and natural design considerations will make hospice climate control different from that of other institutional buildings. Hospices commonly maximize the building's connection to the outdoors with operable windows and make use of natural ventilation more than air conditioning to regulate climate. Hospices using greenhouse windows and extensive south light will experience significant solar gain; natural shading with plants and adaptable solar curtains will be necessary. Clerestories that allow natural ventilation must be operable by convenient means; all solar climate control must be within reach. Double-paned glass will be necessary to minimize drafts, as well as weatherstripping and caulking. Buildings must be airtight, but allow necessary air changes.

The local microclimate should be studied for siting and landscaping possibilities. Natural breezes and other solar tempering aspects of the site should be understood and employed to best advantage. In addition, outdoor seating and recreation areas must be designed with local weather patterns in mind. Too much sun or wind exposure is hard for the sick, so a variety of coverings, including umbrellas and awnings, trellises and trees, are necessary.

Many hospice conversions have used fan-coil heating units. These units allow individual control of room temperature, an important element of hospice care. In addition, the use of task lighting and indirect incandescent fixtures minimizes heat gain from extensive overhead fixtures. Homelike equipment thereby contributes to a deinstitutionalized climate.

Chapter Eight

Conclusion

Architecturally distinct hospice inpatient units are not numerous, nor are they the most common way to provide inpatient hospice beds. However, they are a significant contributor to palliative care for the dying, as well as an image for palliative care.

Architecturally distinct hospices differ in sponsorship, clientele, location, size, and design. They have commonalities within their category, be it parent-based, new construction, remodeled, large or small patient populations. Fundamentally, they display unanimity in their incorporation of homelike, natural, and spiritual elements in design and care.

By providing the dying with compassionate palliative care, the hospice seeks to ameliorate our cultural antipathy toward death. Hospices care for the dying in an atmosphere free of stigma, in an honest attempt to soothe and ease the fears of the dying and their families. Our culture does not easily accept death: Nature may seem uncontrollable; the universe neutral about the importance of mankind. Hospice buildings and units must strive to provide a welcoming, homelike atmosphere while sheltering the dying from the suspicions and fears of society at large.

The use of hotel or school forms is one way in which some hospices diverge from typical health-care designs while adopting a culturally acceptable form. Until society develops consistent, meaningful rituals for death and dying, such duplicity of design and location may continue to be necessary.

However, no physical structure can ensure cultural acceptance of the hospice, or, ultimately, of death and dying. Designers should be aware of this, and not attempt to create panacea architecture. Rather, the first task of hospice planners is to provide homelike elements and connections to nature and the outdoors.

Experimental Design versus Derived Architectural Forms

In the compendium, there are several examples of designs that are unusual or unique. The Connecticut Hospice, for example, designed a rounded scream room, for staff retreat and cathartic purposes, that introduces a womblike or enclosing shape into an otherwise more typical institution. In a search for abstract forms of traditional designs and their psychological or cultural correlates, architects have introduced these designs as a contemporary acknowledgment of natural forms in architecture. In addition, a functional approach to design has led to such experimentation as the circular nursing stations that dominate the patient wings at Calvary Hospital. These design approaches to palliative-care architecture should be recognized as tentative and not adopted wholeheartedly as necessary or even recommended solutions. Moreover, natural or experimental design solutions are precise and programmatic, in a time when hospices are too new to recognize definitive and specific forms. Caregivers have already acknowledged the role of derived architectural forms in deinstitutionalizing the hospice inpatient unit. The use of such derived forms as schools, libraries, or hotels ensures a loose fit and non–medical institution image, as none of the forms was originally planned for hospice or medical use. The use of older derived hospital types, such as the courtyard building at Nathan Adelson Hospice, and associated decorative styles, such as the Spanish mission style used at Rosary Hill, harken back to the original hospital/hospice types and, therefore, to the origins of palliative and holistic care.

Permanent versus Incremental Change

The hospice inpatient unit is more than a temporary home for dying persons who do not need the medical or custodial care provided in hospitals and nursing homes. It is a place that represents a very old and compassionate kind of care; care that the scientific quest for the control of disease has left behind. Palliative care acknowledges that each individual is unique, that his or her problems are timeless and human. Medical science, in contrast, seeks to cure illness; a type of care no longer required by the dying patient.

This individuality and timelessness of palliative care has its environmental correlate in the hospice. In designing a hospice that can be personalized, connected to the outdoors, and that can be changed over time to suit new needs, the hospice planner allows growth and change to be symbolized in the architecture itself. The institutionalized building, on the other hand, is designed to be modified only with difficulty; it does not promote spontaneity, individuality, or change.

The Influence of Hospice Care and Architecture on the Health-care Field

Inpatient hospice care, which is composed of short-term and intermittent stays for respite and pain control, differs from the longer-term palliative care provided by hospitals and nursing facilities, such as Rosary Hill and Calvary, where indigent patients and those without family to support them can stay. However, the architecture of each is not very different except in size; the longer-term palliative facility has greater infrastructure and larger patient populations. Calvary Hospital has witnessed an increase in family participation, however, and commenced a remodel to increase square footage per patient and add family rooms and a larger outpatient and education unit, more in line with hospice goals. The newly remodeled Rosary Hill Home also has more family space than did its previous inpatient unit.

The inpatient hospice unit and the large palliative-care facility represent the continuum of palliative care in the United States, where payment procedures separate health-care types. In Great Britain, the functions of respite, pain control, and long-term care of the dying are provided at the hospice. In this country, however, hospices emphasize home care, and rely on families to shoulder the responsibility of primary caregiving. The indigent and elderly without means of support are left bereft of palliative care, except in areas where the few existing long-term palliative-care facilities are located. Indeed, many of the dying who have limited funds or no surviving spouses are in nursing homes, receiving custodial rather than palliative care. However, the necessarily high ratio of staff to patient, the techniques of pain control, and the interdisciplinary care of hospice palliation make it too expensive for long-term care. Current procedures for palliative care are thus extraordinarily valuable, but limited in breadth.

Hospices have put the dilemma of dying before the American people and offered comfort and support. The rapid growth of hospice care is a sure indicator of the tremendous need that hospices fulfill. However, efforts to legitimize the hospice will also restrict it. The influence of hospice care will depend upon the proponents, legislators, and regulators who are integrating hospice care into the health-care financing system.

The architecture of hospices may also have far-reaching effects on the architecture of other health-care facilities. For example, recognition that such "amenities" as family rooms and connections to the outdoors are instead necessities in hospice architecture establishes priorities for a new kind of health-care facility. Acknowledgment of the palliative effects of homelike design may cause other health-care units to consider this and other issues along with surgery and medicine in the design of new hospitals and nursing units.

Homelike design incorporating natural and spiritual elements need not be expensive design. The design guidelines presented earlier suggest making use of available resources such as ground-floor locations, flexible design, donated furnishings, and volunteer help. Consider how fundamentally this differs from the current approach to the design of most health-care facilities. Honest empathy with the dying and their families, together with knowledge and an open mind, provide the best qualifications for hospice design.

Bibliography

Agee, James. 1965. *A death in the family.* New York: Avon Books.

Ajemian, Ina, and Balfour M. Mount. 1981. *The R. V. H. manual of palliative/hospice care.* New York: Arno Press.

Alper, Bill. 1978. A Thing of Beauty is a Therapeutic Tool. *Argus.* 85(26 May): 7–9.

Alvarez, A. 1972. *The savage god.* New York: Random House.

Annus, George J. 1974. Rights of the Terminally Ill Patient. *Journal of Nursing Administration.* 4(March–April): 40–44.

Aranyi, Laszlo, and Larry L. Goldman. 1980. *Design of long-term care facilities.* New York: Van Nostrand Reinhold.

Aries, Philippe. 1981. *The hour of our death.* New York: Alfred A. Knopf.

———. *Western attitudes toward death.* 1974. Baltimore: Johns Hopkins Univ. Press.

Bell, Nancy, ed. 1981. *Hospice Update* (newsletter) 3(2): 6. Oconomowoc, WI: Rogers Memorial Hospital.

Benoliel, Jeanne Quint. 1978. The Changing Social Context for Life and Death Decisions. *Essence* 2(2): 5–14.

Berrigan, Daniel. 1980. *We die before we live.* New York: Seabury Press.

Bloomer, Kent, and Charles Moore. 1977. *Body, memory, and architecture.* New Haven, CT: Yale Univ. Press.

Cabrini Hospice. *New York Times.* 18 August 1980.

Calvary Hospital in the Bronx. *New York Times.* 28 May 1978.

Carey, Deborah Allen. 1982. Hospice: The place of dying in America. Master's thes., Univ. of Washington, Seattle.

Chan, L. Y. 1976. Hospice: A New Building Type to Comfort the Dying. *AIA Journal.* 65(December): 42–45.

Charles, Eleanor. A Hospice for the Terminally Ill. *New York Times.* 13 March 1977.

Choron, Jacques. 1963. *Death and Western thought.* New York: Collier Macmillan International.

Coffin, Margaret. 1976. *Death in early America.* Nashville: Thomas Nelson.

Cohn, Kenneth P. 1979. *Hospice; prescription for terminal care.* Germantown, MD: Aspen Systems Corp.

Committee on Architecture for Health, AIA. 1982. Proceedings of AIA quarterly conference, March 16–17. Appendices C-4 through C-10.

Connecticut Hospice, Branford. *New York Times.* 30 June 1980.

Consolidated Hospitals. 1981. Certificate of Need, Inpatient Hospice Unit, Tacoma General Hospital.

Cope, Gilbert, ed. 1970. *Dying, death and disposal.* London: Society for Promoting Christian Knowledge.

Davidson, Glen W., ed. 1978. *The hospice: Development and administration.* Washington, DC: Hemisphere Publishing.

Dellabough, Robin. 1980. Four Models of Hospice Care. *Hospital Forum.* 23(January/February): 67.

deVries, Andre, and Amnon Carmi, eds. 1979. *The dying human.* Tel Aviv: Turtledove Publishing.

Dobihal, E. F., Jr. 1974. Talk or Terminal? *Connecticut Medicine.* 38: 364–69.

Donnelley, John, ed. 1978. *Language, metaphysics and death.* New York: Fordham Univ. Press.

Doyle, Derek, ed. 1979. *Terminal care.* New York: Longman, Inc.

Dubois, Paul M. 1980. *The hospice way of death.* New York: Human Sciences Press.

Dubos, Rene. 1980. *The wooing of earth.* New York: Charles Scribner's Sons.

Dupre, Wilhelm. 1975. *Religion in primitive cultures, a study in ethnophilosophy.* Paris: Mouton and Co.

Eaton, Allen H. 1959. *Beauty for the sighted and the blind.* New York: St. Martin's Press.

Eliade, Mircea. 1971. *The myth of the eternal return.* Willard R. Trask, trans. Princeton, NJ: Princeton Univ. Press.

———. 1959. *The sacred and the profane, The nature of religion.* Willard R. Trask, trans. New York: Harcourt, Brace & Co.

Evaluation: Confused, Elderly. 1979. *AIA Journal.* 68(February): 59–61

Feifel, Herman, ed. 1977. *New meanings of death.* New York: McGraw-Hill.

Feigenberg, Loma, and Robert Fulton. 1977. Care of the Dying: A Swedish Perspective. *Omega.* 8(3): 215–28.

Flint, Peter B. Vincent Pulicano Supported Hospices. *New York Times.* 28 February 1981.

Four Winds Hospital, Katonah, New York, Sponsors Hospice Care Seminar with C. Saunders. *New York Times.* 14 June 1982.

Franklin Institute. 1979. Hospices and related facilities for the terminally ill: Selected bibliographical references. Dept. Health & Human Services, pub. no. HRA 79-14022 (January).

Frey, Christine L., et al. 1980. *Aging in culture and society: Comparative viewpoints and strategies.* New York: Praeger Publishers.

Freid, Martha Nenes, and Morton H. Fried. 1980. *Transitions: Four rituals in eight cultures.* New York: Viking Penguin.

Fulton, Robert, and Greg Owen. 1980. Hospice in America: From Principle to Practice. Presented at the International Hospice Conference, 4 June, St. Christopher's Hospice, Sydenham, England.

Geddes, Gordon E. 1981. *Welcome joy, death, in Puritan New England.* Ann Arbor, MI: Research Press.

Glaser, Barney G., and Anselm L. Strauss. 1965. *Awareness of dying.* Chicago: Aldine.

———. 1968. *Time for dying.* Chicago: Aldine.

Goffman, Erving. 1963. *Stigma: Notes on the management of a spoiled identity.* Englewood Cliffs, NJ: Prentice-Hall.

Goldberger, Paul. Architecture: Connecticut Hospice. *New York Times.* 4 December 1980.

Gorer, Geoffrey. 1965. *Death, grief, and mourning.* New York: Doubleday.

Greinacher, Norbert, and Alois Muller, eds. 1974. *The experience of dying.* New York: Herder and Herder.

Grof, Stanislav, and Christina Grof. 1980. *Beyond death.* New York: Thames and Hudson.

Gurewitsch, E. 1978. Calvary Hospital: The Newest Building, the Oldest Organization for the Terminally Ill. *Aging.* 289/290(November/December): 32–37.

Gutheim, Frederick. 1960. *Alvar Aalto.* New York: George Braziller.

Guthmann, Robert F. 1978. *Death, dying and grief: A bibliography.* Lincoln, NE: Pied Publications.

Habenstein, Robert N., and William M. Lamers. 1963. *Funeral customs the world over.* Milwaukee, WI: Bulfin.

Hackley, J. A. 1977. Full Service Hospice Offers Home, Day and Inpatient Care. *Hospitals.* 2(1 November): 84–87.

Hackney's Hospice. 1979. *Architectural Journal.* 169(February): 309.

Hamerton, Philip Gilbert. 1885. *Landscape.* Boston: Roberts Press.

Hamilton, Michael P., and Helen F. Reid. 1980. *A hospice handbook: A new way to care for the dying.* Grand Rapids, MI: Wm. B. Eerdsman Publishing Co.

Hanuman Foundation. Hanuman Foundation Dying Project Newsletter. August 1981. (Sante Fe, NM: Hanuman Foundation).

Harkness, Sarah P., and James N. Groom. 1976. *Building without barriers.* New York: Watson-Guptill.

Health Promotion through Designed Environment: Conference Report. 1978. Dept. of National Health and Welfare of Canada Conference, 5–7 October, Ottawa, Canada.

Hendin, David. 1973. *Death as a fact of life.* New York: Warner Books.

Herzog, Edgar. 1967. *Psyche and Death: Archaic myths and modern dreams in analytical psychology.* New York: G. P. Putnam's Sons.

Department of Health & Human Services, pub. no. HRA 79–14500.

Hinton, John. 1967. *Dying.* Baltimore: Penguin Books.

Horan, Dennis J., and David Mall, eds. 1977. *Death, dying and euthanasia.* Washington, DC: University Publications of America.

Hospice of the Good Shepherd Feasibility Study. 1982. Waban, MA: Hospice of the Good Shepherd. Pamphlet.

Housing the Aged. 1977. *Architectural Record.* 161(May): 123–38.

Ingles, Thelma. 1974. St. Christopher's Hospice. *Nursing Outlook.* 22(December): 759–63.

Jackson, J. B. 1980. *The necessity for ruins.* Amherst, MA: Univ. of Massachusetts Press.

Johnson, Ernest F., ed. 1955. *Religious symbolism.* New York: Harper & Brothers.

Kalish, Richard A., and David K. Reynold. 1981. *Death and ethnicity: A psychocultural study.* Farmingdale, NY: Baywood Publishing Co.

Kastenbaum, Robert. 1977. *Death, society and human experience.* St. Louis, MO: Mosby.

Kohn, J. 1976. Hospice Building Speaks on Many Emotional Levels to Patient, Family. *Modern Health Care.* 6: 56, 57.

Kolbe, Richard. Inside the English Hospice. *Hospitals* (Journal of the American Hospitals Association). 51: 65–67.

Kincelik, Joseph A. 1976. *Designing the open nursing home.* Stroudsburg, PA: Dowden, Hutchinson and Ross.

Krant, Melvin J. 1973. Rights of the Cancer Patient. *The Meadowbrook Staff Journal* (Summer): 24–27.

Kron, Joan. 1976. Designing a Better Place to Die. *New York.* (1 March): 43–49.

Kübler-Ross, Elisabeth. 1969. *On death and dying.* New York: Macmillan Co.

L.A. Sanatorium by Neutra. 1931. *Architectural Record.* 69(June): 210a.

Lamerton, R. C. 1975. The Need for Hospices. *Nursing Times.* 71(4): 55–57.

Langer, Susanne. 1953. *Feeling and form.* New York: Charles Scribner's Sons.

Lerner, Gerda. 1978. *A death of one's own*. New York: Harper & Row.

Leopold, Aldo. 1981. *A Sand County almanac*. New York: Oxford Univ. Press.

Levi-Strauss, Claude. 1962. *The savage mind*. Chicago: Univ. of Chicago Press.

Lindheim, Roslyn, Helen. H. Glaser, and Christie Coffin. 1972. *Changing hospital environments for children*. Cambridge, MA: Harvard Univ. Press.

Lupu, Dale, and Deborah Monahan. 1980. An Evaluation of a Hospice Inpatient Environment: Highlights of Results From a Post-occupancy Evaluation of Hillhaven Hospice. Presented at the 33rd annual scientific meeting of the Gerontological Society of America, 22 November, San Diego, California.

Lynch, Kevin. 1976. *Managing the sense of a region*. Cambridge, MA: MIT Press.

———. 1972. *What time is this place?* Cambridge, MA: MIT Press.

Major Addresses of the institutes on hospices. (Proceedings of the 1978 Institutes on Hospices Conference). St. Louis, MO: Catholic Hospital Association.

Mansell, Pattison E. 1977. *The experience of dying*. Englewood Cliffs, NJ: Prentice-Hall.

Marks, Elaine. 1973. *Simone de Beauvoir: Encounters with death*. New Brunswick, NJ: Rutgers Univ. Press.

Martin, Marian. 1984. Hospice Status Report. *Business Space Design*. Seattle: The NBBJ Group. Pamphlet.

Mills, Edward D., ed. 1976. *Planning buildings for health, welfare and religion*. Huntington, NY: Robert Ekrieger Publishing Co.

Mitford, Jessica. 1978. *The American way of death*. New York: Simon and Schuster.

Moss, Melody Diane. 1981. Development of an Architectural Program for the Design of a Childbirth Center. Master's thes., Univ. of Washington, Seattle.

The National Hospice Organization. 1982–1983. *Hospices coast to coast*. McLean, VA: National Hospice Organization. Directory.

New Haven Hospice. *New York Times*. 12 April 1979.

Newman, Antoinette Barker, et al. 1980. Conversion of Acute General Hospitals to Long Term Care Institutions—The Problems and Possibilities. Presented at the Western Center for Health Planning Conference, San Francisco, California. April.

Nowlis, Elizabeth Ann. 1978. Odyssey to Mare Street; Lessons Learned at St. Joseph's Hospice. In *Current perspectives in oncologic nursing*, vol. 2. St. Louis: Mosby.

Old People's Center, Amsterdam. 1976. *Architectural Record*. 158(February): 68–82.

Osler, Sir William. 1932. *Aequanamitas*. 3rd. ed. New York: McGraw-Hill.

Paige, Roberta, et al. 1977. Hospice Care for the Adult. *American Journal of Nursing*. 77(November): 1812–15.

Pastalan, Leon A., and Daniel H. Carson, eds. 1970. *Spatial behavior of older people*. Ann Arbor, MI: Univ. of Michigan/Wayne State Univ.

Pearson, Leonard, ed. 1969. Death and dying: Current issues in the treatment of the dying person. Cleveland: Case Western Reserve Univ. Press.

Pevsner, Nikolaus. 1976. *A history of building types*, vol. 19, Bolligen Series, no. 35. Princeton, NJ: Princeton Univ. Press.

Plant, Janet. 1977. Finding a Home for Hospice Care in the United States. *Hospitals*. 51(July): 53–62.

A portfolio of architecture for health. 1977. Chicago: American Hospital Association.

Porter, David R. 1982. *Hospital architecture: Guidelines for design and renovation*. Ann Arbor, MI: Univ. of Michigan Press.

Richards, Ian. 1968. *Abbeys of Europe*. London: Hamlyn Publishing Group.

Riverside Hospice, Boonton. *New York Times*. 25 June 1978.

Rose, Mary Ann, and Walter J. Pories. 1977. Some Additional Notes on Hospice. *Ohio State Medical Journal*. 73(6): 379–82.

Rossman, Parker. 1977. *Hospice; Creating new models of care for the terminally ill*. Wilton, CT: Association Press.

Rykwert, Joseph. 1972. *On Adam's house in paradise*. New York: The Museum of Modern Art.

Sanatorium for the National Vaudeville Artist, Saranac Lake, New York. 1930. *Architect*. 14(April): 55–61.

Sartain, Brian. 1978. Continuing Care Unit. *Cancer Nursing*. 1(4): 291–95.

Saunders, Cicely. 1976. Living with Dying. *Man and Medicine*. 1(Spring): 227–46.

Schiff, Harriet Sarnoff. 1977. *The bereaved parent*. New York: Viking Penguin.

Schoenberg, Bernard, et al., eds. 1972. *Psychosocial aspects of terminal care*. New York: Columbia Univ. Press.

Seaside Hospital for Tubercular Children, Waterford, Connecticut. 1934. *Pencil Points*. 15(April): 160.

Sell, Irene L. 1977. *Dying and death: An annotated bibliography*. New York: Tiresias Press.

Shepard, Paul. 1967. *Man in the landscape: An historic view of the esthetics of nature*. New York: Alfred A. Knopf.

Shneidman, Edwin S., ed. 1976. *Death: Current perspectives*. Palo Alto, CA: Mayfield.

Simonson, Harold P., ed. 1970. *Quartet*. New York: Harper & Row.

Sommer, Robert. 1974. *Tight spaces, hard architecture, and how to humanize it*. Englewood Cliffs, NJ: Prentice-Hall.

Sontag, Susan. 1980. *Illness as Metaphor*. New York: Farrar, Straus, and Giroux.

St. Mary's Hospital, Bayside, Queens. *New York Times*. 10 April 1980.

Stannard, David E. 1977. *The Puritan way of death*. New York: Oxford Univ. Press.

Stenfels, Peter, and Robert M. Veatch, eds. 1975. *Death*

inside out: The Hastings Center report. New York: Harper & Row.

Stoddard, Sandol. 1978. *The hospice movement: A better way of caring for the dying.* Briarcliff Manor, NY: Stein and Day.

Summerson, John. 1963. *Heavenly mansions and other essays on architecture.* New York: Norton Library.

Thompson, John D., and Grace Goldin. 1975. *The hospital: A social and architectural history.* New Haven: Yale Univ. Press.

Toynbee, Arnold, et al. 1968. *Man's concern with death.* New York: McGraw-Hill.

Tuberculosis Hospitals with Standards. 1938. *Architectural Record.* 84(August): 97–103.

Twenty-Six Hospice Pilot Program. *New York Times.* 20 December 1979.

Ven den Berg, J. H. 1972. *The psychology of the sickbed.* New York: Humanities Press.

Verderber, Stephen. 1982. *Environment-behavior design factors in the architecture of the hospice.* Houston: College of Architecture, Univ. of Houston. Pamphlet.

Weiss, Joseph Douglas. 1969. *Better buildings for the aged.* New York: McGraw-Hill.

Westchester's United Hospital. *New York Times.* 30 December 1979.

Wheeler, E. Todd. 1964. *Hospital design and function.* New York: McGraw-Hill.

Woodward, Kenneth L., et al. 1978. Living with Dying. *Newsweek.* 91(1 May): 52–61.

Zimmerman, Jack McKay, et al. 1981. *Hospice: Complete care for the terminally ill.* Baltimore: Urban and Schwarbenberg.

Index